Comprehensive

DICTIONARY

of AUDIOLOGY

by

JAMES H. DELK

Fourth Edition
Second Printing

ISBN 0-913775-00-2

Library of Congress Catalog Card Number: 88-81361

The Laux Company, Inc., Maynard, Massachusetts

Printed in the United States of America

Above all to

M'LADY

to whom this book is dedicated

Introduction

It is indeed a pleasure to be a party to the launching of this particular intellectual vessel, not only because of my own interests in the general topic, but because of my lasting regard for the man who, with some considerable help from his helpmate, has put it all together. I do not recall how long I have known the put-togetherer—probably the best part of twenty-five years. I am keenly aware of having known him in various capacities—as a man, a husband, a businessman, a specialist in rehabilitation with particular concern for children, as a doer of things with hearing aids and with those who need them, and mostly as a humanist. For what it is worth, I have known him always as a gentle man with an inquiring mind.

The putting together of any kind of a dictionary that makes sense and reflects the active use of language is a difficult task. This is especially true of the language and meanings of a highly technological field which deeply concerns human welfare. This is a volatile field, complicated with many rapid changes of focus of attention and interest in both instrumentation and in procedures.

In a way this effort is reminiscent of two rather notable figures in the history of dictionary-making: it reflects a Johnsonian spirit with due regard of Isaac Walton—THE COMPLEAT DICTIONARY OF AUDIOLOGY. The first of these, one Samuel by name, evinced major reverence for precise definition of meanings in the language. The second preferred "goin' fishin'", a very important aspect of finding out about the meaning of words. Both are pertinent to the spirit of this book. The author exhibits a profound respect for the semantics of his trade, his range of interests, and the scope of the task. Obviously when one undertakes such a labor in trying to keep up to date with the complexity of meanings, he must have respect for them. And he is always "fishin'" for the new and the better, for freshness and clarity. I know this has been a difficult task. It is well done. One can only wish the put-togetherer and his readers well. This work fills a great need, and should put us all in better communication.

WILLIAM G. HARDY, PhD*
Professor and Director,
Division of Communicative Sciences
and the Hearing and Speech Center,
The Johns Hopkins Medical Institutions

*Dr. Hardy, long a noted figure in the field of audiology, died in January 1980.

Preface

My wife Helen (better known as "M'lady") and I felt the need for a dictionary devoted to audiology from the time of our earliest involvement with hearing problems—over thirty years ago. With that in mind, we began in 1958 to compile a list of terms used in audiologic literature and lectures. Producing an actual dictionary became our objective several years later (and only after entering a wager as to whether the word *audiology* itself was to be found in general dictionaries; it wasn't, we lost, and the seed of this book was planted).

Our early efforts led first to the serialization of a Dictionary of Audiology in the publication then titled the *National Hearing Aid Journal,* then to publication of the hardbound first edition of *The Comprehensive Dictionary of Audiology* in 1973. Now, ten years and several thousand copies later, this fourth edition represents the first complete revision of the *Dictionary's* content—and its greatest expansion, with the addition of more than 700 terms that have become part of the contemporary audiology lexicon.

In scope, we have tried to make the *Dictionary* a complete reference to the field—the only one the student needs before becoming a writer and coining his or her own terms of art. In style, we have tried to use the simplest or most common terms possible in our definitions, and we have included only the audiologic meaning of given words. Pronunciations, where they are indicated, reflect accepted usage in the field (we still hear "hertz" more often than the purist "hairtz," but we haven't given up yet!).

To acknowledge individually all those who have helped and encouraged me in this work and its revision is impossible. I am especially beholden, though, to former *Hearing Aid Journal* publisher Milton Bolstein, who had the courage to undertake his first book publishing venture in order to make this information generally available to the field, and to his successor—*Hearing Journal* publisher Dean M. Laux—for channeling my ongoing collection of new audiologic terms and updating of existing language into this completely revised edition. With his indulgence, I'd like to name several others to whom I'm indebted. . .

Howard Fogel, the late *Hearing Aid Journal* editor, encouraged us to "quit procrastinating and publish" as the first *Dictionary* took shape in the early 1970s, also calling to our attention many words and phrases to be included in the book. Dorothy Reznek, his assistant, cooperated effectively with M'lady to keep me meeting deadlines with as few errors as possible—as has Donna Peterson, editor of this revised edition.

I shall always be grateful to the late William G. Hardy, PhD, the kind words of whose introduction to the original *Dictionary* are retained as they appeared in the first edition.

Kenneth W. Berger, PhD, of Kent State University was most generous in his advice and encouragement. His constructive criticism was invaluable, and I'm sure he will recognize his influence in these pages.

Harold J. Weber, PhD, thoughtfully provided a copy of his extensive glossary to help make this Dictionary as complete as possible.

Various word lists appear as appendices through the courtesy of David H. Barr, PhD, Lawrence J. Deutsch, PhD, Harriet L. Haskins, MA, Louise LaFontaine, MA, Manuel Saavedra, and Jack M. Delk.

In conclusion I must express a special thanks to all our friends and acquaintances in the field who have encouraged us with their expressions of appreciation for the value of the work. Esther R. Daniel, Aram Glorig, MD, and Larry Lovering, PhD epitomize this group. I am also most appreciative of the understanding help and encouragement of my friends and associates in the Audiotone Division of Royal Industries.

Contents

Introduction v

Preface. vii

Guide to Pronunciation. xi

Dictionary of Audiology A–Z 1–161

APPENDICES

I.	Common and Uncommon Abbreviations	163
II.	Guide for the Evaluation of Hearing Handicap	168
III.	Guidelines for Audiometric Symbols	174
IV.	Glossary of Tinnitus Terms.	179
V.	Ototoxic Substances	182
VI.	Parts of the Earmold	183
VII.	Syringe Method of Earmold Impressions	184
VIII.	American Spondaic and PB Word Lists	186
IX.	Speech Discrimination Tests	189
X.	PBK Word Lists.	190
XI.	Spanish Words.	192
XII.	French Words	193
XIII.	German Words	195
XIV.	Portuguese Words	196
XV.	Arabic and Hebrew Words	197
XVI.	Glossary of Computer Terminology	198
XVII.	Glossary of Telecommunications Terms	201
XVIII.	International Standard Manual Alphabet	202
XIX.	One Hand Manual Alphabet.	203
XX.	Bibliography of Hearing-Related Publications	204

Guide to Pronunciation

When the phonetic respelling of a term is given, it appears in parentheses immediately following the main bold face entry. This respelling has been presented in the simplest manner possible, with minimum markings.

The syllable having the greatest stress has one accent mark following it (ab-du′senz). Two accent marks following a syllable indicates the secondary accent (ab′′e-ot′ro-fe). An unstressed syllable is followed by a hyphen.

An unmarked vowel ending a syllable is long (so′nant).

An unmarked vowel in a syllable ending with a consonant is short (kok′le-ah).

A long vowel in a syllable ending with a consonant is marked with a macron (mor′fēm, be-nīn′).

A short vowel ending or constituting a syllable by itself is marked with a breve (jĕ-net′ik, lab′ĭ-rinth).

"ah" is used for the sound of "a" in open, unaccented syllables (ah-kro′mah-tin).

Most consonants are unchanged. "C", however, may be indicated as K or S. "G" may be J, when soft.

A

A. ampere, anode.

a- prefix meaning no, not, lack, or without; e.g., aplasia—lack of development.

A battery *n.* battery used to heat the filaments of vacuum tubes; the only battery needed now that transistors replace vacuum tubes.

A weighted scale. the A weighted scale of a sound level meter attenuates (reduces) the lower frequencies about 5 dB per octave from 1000 Hz down to 250 Hz. Below 250 Hz sounds are attenuated another 10 dB per octave. References to the A weighted scale are commonly noted as dBA.

AA. auditory analysis. Associate in Arts.

AAO-HNS. American Academy of Otolaryngology—Head and Neck Surgery. Formerly AAOO.

AAOO. American Academy of Ophthalmology and Otolaryngology. Now separated into two academies: the American Academy of Ophthalmology and the American Academy of Otolaryngology—Head and Neck Surgery.

AAPM. American Association of Physicists in Medicine.

AAPT. American Association of Physics Teachers.

AARP. American Association of Retired Persons.

AAS. American Auditory Society. Formerly American Audiology Society.

ab- prefix meaning away, from, off; e.g., abnormal—away from the normal.

ABC. absolute bone conduction.

abducens nerve (ab-du'senz). VIth cranial nerve; gives rise to the stapedius and chorda tympani nerves.

abducent (ab-du'sent) *adj.* away from the midline. *ant*: adducent.

aberrant (ab-er'ant) *adj.* deviation from the normal.

aberrant response. unusual or unnatural response; atypical.

ABESPA. American Board of Examiners in Speech Pathology and Audiology.

ABI. auditory behavior index.

abiotrophy (ab"e-ot'ro-fe) *n.* early loss of vitality or degeneration of tissue. *adj*: abiotrophic.

ablation (ab-la'shun) *n.* surgical removal of a part of the body.

ablaut (ab'lowt) *n.* vowel change in the root or stem of a word that indicates difference in use or meaning (as in run, ran).

ABLB. alternate binaural loudness balance test.

abortifacient (ah-bor"tĭ-fa'shent) *n.* drug intended to cause an abortion—sometimes blamed for congenital hearing problems.

ABR. auditory brainstem response.

abrupt high tone loss. hearing pattern that is normal or nearly normal in the low frequencies, but sensitivity drops off abruptly as much as 80 dB per octave; the loss may be total above the abrupt drop.

abscissa (ab-sis'ah) *n.* horizontal coordinate of a graph; e.g., frequencies on an audiogram.

absolute bone conduction test. ABC. 1. test to establish levels of threshold acuity in response to the stimulus of a bone oscillator while the ears are occluded or closed ("relative" bone conduction tests call for the ears to be open or unoccluded). 2. tuning fork test made by comparing the bone conduction of the patient with that of the examiner. The ear canal of the patient is closed by the finger of the examiner and the base of the tuning fork is placed on the mastoid process. If the examiner can still hear the fork in the same manner after the patient has ceased to hear it, this "reduced absolute bone conduction" usually indicates a perceptive impairment. (Compare Bing and Schwabach tests).

absolute pitch. 1. calibrated pure tone. 2. capability of naming or singing a note when heard or requested.

absolute threshold. minimum level of intensity at which a sound can be determined to be present.

absorb *v.* to receive a sound wave without an echo.

absorption *n.* in acoustics, termination of sound waves by material that prevents reflection or echo. *adj*: absorptive.

absorption coefficient. number indicating the fraction of acoustic energy absorbed when sound waves strike a surface; the range from complete reflection to complete absorption would be indicated by figures from 0.00 to 1.00.

AC. 1. air conduction. 2. alternating current.

accent *n.* 1. stress that emphasizes a syllable of a word. 2. manner of speaking distinctive to residents of a given locality.

accent *v.* to emphasize—as a word or letter.

accentual (ak-sen'choo-al) *adj.* distinguished by accent; distinctive because of accent, dialect, or stress. *adv*: accentually.

accentuate (ak-sen'choo-āt) *v.* accent, stress.

accomplishment quotient. achievement quotient.

acculturation (ah-kul"chu-ra'shun) *n.* variation in basic language patterns resulting from intermingling of cultures. *adj*: acculturational, acculturative.

accumulator (ah-ku'mu-la"ter) *n.* storage cell for electrical energy, especially a rechargeable battery.

acetylcholine (as"ĕ-til-ko'lēn) *n.* chemical transmitter that triggers nerve impulses.

1

achievement quotient. AQ. number given to represent the relationship between chronological age (set as 100—or 100%) and the skills exhibited.

achondroplasia (ah-kon″dro-pla′ze-ah) *n.* abnormal cartilage development—failure to turn into bone.

achromatin (ah-kro′mah-tin) *n.* nonstainable portion of a cell nucleus (the stainable part is chromatin).

acid, nicotinic (nik″o-tin′ik) **niacin** (ni′ah-sin). an acid of the vitamin B complex used to dilate blood vessels (a vasodilator).

ACLC. assessment of children's language comprehension test.

acouesthesia (ah-koo″es-the′ze-ah) *n.* acute sensation of hearing.

acoualion (ah″ku-la′le-an). instrument similar to a speaking tube in teaching speech to the deaf.

acoumeter (ah-koo′met-er) *n.* **acouometer** (ah-koo-om′et-er) **acoutometer** (ah-koo-tom′e-ter). predecessors of the audiometer used in measuring hearing acuity. (Hartmann 1878). *n:* **acoumetry**; *adj:* **acoumetric, acoumometric.**

acoupedic method (ah-koo-pēd′ic). system of teaching the hearing-impaired infant to hear and to speak by concentrating on acoustic stimulation of the residual hearing. First introduced by Professor Henk Huizing in 1953 at Groningen Conference on Paedo-Audiology and expanded in 1959 as acoupedic method.

acouphone (ah′koo-fōn) *n.* early generic name for electric hearing aid either resulting from or inspiring the trademark "Akouphone" (1902).

acousia, acousis (ah-koo′ze-ah, ah-koo′sis) *n.* hearing sense, usually used as a combining form.

acousma (ah-kōōz′mah) *n.* tinnitus, head noises, esp. when considered an auditory hallucination.

acousmatagnosis (ah-kōōz′ma-tag-no′sis). auditory aphasia: a form of central deafness. Auditory pathways are intact but there is no understanding of the spoken word.

acousmatamnesia (ah-kōōz′-mat-am-ne″ze-ah) *n.* auditory amnesia or loss of memory for sounds.

acoustic (ah-kōōs′tĭk) *adj.* pertaining to the science of sound, or to the sense of hearing. *adj:* **acoustical;** *adv:* **acoustically.**

acoustic admittance. flow of sound pressure waves through the middle ear mechanism—especially as measured by an "oto-admittance" meter.

acoustic agnosia (ag-no′se-ah). loss or impairment of ability to identify objects and noises by sound alone although the sensory sphere is intact. *syn:* auditory agnosia, auditory deafness, cerebral deafness, mind deafness, psychic deafness.

acoustic agraphia (ah-graf′e-ah). inability to write from dictation. *syn:* auditory agraphia.

acoustic aphasia (ah-fa′ze-ah). inability to understand spoken language. *syn:* auditory aphasia, auditory agnosia.

acoustic area. area within cortex of the temporal lobe of the cerebrum to which sound is referred. Also referred to as the acoustic center.

acoustic axis. direction of greatest intensity of sound as produced by a tuning fork. It can be represented by a straight line drawn through the ends of both prongs of the fork.

acoustic cell. one of the hair cells of the organ of Corti.

acoustic center. area within cortex of the temporal lobe of the cerebrum to which sound is referred.

acoustic compliance. another term for acoustic admittance.

acoustic cortex *pl.* **cortices, cortexes.** also known as the acoustic center: the area in the temporal lobe of the cerebral cortex that serves as the terminus for the afferent nerve fibers of the inner ear.

acoustic coupler. 1. earmold that connects the hearing aid with the ear canal. 2. device that converts teletypewriter signals into tones compatible with the voice band of the telephone lines and vice-versa at the receiving end.

acoustic crest. thickened section of lining of the bulbous portion (ampulla) of each semicircular canal. Fibers of the vestibular nerve pass through the crest of the hair cells. *syn:* ampullary crest.

acoustic cue. portion of a speech sound or formant considered most important in identifying the speech signal.

acoustic duct. external ear canal. *syn:* acoustic meatus.

acoustic energy. the power generated by sound waves.

acoustic feedback. howl or whistle caused by the recirculation of acoustic output of an amplifying system. In a hearing aid the sound emanating from the receiver may reach (or feed back into) the microphone and be reamplified until it builds up into a high-pitched whistle.

acoustic field. area in which sound pressure waves are moving unimpeded from their source. *syn:* free field.

acoustic filter. a device or material (e.g., lamb's wool) used to alter the acoustic response of an amplifier.

acoustic gain. increase in sound output (intensity or volume) resulting from the amplification of the sound entering the microphone. It is calculated by subtracting the input in dB from the output in dB.

acoustician (ah-kōō-tish'un) *n.* one who specializes in acoustics. A title used in Europe (especially West Germany) by a specialist in fitting and selling hearing aids.

acoustic impedance. resistance to the flow of sound pressure waves through a medium. In audiology, the term has come to refer more specifically to the resistance of the eardrum and middle ear to the transmission of sound.

acoustic impedance audiometry. impedance audiometry.

acoustic inertance. resistance to the movement of sound pressure waves in a tube. More frequently referred to as inertance. *syn*: acoustic mass.

acoustic insulation. material designed to absorb sound waves.

acoustic interferometer. instrument designed to utilize lights and mirrors in the measurement of sound wavelengths and velocities.

acoustic mass. resistance to movement of sound pressure waves in a tube. *syn*: acoustic inertance or, simply, inertance.

acoustic meatus (meatus acusticus externus), (me-a'tus). external—ear canal from ear flap to eardrum. *syn*: external auditory meatus or porus. internal—auditory canal through which the auditory and facial nerves pass on their way to the brain. *syn*: internal meatus or porus.

acoustic meatus cartilage. the cartilage that forms part of the wall of the external ear canal.

acoustic MHO, moh. unit of measurement of conductance of the flow of sound pressure waves through a medium. The reciprocal of the acoustic ohm.

acoustic microtrauma. damage to the ear resulting from the cumulative effect of minute injuries. Noise-induced hearing loss.

acoustic muscle reflex. AMR. the reflex contraction of the intra-aural muscles (tensor tympani and stapedius) in response to a stimulus. Also known as intra-aural reflex and more simply as acoustic reflex.

acoustic nerve. the VIIIth cranial nerve, combining the nerves of hearing (cochlear) and balance (vestibular). *syn*: auditory nerve, vestibulocochlear nerve.

acoustic neurinoma. tumor of the VIIIth cranial nerve. Acoustic neuroma.

acoustic neuroma (nu-ro'mah). tumor of the VIIIth cranial nerve.

acousticofacial ganglia. embryonic cell mass that develops into the VIIth (facial) and VIIIth (acoustic) nerve.

acousticolateral *adj.* concerning the lateral-line organs and their central connections with the ear.

acoustic ohm. unit of measurement of resistance to the flow of sound pressure waves through a medium. The unit is equal to a pressure amplitude of one dyne per square centimeter per second of flux amplitude.

acoustico-orbicular reflex. auropalpebral reflex; cochleo-orbicular reflex.

acousticophobia (ah-kōōs'tĭ-co-fo'be-a) *n.* morbid fear of sounds.

acoustic organ. uncommon name for the organ of Corti.

acoustic output. sound pressure resulting from the increase in intensity of an input signal as measured at the speaker, earphone, or receiver of an electronic amplifying system.

acoustic papilla. the organ of Corti. *syn*: organum spirale.

acoustic paralysis. sensorineural deafness.

acoustic power. square root of the pressure generated by a tone or combination of tones.

acoustic probe. device designed to test the ability of various portions of the ossicular chain to transmit sound pressures.

acoustic pulse. sound of limited duration—one which begins and ends abruptly; a click, gunshot, burst of noise, tone pip, etc. *syn*: acoustical pulse.

acoustic radiation pressure. tiny increase in atmospheric pressure on a surface resulting from sound waves.

acoustic reactance. portion of acoustic impedance that results from a combination of the stiffness and mass of the eardrum and middle ear mechanism.

acoustic reflex. reflex contraction of the intra-aural muscles (tensor tympani and stapedius) in response to sound. *syn*: intra-aural reflex, cochlear reflex.

acoustic resistance. acoustic impedance measured in acoustic ohms. It differs in phase from acoustic reactance by one-quarter cycle.

acoustics. 1. study of the physical properties of sound. 2. architectural arrangement of an auditorium, sanctuary, or theater that determines ability to hear from any location.

acoustic shadow. 1. reduction of sound resulting from interposition of head—especially when sound comes from the side. *syn*: head shadow effect. 2. reduction of sound in any field caused by an obstacle.

acoustic shock. a sudden and violent movement of air—as from an explosion—which may damage the hearing (causing acoustic trauma).

acoustic signature. the different characteristics of each combination of sounds that make the signal distinctive.

acoustic spectrum. distribution of frequency and pressure of waves within an envelope of sound.

acoustic tile. tile made of material designed to absorb sound waves.

acoustic trauma. loss of hearing as a result of relatively short exposure to noise (usually explosive).

acoustic tumor. growth (either benign or malignant) on the sheath of the auditory (VIIIth) nerve. *syn:* acoustic neuroma.

acoustic window. range of frequencies necessary to make a particular speech sound intelligible.

acoustopalpebral reflex. rapid and distinct closing of the eyelids or twitch at the corner (canthus) of the eye resulting from a sudden sound stimulus. *syn:* auropalpebral reflex; cochleopalpebral reflex.

acromania (ak″ro-ma′ne-ah) *n.* mania accompanied by excessive motor activity and sometimes by loss of ability to speak.

ACTH. adrenocorticotropic hormone.

action potential. AP; change in electrical potential of the cochlea in response to an auditory stimulus.

actuarial hearing thresholds. average hearing sensitivity of normally hearing persons according to age and sex.

ACU. automatic control unit.

acuity (ah-ku′ĭ-te) *n.* sharpness, clearness, distinctness, or keenness of a sense. Auditory acuity: degree of clearness of hearing. Threshold of minimal acuity: point where pure tone is heard at 50% of presentation. This word is being replaced in the latter usage by the word *sensitivity.*

acumeter (ak′u-me-ter) *n.* early device for measuring hearing that made a ticking sound similar to that of a watch.

acuphenes (ah-ku-fe′nis) *n.* tinnitus.

acusis (ah-ku′sis) *n.* hearing.

acusticus (ah-kōōs′tĭ-kus) *n.* the auditory or VIIIth cranial nerve.

acute. 1. sharp or especially sensitive when related to hearing. 2. severe and painful but of short duration when related to disease.

acute eustachian salpingitis (u-sta′ke-an salpin-ji′tis). closure of the eustachian tube by inflammation.

acute otitis media (o-ti′tis me′de-ah). active inflammation of the middle ear.

acute serous otitis media (ser′us). accumulation of fluid within the middle ear cavity, accompanied by severe pain.

acute suppurative otitis media (sup′u-ra″tiv). disease of the ear characterized by discharge emanating from the middle ear cavity.

AD. auricula dexter, auris dextra (right ear) (AS—left ear. AU—both ears.)

ADA. Academy of Dispensing Audiologists.

Adam's apple *n.* part of the larynx; the protruding thyroid cartilage.

adaptation, auditory. phenomenon exhibited by some ears by which an audible tone or

sound may become inaudible within a short time (tone decay).

aden- medical prefix indicating a gland.

adenoidectomy (ad″ĕ-noid-ek′to-me) *n.* surgical removal of the adenoids.

adenoids (ad′ĕ-noid) *n.* lymphoid tissue growing around the nasopharyngeal opening of the eustachian tube. *syn:* pharyngeal tonsil.

adenoma (ad-ĕ-no′mah) *n.* glandular-shaped, usually benign, tumor within the epithelium.

adhesive otitis media. glue ear (may damage or destroy ossicles).

adiadochocinesia, adiadochocinesis, or **adiadochokinesia, adiadochokinesis** (ah-di″ah-do″ko-sĭ-ne′se-ah) *n.* lack of ability to perform rapidly alternating movements.

adipose (ad′ĭ-pōs) *adj.* relating to fatty tissue or connective tissue containing fat cells.

aditus (ad′ĭ-tus) *n.* opening or passage.

aditus ad antrum (ad-an′trum). passage leading from the attic of the middle ear to the mastoid cavity. Head of the malleus and greater part of the incus are located in the attic section.

admittance *n.* ease of flow of sound pressure waves. Reciprocal of impedance in tympanometry.

adrenocorticotropic hormone. ACTH.

adventitious (ad-ven-tish′us) *adj.* occurring after birth; e.g., a hearing loss as a result of disease or accident. *adv:* **adventitiously,** *n:* **adventitiousness.**

aero-otitis (a″er-o-o-ti′tis). dysfunction of the middle ear caused by the changes of atmospheric pressure while flying. *syn:* barotrauma.

adult growth examination. measurements of auditory thresholds, close-up vision, and blood pressure are combined to arrive at an estimated biological age.

advantage, ear. the right ear, stimulating the left hemisphere of the brain, is considered the better ear for speech discrimination. The left ear, stimulating the right hemisphere, responds better to environmental sounds and music.

AERA. average evoked response audiometry.

AF. audiofrequency.

afferent (af′er-ent) *adj.* portion of a nervous system that conveys the impulses inward, e.g., the afferent auditory nervous system conveys impulses from the inner ear toward the cortex of the brain. *adv:* **afferently.**

AGC. automatc gain control. Same as AVC.

AGE. adult growth examination.

age, chronological. CA. Length of time an entity has lived from birth to current date; *syn:* actual age.

age, hearing. ability of a congenitally hearing-impaired child to understand speech when compared with the chronological age of a child hearing normally from birth. It is governed by the period of time the congenitally impaired child has had adequate personal amplification and aural rehabilitation (auditory training).

age, language. ability of a congenitally hearing-impaired child to understand and communicate ideas by gestures or signs when compared with the chronological age of a child hearing normally from birth. The innate intelligence of an infant may obscure a hearing impairment when this language alone is considered.

age, mental. MA. numerical expression of individual intellectual age when compared with the norm for the same chronological age.

agenesis (ah-jen′ĕ-sis) *n.* incomplete or lack of development; e.g., a missing or rudimentary imperfect pinna; *syn*: aplastic.

agnosia, auditory (ag-no′ze-ah). form of receptive aphasia in which sounds are not recognized—heard but not understood.

agraphia (ah-graf′e-ah) *n.* loss of ability to write—due to a lesion of the cerebral cortex or to lack of muscular coordination. Writing from dictation may still be possible. If one cannot write from dictation, the dysfunction is known as acoustic or auditory agnosia.

AHRF. American Hearing Research Foundation.

AHS. American Hearing Society—now National Association of Hearing and Speech Agencies (NAHSA).

AI. articulation index.

aid, hearing. electric amplifying device to make sounds audible to the individual with a hearing loss. Sound pressure waves are converted into electricity by a microphone. The electric impulses are then amplified through controlled electronic circuitry. The amplified electric impulses are then reconverted by a receiver (earphone) to pressure waves at a much more intense level to be presented to the impaired ear.

aided threshold. the point at which a listener can first determine that a sound is becoming audible when an amplifier is used (usually a hearing aid).

AIP. American Institute of Physics.

air-bone gap. difference in hearing sensitivity as measured by air conduction and bone conduction.

air cell. popular name for zinc-air hearing aid battery.

air conduction. transmission of sound pressure waves through the air to the eardrum, thence by way of the ossicular chain to the inner ear.

air conduction receiver. device (transducer) that receives the amplified electronic signal of the hearing aid circuit and converts it into sound pressure waves (acoustical energy) that activate the eardrum and start the hearing process.

AL. annoyance level.

Albers-Schönberg disease. characterized by brittle bones that may result in spontaneous fractures, this condition may be responsible for a disarticulation of the ossicular chain. *syn*: osteopetrosis.

Albrecht effect (Karl Albrecht, German anatomist, 1851-1894). fast adaptation, fast auditory fatigue, or tone decay. This phenomenon is evidenced by the inability of an impaired ear to hear a continuous tone presented at successively higher (5 dB) levels of intensity as the tone appears to the listener to fade out.

alexia (ah-lek′se-ah) *n.* inability to read.

alexia, auditory. inability to learn to read (e.g., by the phonics approach) due to failure to recognize differences and similarities in voiced sounds; *syn*: : verbal alexia.

alexia, verbal. alexia, auditory.

algophobia (al-go-fo′be-ah) *n.* extreme fear of pain.

allergen (al′er-jen) *n.* any substance that produces an allergic reaction.

allergy (al′er-je) *n.* reaction to a substance or condition that is different from that of most individuals; e.g., sneezing, skin rashes, or itching; *adj*: **allergic.**

all-in-the-ear-earmold. designed to hold an all-in-the-ear hearing aid in the ear. The term usually refers to an earmold fabricated to hold a modular type instrument.

allophone (al′o-fōn) *n.* speech sound that is a variant of a phoneme—one of the smallest units of speech.

alloquism (al′o-kwism) *n.* communication by speech.

alphabet, initial teaching. ITA. alphabet in which each symbol represents only one sound. It is designed to stimulate early reading skills.

alphabet, international phonetic. IPA. a system of symbols for speech sounds adopted by the International Phonetic Association. Each speech sound is represented by a distinctive symbol.

alpha rhythm. a basic brainwave pattern of about 10 peaks per second on an electroencephalogram.

alpha wave. alpha rhythm.

Alport's syndrome. deafness associated with hereditary kidney disease (nephropathy) and mental retardation.

alternate binaural loudness balance test. test for recruitment in which the patient is asked to balance the sensation of loudness experienced in a normal ear and an impaired ear.

5

Using a dual-channel audiometer (or two balanced audiometers) a pure tone is introduced in the normal ear at a level above threshold; e.g., 20 dB. The patient is asked to indicate when the tone presented alternately to the affected ear is equally loud. This point is noted on a chart and the intensity of the tone in the normal ear is increased 10 or 20 dB and the first step is repeated.

These steps are continued and a laddergram constructed until the points on the chart are even—complete recruitment—or pass each other—over recruitment. If the differences remain constant there is said to be no recruitment.

alternate monaural loudness balance test. AMLB. see monaural loudness balance test.

alternating current. AC or ac. electric current that flows first in one direction—then in the other. When this reversal occurs sixty times in one second, it is called sixty-cycle current.

alternating pulses. series of short bursts of pure tones that vary in amplitude in regular cycles.

AM. amplitude modulation.

AMA. American Medical Association.

AMA hearing impairment formula. see hearing loss (percentage of impairment).

ambient (am′be-ent) *adj.* pertaining to surrounding sounds of the environment or to sounds in an amplifying system that are not part of the wanted signal. *syn:* ambient noise.

amblyacousia, amblyacusia (am-ble-ah-koo′se-ah) *n.* **amblyfonia, amblyphonia** (am-ble-fon′i-a). blunt (ambly) hearing—loss of hearing sensitivity.

ameliorate (ah-mēl′yo-rāt) *v.* to improve. **amelioration** (ah-mēl″yo-ra′shun) *n.* improvement.

American Hearing Society. formerly AHS—now NAHSA; National Association of Hearing and Speech Agencies.

AMESLAN. American Sign Language.

AMLB. alternate monaural loudness balance test. Same as MLB: monaural loudness balance test.

ammeter (am′me-ter) *n.* device to measure electric current in amperes.

amnesia, auditory (am-ne′ze-ah). loss of memory for speech.

amniocentesis (am″ne-o-sen-te′sis) *n.* process of removing amniotic fluid by suction from the uterus during pregnancy for diagnostic purposes.

amperage (am′per-ij) *n.* the power of a current of electricity expressed in amperes.

ampere (am′pēr) *n.* unit of electricity equal to the steady current produced by one volt applied across a resistance of one ohm.

amplification (am″plĭ-fĭ-ka′shun) *n.* a magnification or increase in intensity of sound. Also referred to as gain.

amplification, selective. the amplification of certain frequencies more than—or to the exclusion of—other frequencies.

amplification, split band. presentation of lower frequencies to one ear and higher frequencies to the other through hearing aids. This system is advocated by Barbara Franklin, PhD, especially for children. Some adults with difficult hearing problems also benefit. The higher frequencies should usually be applied to the right ear and the lower frequencies to the left.

amplifier *n.* any device, usually electronic, that magnifies the intensity of a sound wave (or electrical impulse).

amplify *v.* to increase or magnify; e.g., the intensity of sound waves.

amplitude *n.* range of movement of a wave from its mean value. Directly related to intensity.

amplitude distortion (or nonlinear distortion). when the output of an electroacoustic system is not proportional to the input. Frequencies not present in the input are produced in the output, thus making the forms of the output wave different from that of the input wave.

amplitude modulation. variation of the amplitude of a radio carrier wave in relation to the strength of the audio or other signal.

ampulla (am-pul′lah) *pl.* **ampullae** (am-pul′le) *n.* a swelling or pouch in an anatomical canal, esp. the semicircular canals of the ear.

ampullary crest. thickened section of lining of the bulbous portion (ampulla) of each semicircular canal. Fibers of the vestibular nerve pass through the crest of the hair cells; *syn:* acoustic crest.

ampullated (am′pul-la-ted) *adj.* dilated into the shape of a flask.

AMR. acoustic muscle reflex.

amusia (ah-mu′ze-ah) *n.* musical deafness; inability to produce or understand music or musical sounds.

amyloidosis (am″ĭ-loi-do′sis) *n.* accumulation of nodules made up of deposits of an abnormal protein (amyloid) that may affect tissues or nerves of the organ of hearing.

ANA. Acoustic Neuroma Association.

anabolism (ah-nab′o-lizm″) *n.* synthetic or constructive metabolism. A process by which a cell converts nutritive material into more complex living matter.

anacousia, anacusia (an″ah-ku′ze-ah). total lack of hearing. Deafness.

anacousis, anacusis, anakusis (an″ah-koo′sis). total deafness.

analog (variation of analogue). device designed to simulate the action of the ear or voice for study purposes.

analog computer. computer designed to average out measurably different electrical voltages or resistances resulting from ongoing brain activity.

analysis, phonemic. study of speech sounds.

analyzer, noise. instrument designed to determine the frequency components of a particular noise; e.g., the sound levels in bands, one-third, one-half, or one octave, in width, may be measured.

anaphylactic (an″ah-fĭ-lak′tic) *adj.* pertaining to the hypersensitive reaction to a foreign protein or drug.

anaphylaxis (an″ah-fĭ-lak′sis) *n.* hypersensitivity that develops from contact with a foreign protein or drug—to the degree that a second dose brings about an acute reaction; e.g., sudden deafness

anastomose (ah-nas′to-mos) *v.* to form an interconnection by anastomosis.

anastomosis (ah-nas″to-mo′sis) *pl.* **anastamoses** *n.* interconection of normally distinctive parts, organs, or spaces surgically or pathologically. Lack of such safety-valves between arteries may cause deafness by obstruction of the flow of blood through one or the other.

anastomotic (ah-nas-to-mot′ik) *adj.* pertaining to anastomosis.

anechoic (an-ĕ-ko′ik) *adj.* without echoes or reverberations.

anechoic chamber. room especially built so that the sound waves generated within are almost totally absorbed by the material used to cover walls, ceiling, and floor. The material must not only be highly absorbent but it is usually arranged in wedges with the thin edges pointed inward. Wire mesh suspended above the bottom wedges serves as a floor in the typical chamber. There must also be a high degree of isolation from external sounds to allow measurements to be made of sound waves generated within the room without interference from outside noises as well as sound wave reflection within the room.

aneneia (ah-nĕ-ne′ya) *n.* condition of being without speech because of deafness; *syn:* surdomute.

anesthesia (an″es-the′ze-ah) *n.* loss of sensation as a result of injury, disease, or the administration of a gas or drug. In general anesthesia, hearing is the last sense to be lost and usually the first to return.

angioma (an″je-o′mah) *n.* tumor involving blood vessels; *syn:* vascular tumor.

angiopathy (an-je-op′ah-the) *n.* any disease of the circulatory or lymphatic systems.

angiosclerosis *n.* hardening of the walls of blood vessels.

angiospasm (an′je-o-spazm″) *n.* blood vessel contraction (sometimes considered responsible for sudden loss of hearing).

angiotitis (an″je-o-ti′tis) *n.* inflammation of blood vessels in the ear.

ankylose (ang′kĭ-lōz) *v.* to immobilize by ankylosis.

ankylosis (ang″kĭ-lo′sis) *n.* immobilization of a joint by disease or surgery. In audiology, specifically referring to the immobilization of the footplate of the stapes by disease.

ankylotia (ang″kĭ-lo′sha) *n.* closure of the external auditory canal. *syn:* atresia.

anlage (ahn′lah-geh) *n.* first recognizable embryonic cells from which an organ or part develops.

annoyance level. AL. 1. subjective judgment of noise as disturbing or a nuisance. The unit of measurement is the "noy." 2. point at which ambient noise interferes with speech understanding. This is more commonly known as speech interference level (SIL).

annular cartilage. a ring composed of cartilage, e.g., the ring that holds the eardrum in place.

annular ligament (an′u-lar lig′ah-ment). ring-like ligament. In audiology, the tendon that holds the footplate of the stapes in the oval window.

annular ring. annular ligament.

annulus, anulus* (an′u-lus) *pl.* **annuli** *n.* ring-shaped structure of tissue surrounding an opening.* Nomina Anatomica (1960 revision) dropped one n—although it is not commonly used.

annulus tympanicum. the tympanic ring; a tough fibrous ring holding the eardrum in place.

anode *n.* 1. the positive electrode in a vacuum tube that collects the free electrons released by the negative electrode (cathode). 2. the positive electrode of a hearing aid cell.

anomalous (ah-nom′ah-lus) *adj.* differing from what would naturally be expected; *syn:* irregular. *adv:* **anomalously;** *n:* **anomalousness.**

anomaly (ah-nom′ah-le) *n.* 1. an abnormality. 2. an unusual or unexpected result or development.

anotia (an-o′she-ah) *n.* congenital absence of the pinna or external ear.

anotus (an-o′tus) *n.* a person without external ears.

anoxia (ah-nok′se-ah) *n.* lack of oxygen to a degree that may produce permanent damage (more severe than hypoxia).

ANS. autonomic nervous system.

ANSI. American National Standards Institute. Successor to USASI—United States of America Standards Institute. Successor to ASA—American Standards Association.

antepenult (an″te-pen-ult′) **antepenultima** (an″te-pen-ul′tĭ-ma) *n.* syllable before the next to last syllable of a word, e.g., "di" in auditory.

7

anterior (an-ter′e-or) *adj.* forward or toward the front.

anterior transverse temporal pyrus (pi′rus). auditory area in the cerebral cortex.

anterior vertical canal. one of the semicircular canals of balance; *syn:* superior semicircular canal.

anti- (an′tĭ). prefix indicating opposite, against or preventive.

antibiotic (an″tĭ-bi-ot′ik) *n.* product of a microorganism that may weaken or kill harmful microorganisms.

antibiotic *adj.* tending to weaken or destroy life.

antibody. a substance in the body that weakens or destroys bacteria or viruses.

anticholinergic drugs (an″tĭ-ko″lin-er′jik). those that block stimulation of the nerve endings in the ear. Used as a preventive treatment for motion sickness.

antigen (an′tĭ-jen) *n.* substance that stimulates the formation of antibodies.

antihelix (an″tĭ-he′liks) *n.* curved ridge of cartilage above the concha and in front of the helix or outer cartilage of the external ear.

antihistamine (an″tĭ-his′tah-mēn) *n.* agent used to treat allergic reactions and cold symptoms by counteracting histamine.

antilobium (an″tĭ-lo′be-um) *n.* the tragus—a small stiff ridge in front of the external opening of the ear canal.

antinode (an′tĭ-nōd″) *n.* point, line, or surface between the nodes of a vibrating system or standing wave where some characteristic has maximum amplitude.

antiphasic (an-tĭ-fa′sik) *adj.* reversed in phase in relation of one ear to the other.

antitragicus (an″tĭ-traj′ĕ-kus) *n.* vestigial muscle attached to the antitragus in the pinna of the ear.

antitragus (an″tĭ-tra′gus) *n.* projection on the ridge of cartilage opposite the tragus. It is just below the antihelix of the external ear. *adj:* **antitragic.**

antrotympanic (an″tro-tim-pan′ik) *adj.* pertaining to the tympanic or mastoid antrum and the middle ear cavity.

antrotympanitis (an′tro-tim-pah-ni′tus) *n.* inflammation of the middle ear and mastoid antrum.

antrum (an′trum) *n.* any nearly closed cavity or hollow space in a bone.

antrum auris (aw′ris) *n.* external auditory canal.

antrum, mastoid. (mas′toid) *n.* space in temporal bone, posterior to the tympanic cavity; *syn:* tympanic antrum; mastoideum; tympanicum.

antrum tympanicum (tim-pan′ik-um) *n.* space in bone posterior to the tympanic cavity. *syn:* mastoid antrum.

anvil (an′vil) *n.* the incus. Popular name for the middle bone of the ossicular chain.

AOR. auditory oculogyric reflex.

AP. action potential.

APA. American Psychological Association.

aperiodic (ah″pe-re-od′ik) *adj.* occurring at irregular intervals. *syn:* nonperiodic.

aperiodic wave. wave form that does not repeat itself in a regular pattern; *syn:* nonperiodic wave.

Apert's syndrome (Eugene Apert, French pediatrician, 1868-1940.) an unusual congenital group of symptoms including a peaked head (associated with achondroplasia) and webbed fingers.

aphaeresis, apheresis (ah-fer′ĕ-sis) *n.* omission of one or more sounds at the beginning of a word. *adj:* **aphaeretic.**

aphasia (ah-fa′ze-ah) *n.* breakdown or lack of power to use language—the result of congenital or adventitious brain damage. There is hearing but not understanding; *syn:* dysphasia. *adj:* **aphasiac, aphasic.**

aphasia, acoustic. inability to understand spoken language; *syn:* auditory aphasia, auditory agnosia, acousmatagnosis.

aphasia, auditory. inability to understand spoken language; *syn:* acoustic aphasia, auditory agnosia, acousmatagnosis.

aphasia, formulative. a type of aphasia characterized by inability to join words and phrases into connected language.

aphasia, functional. symptoms of aphasia resulting from hysteria or toxins. No cerebral lesion is present.

aphasia, receptive. lack of ability to understand spoken or written language.

aphemesthesia (ah″-fe-mes-the′ze-ah) *n.* word deafness or word blindness.

aphesis (af′es-is) *n.* a type of aphaeresis consisting of the dropping of a short unaccented vowel at the beginning of a word. *adj:* **aphetic;** *adv:* **aphetically.**

aphonia (ah-fo′ne-ah) *n.* inability to speak except in whispers. *adj:* **aphonic.**

aplasia (ah-pla′zhe-ah) *n.* lack of development of an organ or part of the body.

aplastic *n.* having deficient or arrested development; *syn:* agenesis.

apnea *n.* temporary halt in breathing. In the newborn the resultant lack of oxygen may cause hearing deficits among other problems.

apoplexy (ap′o-plek″se) *n.* bursting or clotting of a blood vessel in the brain (called a cerebral vascular accident, CVA) causes sudden loss or lowering of consciousness and loss of voluntary muscular control. More lasting physical problems and speech and language disorders may result.

APR. auropalpebral reflex.

Apriton (Ap′ri-ton) *n.* device developed by Marion Downs (University of Colorado Medical Center) to use in screening the hearing of newborn babies.

aprosexia (ap″ro-sek′se-ah) *n.* unintentional inattention; e.g., from defective hearing.

APS. American Physical Society.

AQ. achievement quotient. accomplishment quotient.

aqueduct, fallopian. bony passage through which the facial nerve traverses the middle ear into the internal auditory canal. *syn*: fallopian canal.

aqueduct, vestibular. portion of the bony endolymphatic canal through which passes the membranous tube containing endolymph.

arachnoid (ah-rak'noid) *n.* delicate, weblike, middle membrane surrounding the brain and spinal cord. *adj*: **arachnoid.**

arches, Corti's. meeting points of the inner and outer rods of Corti that form the tunnel of Corti.

arcus senilis. white opaque ring at the periphery of the drumhead due to deposit of fat, similar to the opaque white ring about the corneal periphery seen in aged persons.

area, acoustic. area within cortex of the temporal lobe of the cerebrum to which sound is referred; *syn*: acoustic center.

areal *adj.* pertaining to area, as in air conduction, the areal and lever relationships of the ossicular chain and tympanic membrane that results in about 26 dB gain.

Argand diagram. graph that shows a complex number in relation to rectangular coordinates x (horizontal) and y (vertical).

argument *n.* angle that determines the direction of a complex number (a combination of a real and an imaginary number).

armamentarium (ar"mah-men-ta're-um) *pl.* **armamentaria** *n.* equipment and methods used in any field of activity—especially in medicine.

arousal response. increase in activity level as a result of stimulation, e.g., neonatal response to narrow-band noise.

arrhythmic *adj.* without regularity or rhythm.

arsenic *n.* a very poisonous grayish white metal used in the manufacture of medicines. Sometimes ototoxic in its residual effect.

ART. acoustic reflex threshold.

arterial or venous tinnitus. head noises believed to result from blood-flow disturbances within the external or middle ear. Type of objective tinnitus.

arteriosclerosis (ar-te"re-o-sklĕ-rɔ'sis) *n.* thickening of the arterial walls accompanied by loss of elasticity, and contractility. Said to contribute to presbycusis—the loss of hearing as part of the aging process.

artery, internal auditory. artery that supplies blood to the inner ear. *syn*: labyrinthine artery.

arthritides (ar-thrit'ĭ-dēz) *n.* plural of arthritis.

arthritis (ar-thri'tis) *n.* inflammation of a joint. Tinnitus may accompany this disease.

arthritis, pneumococcic (nu-mo-kok'sik) *n.* an arthritis sometimes following lobar pneumonia, affecting one or more joints and the middle ear.

articular (ar-tik'u-lar) *adj.* relating to structures that meet to form a joint.

articulate (ar-tik'u-lat) *adj.* able to speak clearly and effectively. *n*: **articulateness, articulation,** *adv*: **articulately.**

articulate (ar-tik'u-lāt) *v.* 1. to pronounce clearly. 2. to join together and move—as a joint. *n*: **articulator.** *adj.* **articulative.**

articulation *n.* 1. act or manner of speaking. 2. understanding of speech. 3. connection of bones in a movable joint. *adj*: **articulatory.**

articulation curve. curve that results when an articulation score is plotted on a graph; *syn*: discrimination curve.

articulation index. AI. number that represents the ability to understand speech in the presence of noise. It is based on measurements made with 20 controlled noise frequency bands.

articulation score. rating of ability to understand speech based on comparison of similar word lists (see articulation test) presented at 10 dB increases in intensity. Results are given in percentage of articulation (intelligibility) at stated dB of increase over speech reception threshold. When the results are displayed in graphic form, it is known as an articulation curve.

articulation test. hearing test designed to measure the intelligibility of speech or of speech sounds. There are tests for individual sound articulation, syllable articulation, vowel or consonant articulation, initial or final consonant articulation.

artificial ear. device using a microphone in a cavity for the measurement of the acoustic output of an earphone. The cavity (6 cc in volume) is designed to present an acoustical impedance to the earphone equal to the impedance of the average human ear.

artificial eardrum. paper or plastic device designed to convey sound vibrations to the oval window through a reed—also of plastic.

AS. auricula sinister, auris sinistra (left ear). AD—right ear. AU—both ears.

ASA. Acoustical Society of America. American Standards Association—now ANSI.

ascending method. determining an audiometric threshold by increasing the intensity of the stimulus until it is identified. Opposite: descending method.

ASHA. American Speech and Hearing Association. New name: American Speech-Hearing-Language Association.

ASL. American Sign Language.

ASLHA. American Speech-Language-Hearing Association. Successor to

ASHA—American Speech and Hearing Association. (The association is still referred to as ASHA in common usage).

Aspergillus (as″per-jil′us) *n.* species of mold that sometimes affects the external ear canal.

Aspergillus auricularis. species of mold found in the external ear canal.

Aspergillus fumigatus. species of mold found in the ears, nose, and lungs.

Aspergillus glaucus. bluish-colored mold found on dried fruit and sometimes in the human ear.

Aspergillus niger. form of mold with black spores that is found in the external ear canal.

Aspergillus repens. species of mold found in the external auditory canal.

aspirate (as′pĭ-rāt) *n.* 1. consonant or other speech sound having a breathy quality. 2. product removed by suction from a body cavity.

aspirate *v.* 1. to produce a sound with breath. 2. to remove a fluid from a body cavity by suction, e.g., mucous or pus from the middle ear.

aspiration (as″pĭ-ra′shun) *n.* 1. act of producing a sound with breath. 2. removal of a fluid or foreign body from a body cavity.

aspirin (as′pĭ-rin) *n.* salicylic acid. Drug used for the relief of pain. It is ototoxic for some individuals. Tinnitus may be the first indication of sensitivity.

ASR. automatic send and receive—optional part of a TDD (telecommunications device for the deaf).

association method. teaching method concentrating on a close association of the essential processes of learning, i.e., attention, retention, and recall in a repetitive manner—of special value in aphasia.

assonance (as′o-nans) *n.* 1. similarity of sounds in words or syllables. 2. relative closeness of similar sounds, esp. of vowels. *adj.* or *n:* assonant, ent.

assortative mating pattern (ah-sor′ta″tiv). tendency of deaf persons to marry deaf mates.

ASTM. American Society for Testing and Materials.

astrocyte (as′tro-sīt) *n.* star-shaped nerve cell.

astrocytoma (as″tro-si-to′mah) *n.* tumor involving the astrocytes of the nervous system.

asylum-ear. bloody tumor of the ear sometimes found in the insane; *syn:* hematoma auris.

asymmetric (a″sim-met′rik) *adj.* not equal. Not of equal proportions.

asymptote (ah′sim-tōt) *n.* level of expected performance.

asymptotic localization. method of measuring auditory adaptation.

ATA. American Tinnitus Association.

ataxia (ah-tak′se-ah) *n.* lack of ability to coordinate voluntary muscular activity.

atelectasis (at″e-lek′tah-sis) *n.* lack of air in the middle ear or in the mastoid air spaces.

atelolalia. delay in development of speech due to hearing impairment. *syn:* hearing mutism.

athetoid (ath-ĕ-toid) *adj.* affected with athetosis.

athetosis (ath″ĕ-to′sis) *n.* condition, caused by a brain lesion, where involuntary movements interfere with voluntary movements in children.

atonic (ah-ton′ik) *adj.* spoken without accent or stress. Also used as a noun to designate an unaccented or unstressed word. *n:* **atonicity.**

atoxic (ah-tok′sik) *adj.* not toxic.

atresia (ah-tre′ze-ah) *n.* 1. closure of the ear canal or esophagus. 2. congenital absence of any normal anatomical opening.

atresic (ah-tre′zik) *adj.* concerning atresia: closed, e.g., an ear canal. *adj:* **atretic** (ah-tret′ik).

atrium (a′tre-um) *n.* 1. portion of the middle ear cavity lying below the malleus. 2. tympanic cavity. 3. any body cavity or passage, e.g., the auricle of the heart.

atrophy (at′ro-fe) *n.* wasting away from disuse or lack of nourishment. *adj:* **atrophied.**

attentive response. decrease in general activity level upon sound stimulation; e.g., in neonatal screening.

attenuate (ah-ten′u-āt) *v.* to reduce intensity or power.

attenuation (ah-ten″u-a′shun) *n.* weakening or lessening of intensity.

attenuation, interaural. the lessening of intensity that occurs as a sound stimulus passes through the head from one ear to the other.

attenuation, real-ear. measurement of the amount by which ear protectors lessen sound pressure reaching the eardrum of a particular observer. It is expressed in decibels of difference between thresholds of audibility when the ears are open and when they are protected.

attenuator (ah-ten′u-a″tor) *n.* device designed to diminish the intensity of a tone or signal, e.g., the hearing level control of the audiometer.

attic *n.* portion of the middle ear cavity above the eardrum occupied by the head of the malleus and the body and short process of the incus. *syn:* epitympanic recess.

atticitis. inflammation of attic or epitympanic recess.

atticoantrotomy (at″ĭ-ko-an-trot′o-me) *n.* operation to correct problems in the attic and mastoid antrum.

atticotomy (at″ĭ-kot′o-me) *n.* surgical opening of the attic of the middle ear.

atypical (a-tip'ĭ-kal) *adj.* not normal or typical.

AU. auris uterque. both ears. AD—right ear. AS—left ear.

audi, audio. combining form pertaining to hearing or the transmission, reception, or reproduction of sound.

audible (aw'di-bil) *adj.* heard or loud enough to be heard. *adv:* **audibly.**

audible frequency range. the most sensitive young ear has a hearing range from about 15 Hz to 20,000 Hz. The normal young ear with no history of disease has a range closer to 15-15,000 Hz.

audibility (aw"di-bil'-ĭ-te) *n.* capability of being heard.

audicle (aw'di-kul) *n.* early name for hearing aid.

audience *n.* act of hearing or paying attention.

audient *adj.* hearing, listening.

audile (aw'dil) *n.* person who has a tendency to derive mental images from sounds. *adj:* **audile.** 1. concerning hearing. 2. earminded as opposed to visual-minded.

auding *n.* perception and comprehension of speech.

audioanalgesia (aw"de-o-an"al-je'ze-ah) *n.* loss of pain sensation in the presence of loud or soothing sounds.

audiofrequency. a sound wave frequency within the so-called audible range: 15 Hz to 20,000 Hz.

audiodontic *adj.* concerning the concept of planting a hearing aid in a tooth.

audiogenic (aw"-de-o-jen'ik) *adj.* resulting from frequencies similar to sound waves. Usually referring to brain waves that cause epileptic type responses.

audiogram (aw'de-o-gram") *n.* record of the threshold of sensitivity of hearing measured at several different (usually discrete) frequencies.

audiogram, baseline. audiogram that represents the hearing of a worker before exposure to noise (or after at least 12 hours of quiet).

audiogram classifications. audiogram charts are broadly divided into the following categories:

flat curve: hearing loss is approximately equal at all frequencies.

gradually rising or falling curve: the loss falls or rises at approximately 5-10 dB per octave.

sharply falling or marked falling curve: loss increases about 15 to 20 dB per octave at higher frequencies.

saddle, dipper, trough or U-shaped curves: denotes less hearing loss at the low and high frequencies than in the middle range.

steep drop, ski-slope, waterfall, precipitous or sudden drop curves: usually denote nearly normal hearing in lower frequencies (sometimes as high as 2000 Hz) followed by a precipitous drop of 25 dB or more per octave.

audiogram, diagnostic. diagnostic audiograms usually include measurements at the half-octaves of 750 and 1500 Hz as well as lower frequencies, and higher frequencies.

audiogram, industrial. industrial audiograms commonly include measurements of thresholds at 500, 1000, 2000, 3000, 4000 and 6000 Hz.

audiogram, masking. graphic representation, in the form of a laddergram, of the masking effect of a lower frequency on a higher frequency at increasing levels of intensity. It is a seldom-used technique for differential diagnosis of sensorineural and conductive lesions.

audiogram, noise. audiogram based on the use of narrow bands of white noise.

audiogram, preplacement. in industrial audiometry, an audiogram resulting from a hearing test that precedes placement in a position.

audiogram, reference. 1. pre-employment audiogram. 2. any base audiogram.

audiograph (aw'de-o-graf) *n.* graphic chart showing the relationship between hearing loss and frequency. *syn:* audiogram.

audiography. audiometry.

audiogravic illusions. mistakes in auditory localization resulting from errors in perception of body position.

audiokinetic nystagmus (aw"de-o-kĭ-net'ik nis-tag'mus) *n.* involuntary movements of the eyeball that may result from sudden loud sounds, or the touching of the canthus (corner) of the eye.

audiologist (aw"de-ol'o-jist) *n.* person trained in audiology—a specialist in the problems of hearing and deafness—in America and Canada excluding the field of medicine.

audiologist, clinical. one who practices audiology in a clinic or doctor's office.

audiologist, pediatric. one engaged primarily with hearing problems of infants and children. *syn:* paedoaudiologist.

audiologist, research. one engaged primarily in research in regard to the function of the auditory system.

audiology (aw"de-ol'-o-je) *n.* study of hearing and hearing impairment. In Europe the term usually includes the study of the nature, causes, and treatment of diseases of the ear.

audiology clinic. facility or center, usually connected with a hospital or university, devoted to the analysis of hearing problems and offering advice and rehabilitative programs.

audiology, pediatric. specialty devoted to the hearing problems of infants and children; *syn:* paedoaudiology.

audiogyral illusions. mistakes in auditory localization resulting from rapid rotation of the body with the eyes closed.
audiometer (aw″de-om′ĕ-ter) *n.* instrument designed to measure the sensitivity of hearing. (See American National Standard Specification (ANSI) for Audiometers effective September 1, 1970). *adj:* **audiometric;** *n:* **audiometry.**
audiometer, automatic. audiometer that produces a pure tone, either continuous or pulsed, whose frequency is slowly changed (either continuously or at intervals from the lowest to the highest of the frequency testing range). The patient himself controls the intensity by pressing a button that engages a motor-driven attenuator to reduce the intensity of the tone until it fades below his threshold. By releasing the button the intensity of the tone is automatically raised again. The procedures may be reversed. The changes are recorded by a stylus on a moving chart. Thus the patient traces his own audiogram. *syn:* Bekesy audiometer.
audiometer, Bekesy. type of automatic audiometer.
audiometer, clinical. now called a "wide range audiometer."
audiometer, continuous frequency. one whose output frequency may be varied in steps of 1 cycle per second throughout the frequency range of the instrument.
audiometer, discrete frequency. one that generates pure tones at preselected individually distinct (discrete) frequencies. The frequencies usually selected are at octave or half-octave intervals rounded off from middle C (250 Hz scientific and tuning fork; 261.6 Hz musical). The full range of a diagnostic audiometer may include 125, 250, 500, 750, 1000, 1500, 2000, 3000, 4000, 6000, and 8000 Hz.
audiometer, extended high frequency. audiometer designed to generate frequencies from 8000 to 20,000 Hz.
audiometer, group. audiometer with a number of headsets designed to check the hearing of several people at the same time. One type uses live voice or a phonograph record giving numbers progressively softer. The last number heard by the listener indicates his *threshold.*
audiometer, limited range. one designed to test by air conduction limited ranges of frequency and sound pressure level. Pure tone frequencies of 500, 1000, 2000, 3000, 4000, and 6000 Hz are included. Sound pressures may be limited to 0 to 70 dB re standard audiometric zero.
audiometer, narrow range. one designed to test the response to one, two, or three pure tone frequencies at limited sound pressure levels for hearing screening purposes.

audiometer, pure tone. basic type of audiometer. An instrument that generates pure tones of various frequencies and ranges of intensity that can be controlled to measure hearing acuity or sensitivity.
audiometer, screening. any audiometer utilizing limited frequencies and intensities to make quick checks for hearing loss. For example, the audiometrist may "sweep" through selected frequencies at a preset level of intensity to determine the listener's ability to hear. Failure to hear one, two, or more tones is usually followed by referral for more complete testing.
audiometer, speech. an audiometer utilizing an amplifying circuit capable of presenting speech levels in graduated steps. It is used to determine individual thresholds of speech understanding—the speech reception threshold (SRT). Also used to determine the PB score, i.e., the percentage of words understood when a phonetically balanced word list (of monosyllables) is presented at a comfortable listening level. A masking circuit must also be included.
audiometer, tinnitus research (TRA). term applied to an instrument designed to determine the pitch and intensity of the individual's tinnitus.
audiometer, wide range. one designed to test, both by air and bone conduction, most of the auditory range in regard to both frequency and sound pressure level. A masking circuit must also be included. Formerly known as a clinical audiometer.
audiometric (aw″de-o-met′rik) *adj.* pertaining to audiometry.
audiometric assistant. person who has been trained in a special program to perform hearing tests, provide care for those with hearing handicaps, handle medical records, and work with other health care personnel.
audiometric curves. suggested revision by AAOO. 1. ascending—greater loss in low frequencies. 2. descending—greater loss in high frequencies. 3. abrupt drop—change of 40 dB or more in one octave. 4. basin—greater loss in middle frequencies. 5. dip—a depression of 10 dB or more and subsequent return to former level. 6. peak—elevation of 10 dB or more and subsequent return to former level.
audiometric nomograph (nom′o-graf). graphic representation of the audiometric results to be expected from a surgical procedure.
audiometric technician. person trained and qualified to administer audiometric tests and usually works under the supervision of an audiologist or otologist.
audiometric zero. zero level of a pure tone audiometer varies at each frequency in sound pressure level; that is re 0.0002 dyne per square centimeter (cm²). Zero represents the average threshold of hearing sen-

sitivity at each frequency of otologically normal young people between 18 and 30 years of age.

New studies brought about a change in reference levels from those in use since 1939 and officially adopted in 1951 by the American Standards Association (ASA).

The ANSI (American National Standards Institute) is now in agreement with the 1964 ISO (International Organization for Standardization).

The following table gives a comparison of reference threshold levels:

Table 1. Reference Threshold Level

1969 ANSI*

freqc'y	1951 ASA	1964 ISO	Diff.	**
125	54.5dB	45.5dB	9dB	
250	39.5	24.5	15 ⎫	15
500	25	11	14 ⎭	
1000	16.5	6.5	10	
1500	16.5	6.5	10 ⎫	
2000	17	8.5	8.5 ⎬	10
3000	16	7.5	8.5 ⎭	
4000	15	9	6	5
6000	17.5	8	9.5 ⎫	10
8000	21	9.5	11.5 ⎭	

* ANSI S3.6—1969 adopts the same sound pressure level base as ISO but changes the SPL calibration for different earphones (made by various manufacturers) to reach that standard.

** Since most audiograms are plotted in 5dB steps, it is more convenient to use the approximate values in column 5 to convert individual audiograms.
Add the figures to ASA 1951 Audiograms to compare them to ISO or ANSI graphs.
Subtract the figures to convert ISO to ASA.

audiometrist. audiometric technician. Some states license audiometrists to screen hearing in public schools.

audiometry. technique of measuring the sense of hearing by means of an audiometer.

audiometry, automatic. technique of administering hearing tests by means of an automatic audiometer and quantifying and classifying the results.

audiometry, behavioral. any audiometric procedure utilizing either a motor or verbal response to auditory stimulation, especially play audiometry.

audiometry, Bekesy. type of automatic audiometry. It is diagnostically important from the classification of the results into

one of five types (after Jerger, et al) when responses to continuous and pulsed tones are compared.

Type 1. pulsed and continuous tone tracings are intermingled; typical of normal ears or conductive hearing losses.

Type 2. continuous tone tracing drops 5 to 20 dB below pulsed tone tracing in the middle and upper frequencies: noted in cochlear lesions.

Type 3. continuous tone tracing drops abruptly by as much as 40 to 50 dB below tracing for pulsed tone: noted in lesions of the eighth nerve.

Type 4. similar to Type 2 except that the continuous tone tracing drops below the pulsed tone tracing at frequencies below 500 cps: noted in eighth nerve lesions.

Type 5. continuous tone tracing better than pulsed tone: indicative of nonorganic hearing loss.

audiometry, brainstem. shortened term for brainstem electric (or evoked) response audiometry (BSER, BERA) or auditory brainstem response (ABR) testing.

audiometry, cardiac evoked response. CERA. measurements are made of changes in heart activity that result from sound stimulation. A form of electrophysiologic audiometry.

audiometry, conditioned audio-visual response. CAVR. version of play audiometry that utilizes the lighting of a plastic toy to heighten the child's interest. Devised by Rayford C. Reddell and Donald R. Calvert.

audiometry, conditioned orientation reflex. CORA. version of play audiometry devised by Tokuro Suzuki and Yoshio Ogiba. It relies on an assessment of the child's localizing ability as lighted toys are coordinated with two loudspeakers.

audiometry, delayed feedback. DFA. method of estimating a speech reception threshold by determining the amount of intensity of a delayed speech signal required to cause a change in the voice pattern of the person being tested.

audiometry, detection. screening audiometry.

audiometry, electrodermal. EDA. method of determining hearing thresholds by measuring changes in skin resistance, associated with a conditioned response to sound stimulus. *syn*: electrodermal response audiometry (EDR); psychogalvanic audiometry (PGA); psychogalvanic skin response (PGSR).

audiometry, electroencephalic. EEA. type of electrophysiologic audiometry. The electroencephalic response (EER), resulting from sound stimulation, causes changes in the pattern of the electroencephalogram (EEG). These changes are measured and quantified.

audiometry, electrophysiologic. inclusive term covering many types of so-called objective audiometry designed to measure the individual's response to a sound stimulus without subject cooperation being necessary.

An instrument is used that records changes in brain waves, heart rate, or skin resistance in response to sound stimuli. The response may be pre-conditioned or reinforced by mild electric shock which follows the sound stimulus at an interval of about 0.6 second. See: evoked (or electric) response aud. (ERA); cardiac evoked response audiometry (CERA); electrocardiographic response (ECR); electrodermal audiometry (EDA); electroencephalic audiometry (EEA).

audiometry, evoked response. ERA. form of electrophysiologic audiometry in which an analog computer is included in the circuit to average out ongoing or spontaneous brain wave activity.

A characteristic pattern of response to a sound stimulus may then become evident. *syn*: electric response audiometry.

audiometry, group. method of checking the hearing of several people at once by means of a group audiometer.

audiometry, identification. screening audiometry.

audiometry, impedance. not fully accepted, this term is used by many authorities to cover the measurements made through the use of an electroacoustic bridge: tympanometry, acoustic impedance, and acoustic reflex threshold.

audiometry, industrial. audiometry concerned with monitoring or periodically checking the effects of industrial noise exposure.

audiometry, monitoring. periodic retests of hearing to detect possible hearing loss from noise exposure, ototoxic drugs, or other causes.

audiometry, physiological. test of hearing that depends upon the measurement of changes in electrical from either the skin (electrodermal) or the brain (electroencephalic).

audiometry, play. technique for measuring the hearing of young children by rewarding a correct response to an auditory stimulus by allowing the child to see a picture, or to activate a mechanical toy, or do something equally interesting.

audiometry, psychogalvanic. PGA. commonly called PGSR (psychogalvanic skin response). A method of determining hearing thresholds by measuring changes in

skin resistance, associated with a conditioned response to sound stimuli. *syn*: electrodermal audiometry.

audiometry, pure tone. audiometry based on the use of pure tones of various frequencies and intensities as auditory stimuli to measure hearing. Included are comparisons of responses to pulsed and continuous tones and comparisons of results with earphones and bone oscillators.

audiometry, respiration. audiometry based on a recording of changes in respiration in response to sound stimuli. See Crib-O-Gram.

audiometry, screening. technique involving checking large groups of people rapidly against a pre-established limit of normalcy as far as hearing is concerned. *syn*: identification audiometry.

audiometry, speech. technique of measuring ability to understand speech under various conditions of intensity and noise interference using sound field as well as earphones and bone oscillators.

audiometry, sweep frequency. screening test in which the examiner uses a fixed level of intensity and a limited number of frequencies.

audiometry, toddler. variation of behavioral audiometry reserved for younger children. It is dependent upon observation of the child's reaction (other than infant startle response) to stimuli presented in sound field. A method devised by Anne Harrison.

audiophile (aw'de-o-fīl') *n.* enthusiast of high-fidelity sound reproduction.

audioprosthetist (aw''de-o-pros'the-tist) *n.* specialist in the fitting and sale of hearing instruments.

audioprosthologist *n.* alternative title for a hearing aid-fitting specialist who has completed a course in audioprosthology.

audioprosthology (aw''de-o-pros-thol'oj-e) *n.* word coined by Harold N. Williams, PhD, to apply to a special course devoted to the study of hearing aid fitting.

audioreflexometry (aw''de-o-re-flex-om'ĕ-tre) *n.* the measurement of levels of hearing through observation of involuntary responses to acoustic stimulation.

audiotherapy. application of therapeutic techniques to help an individual use his residual hearing to maximum advantage; *syn*: auditory training, aural rehabilitation.

audiovestibular *adj.* concerning the function of the vestibular system as related to hearing.

audiovision or audivision. 1. sending of pictures, print, or symbols to accompany sounds on the telephone. Sometimes referred to as phonovision. 2. addition of signs or print (subtitles) to television pictures for the benefit of those with impaired hearing. Now more commonly referred to as captioned television.

audiovisual *adj.* pertaining to both hearing and sight, especially in forms of instruction.

audiphone, audiophone *n.* early device for conveying sound to the auditory nerve through the bones of the head. Often shaped like a fan, it was sometimes held in the teeth. Both names were used as trade names for early hearing aids.

audist *n.* uncommon name for audiologist.

audit *v.* to attend a course as a listener only, without expecting formal credit.

audition *n.* sense of hearing or the act of hearing.

auditive *adj.* auditory.

auditive *n.* auditory-minded person or one who depends upon hearing in learning or recall.

auditognosis (aw″dĭ-tog-no′sis) *n.* understanding and interpretation of body sounds as a method of diagnosis.

audito-oculogyric reflex (aw″dĭ-to-oc″-ul-o-ji′rĭk). quick movement of the head and eyes in the direction of a sudden loud sound.

auditor (aw′dĭ-ter) *n.* 1. one who hears or listens. 2. one who attends classes without earning formal credit.

auditorally. executed as an auditor.

auditorially. 1. in an auditory manner. 2. as in auditing accounts.

auditory (aw′dĭ-to″re) *adj.* pertaining to the ear and the sense of hearing.

auditory adaptation. phenomenon exhibited by some ears by which an audible tone or sound may become inaudible within a short time (tone decay).

auditory agnosia (ag-no′ze-ah). loss or impairment of auditory sensation although the sensory tract is relatively intact. *syn:* acoustic agnosia.

auditory alexia. inability to learn to read (e.g., by the phonics approach) due to failure to recognize differences and similarities in voiced sounds. *syn:* verbal aphasia.

auditory aphasia. inability to understand spoken language. *syn:* acoustic aphasia, auditory agnosia, acousmatagnosis.

auditory behavior index. ABI. classification of responses to auditory stimuli to be expected of the infant from birth to two years.

auditory brainstem response. ABR. an electronic method of making an objective measurement of response to acoustic stimuli used chiefly with infants; *syn:* brainstem response audiometry, brainstem evoked (or electric) response (BSER).

auditory canal. external: opening or passageway that allows sound waves to reach the eardrum. The external auditory meatus or porus (**meatus acusticus externus**). Internal: sheath through which the auditory nerve passes on its way from the cochlea to the brain. The internal auditory meatus or internal acoustic meatus or porus (**meatus acusticus internus**).

auditory capsule. cartilaginous capsule in the embryo that becomes the external ear. *syn:* auditory cartilage.

auditory cartilage. auditory capsule or auricular cartilage.

auditory closure. recognition of complete words when only parts are spoken or heard.

auditory cortex. portion of the outer layer of the brain that serves as the terminus of nerve impulses from the ear.

auditory discrimination. 1. ability to distinguish various sounds and relate them to their source. 2. ability to distinguish between words by sound alone.

auditory dysiconia (dis-ĭ-ko′ne-ah). defective ability to formulate auditory images.

auditory fatigue. the higher threshold of hearing that may result from continuous exposure to sound. It is expressed in dB per frequency and related to exposure time; *syn:* temporary threshold shift (TTS).

auditory feedback. nearing of one's own vocalizations.

auditory flicker. recognition of the discontinuity of an interrupted sound; *syn:* auditory flutter.

auditory flutter. auditory flicker.

auditory flutter fusion. loss of recognition of discontinuity of an interrupted sound due to increased rapidity of the interruptions.

auditory fusion. the apparent blending of a series of short pulses of sound into one sound; *syn:* aural fusion.

auditory hallucination. sensation of hearing something when there is no external auditory stimulus. Sometimes considered a form of tinnitus.

auditory irreminiscence (ir-rem-in-ĭs′ens). loss of ability to recall auditory memories.

auditory lateralization. determination by the listener that a sound is more from one side than the other.

auditory localization. determination of the source of a sound made possible partly by the difference in loudness and partly by the difference in time of reception between the two ears.

auditory meatus (me-a′tus). external: auditory canal from orifice to eardrum. *syn:* external acoustic meatus. internal: auditory canal in the petrous portion of the temporal bone through which pass the facial and auditory nerves and vessels. *syn:* internal acoustic meatus.

auditory memory span. ability to recall vocal sounds, usually tested by presenting a series of phonetic vowel sounds spoken at the rate of one per second. At the conclusion of the series, the subject tries to repeat the vowels in the order given.

15

auditory nerve. eighth cranial nerve. It leads from the inner ear to the brain. It is formed by a merger of the cochlear (hearing) nerve and the vestibular (balance) nerve. *syn*: acoustic nerve.

auditory oculogyric reflex. AOR. more commonly known as auditory reflex—brief closure of the eyes as a result of sudden sound.

auditory ossicles. small bones of the middle ear that convey sound impulses from the eardrum to the oval window. They are known as the hammer (malleus), anvil (incus), and stirrup (stapes).

auditory pit. 1. depression on either side of the head of the embryo where the ear will develop. 2. depression in front of the ear indicating a preauricular sinus which may be a site of infection.

auditory placode (plak'ōd). collection of embryonic cells that develop into the internal ear.

auditory plate. bony roof of the external ear canal.

auditory point *n.* the lowest point of the notch between the tragus and the rim of the concha.

auditory process. the edge of the tympanic plate to which is attached the cartilage of the external ear canal.

auditory receptor. hair cell in the inner ear.

auditory reflex. brief closure of the eyes as a result of a sudden sound.

auditory sensation area. 1. region on a graph of frequency of pure tones versus intensity of pure tones between the curve representing the threshold of audibility and the curve representing the threshold of tickle. 2. portion of the temporal lobe of the cortex of the brain that responds to sound.

auditory space. area within which sounds may be localized.

auditory synthesis. ability to integrate separately presented phonemes into syllables and words.

auditory teeth. minute toothlike projections along the free margin of the labium vestibulare of the cochlea; *syn*: Huschke's auditory teeth.

auditory threshold. sound pressure level of the minimum acoustic signal that causes an auditory sensation for the specified percentage of the number of times the signal is presented to the ear. The auditory threshold for spondees, for example, is defined as the minimum sound pressure level at which a subject can repeat correctly 50% of the spondaic words presented to him. Auditory thresholds vary with different stimuli, and the particular stimulus must be specified.

auditory threshold of sensitivity. point on a sound pressure level scale at which 50% of the stimuli presented to the ear are heard; *syn*: threshold of audibility, threshold of detectability.

auditory trainer. amplifying instrument designed for use in helping the hearing-impaired learn to hear.

A hard-wire system has wired connections from the teacher's microphone and amplifer to desk units and receivers (headphones) controlled by the pupils.

An induction loop system utilizes a magnetic field activated by a microphone and amplifier at the teacher's control and received by a telephone coil on the pupil's hearing aid.

More recently, wireless FM systems have come into use. These utilize a frequency-modulated radio signal between teacher and pupil.

auditory training. lessons or vocal experience exposure designed to help a person with impaired hearing make best use of his remaining hearing; *syn*: aural rehabilitation.

auditory trauma. loss of hearing from any kind of damage: burns, head injury, pressure changes, as well as noise.

auditory tube. eustachian tube.

auditory tube cartilage. tough connective tissue that forms part of the roof of the eustachian tube.

auditory vesicle. embryonic cell body from which the ear develops; *syn*: otocyst.

aur-, auri- combining form from the Latin: ear.

aural (aw'ral) *adj.* concerning the ear or sense of hearing.

aural adaptation. phenomenon exhibited by some ears by which an audible tone or sound may become inaudible within a short time; *syn*: tone decay, auditory adaptation.

aural calculus. thickened wax in the external ear canal.

aural fusion. apparent blending of a series of short bursts of sound into one sound; *syn*: auditory fusion.

aural harmonics. type of distortion generated within the ear itself. Increasing the intensity may cause pitches to be heard that are harmonics of the stimulating frequency.

aural microphonic. electrical voltage produced by the hair cells of the cochlea. The electrical response follows the wave form of the acoustic stimulus in a manner similar to the action of a microphone; *syn*: cochlear microphonic.

aural murmurs. tinnitus. Noises originating within the ear itself.

aural nystagmus (nis-tag'mus). nystagmus resulting from labyrinthine disturbances; characterized by involuntary eyeball movements—first rather slowly in one direction, then by quick jerking movements in the opposite direction.

aural overload. distortion of a sound signal by the ear itself when the intensity of the sound exceeds the limit of the individual's hearing mechanism.

aural reflex. involuntary reaction to an auditory (sound) stimulus.

aural rehabilitation. re-education in the use of the sense of hearing either with or without the help of amplification; syn: auditory training.

aural speculum. a short, funnel-shaped device for inspecting the external ear canal and eardrum—or into the middle ear when the eardrum is removed or missing.

auralism (aw'ral-izm) n. system of teaching the deaf that emphasizes the oral approach.

aurally adv. by ear.

auricle (aw'rĕ-kl) n. 1. external ear or pinna. 2. early type of hearing aid (nonmechanical).

auricula (aw-rik'u-lah) n. external ear, auricle, or pinna.

auricula dexter, auris dextra. AD. right ear.

auricula sinister, auris sinistra. AS. left ear.

auriculae uterque, auris uterque. AU. both ears. (To each one).

auricular. 1. concerning the ear or the sense of hearing. 2. pertaining to an auricle. 3. received by the ear. 4. ear-shaped.

auricular cartilage. auditory capsule or cartilage.

auricular ligaments. ligaments that attach the external ear to the temporal bone. Valsalva's ligaments.

auricular point. center of external entrance to auditory canal.

auricular therapy. acupuncture at the pinna to affect other parts of the body or psychological problems (such as overeating or smoking). syn: auriculotherapy.

auriculare, pl. **auricularia** n. point at center of opening of external auditory canal; syn: auricular point.

auricularis, Aspergillus (aw"rik-u-la'ris as"per-jil'us). species of mold sometimes found in the external auditory canal.

auriculate adj. 1. having ears or ear-shaped projections. 2. like an ear.

auriculopalpebral-reflex (aw-rik"-u-lo-pal-pe'bral). closure or blink of an eye resulting from stimulation by sudden sound, heat, or some irritant touching the external auditory canal. syn: Kisch's reflex, auropalpebral reflex, audito-oculogyric reflex.

auriculostomy n. surgical operation by which a hole is made in the lower part of the external ear (into the concha) to allow passage of a plastic tube or cord in an effort to make the wearing of a hearing aid less conspicuous or to improve sound pressure to the eardrum.

auriculotemporal syndrome. sweating and flushing of the ear as a result of jaw movement while eating.

auriculotherapy (aw-rik"u-lo-ther'ah-pe) n. method of treating disease by the use of acupuncture and acupressure at various points of the pinna; syn: auricular therapy.

auriform. shaped like an ear.

aurilave (aw'ri-lav) n. device for cleansing the external ear with water.

auripuncture. puncture of the eardrum; syn: myringotomy.

auriscalp, auriscalpium n. instrument used to scrape foreign matter from the ear.

auriscope n. instrument for making a visual examination of the external ear canal and eardrum; syn: otoscope.

auris (aw'ris) n. the ear.
  dextra: right ear (AD).
  externa: external ear, auricle, pinna.
  interna: internal ear, labyrinth.
  media: middle ear, tympanic cavity.
  sinistra: left ear (AS).
  uterque: both ears (AU). (To each one).

aurist n. seldom used term for specialist in diseases of the ear; syn: otologist.

auristics n. treatment of ear diseases.

aurometer n. predecessor of audiometer.

auropalpebral reflex (aw"ro-pal-pe'bral). rapid and distinct closing of the eyelids, or twitch at the corner (canthus) of the eye resulting from a sudden sound stimulus. It is said to be closely related to the stapedius muscle reflex in the middle ear. syn: acousticopalpebral reflex, cochleopalpebral reflex.

auscultate (aws'kul-tāt) v. to examine by listening to body sounds.

auscultatory adj. pertaining to auscultation.

auscultation n. act of listening, usually with a stethoscope, to sounds arising within the body.

auscultation tube. tube designed for listening to sounds within the patient's ear.

autism (aw'tizm) n. unnaturally extreme concentration on oneself. Self-centered day-dreaming and wishful thinking unduly influencing ability to cope with reality; syn: childhood schizophrenia. adj: autistic.

autogenesis (aw"to-jen'ĕ-sis) n. self-produced. This phenomenon forms the basis for biofeedback—sometimes used to treat tinnitus. adj: autogenic.

automatic control unit. device that may be connected to a telecommunications device for the deaf (TDD) to automatically turn on the acoustic coupler of the TDD after a preset number of rings.

automatic gain control. AGC. another term for automatic volume control. In hearing aids, a special circuit designed to prevent sounds from being amplified too much for the impaired ear.

automatic send and receive. portion of a telecommunications device for the deaf

(TDD) that consists of a teletypewriter unit that can be activated by prepunched tape.

automatic volume control. AVC. In hearing aids, a special circuit designed to prevent sounds from being amplified too much for the impaired ear; syn: automatic gain control (AGC).

autonomic (aw"to-nom'ik) adj. refers to a part of the nervous system not consciously controlled by the brain.

autophony (aw-to'fo-ne) n. ability of a person to hear his own voice louder than normally when the eustachian tube is abnormally open; syn: tympanophonia.

autotelic (aw-to-tel'ik) adj. concerning a method of teaching reading to young deaf children.

AV. international hearing aid symbol for automatic volume control.

AVC. automatic volume control.

average, pure tone. PTA. average of the pure tone thresholds at 500, 1000, and 2000 Hz.

aviator's ear. pain in the ear resulting from unequal balance between the middle and outer ear; syn: aero-otis media, barotrauma.

avulsed (ah-vulsed') v. forcibly torn away; e.g., the eardrum separated from the annular ring by the force of an explosion.

axion (ak-se'on) n. cerebrospinal axis; the brain and spinal cord.

axon, axone n. central process of a nerve cell or neuron usually conducting impulses away from the cell body. adj: **axonal, axonic.**

Aztec ear. an outer ear with no lobe; syn: Cagot ear.

B

B battery n. battery made up of several cells, connected to the plate circuit of a vacuum tube to cause flow of electron current in the tube. Used in old style vacuum tube hearing aids.

B scale. the B scale of a sound level meter is weighted (sounds are filtered) to cut the frequencies below 300 Hz—increasing from about 4 dB per octave.

babble v. to utter meaningless sounds with no attempt to make conventional speech sounds or to communicate with others. A normal stage in the development of speech. Lack of or early cessation of babbling may be indicative of hearing impairment in the infant. syn: psopholalia. n: **babble,** n: **bab-blement,** n: **babbler.**

background noise. 1. intrusive circuit sounds that interfere with electronic signals. 2. surrounding sounds of the environment—ambient noise.

backward masking. a louder noise is introduced within 100 milliseconds after a short pure test tone is presented. The louder noise masks out (makes inaudible) the pure tone even though the louder sound is presented after the test tone.

badge test. Bekesy ascending and descending gap evaluation.

baffle n. device designed to prevent sound waves from interfering with each other; e.g., the wedge-shaped pieces of absorbent material in an anechoic chamber, or the partition or cabinet between front and back of a loudspeaker. n: **baffler,** v: **baffle.**

bag, Politzer. pear-shaped rubber bulb used for forcing air through the eustachian tube into the middle ear.

balance nerve. vestibular nerve that joins with the cochlear nerve to become the auditory or acoustic nerve (VIIIth cranial nerve).

balance, organ of. semicircular canals of the internal ear. Situated at right angles to each other in three planes, movement of the fluid (endolymph) within the canals activates the hair cells that initiate nerve impulses. These nerve impulses are conducted along the vestibular nerve to the cortex to be interpreted by the brain for orientation in space and thus help to maintain equilibrium.

band, critical. narrow range of frequencies that are most effective in masking a particular pure tone.

band-pass filter. electrical filter that allows a fixed or pre-selected band of frequencies to pass—to be transmitted. Acoustic signals or frequencies above or below the band-pass filter are rejected—not transmitted or amplified.

band pressure level. sound pressure level for a spectrum of specified frequencies within a restricted band.

band spectrum pl. **spectra.** sound pressure levels of each octave (or narrower) component of a complex noise are measured and presented in diagrammatic form to show comparative relationships.

bandwidth. frequencies included between specified cut-off frequencies. For example: the octave band width with 1000 Hz as its geometric midfrequency has cut-off frequencies at 710 and 1400 Hz.

BAP. best audible pressure.

Barany's caloric test (bah-rah'nē). (Robert Barany—Viennese otologist 1876-1936). Water, either above or below body temperature, is used to irrigate the external auditory canal. This stimulates the vestibular portion of the ear and results in more or less rapid eye movements (nystagmus).

Barany chair. chair designed to allow the patient to be turned in a circular motion to test the effect on equilibrium.

Barany noise box. device operated by a key-wound spring to produce "white noise" for masking purposes.

barbula hirci (bar'bu-lah hir'se). (Goat's beard) hairs growing at the outer opening of the external auditory canal.

barotitis media (bar"o-ti'tis). (bar—weight or pressure) damage to the middle ear caused by changes in barometric pressure (aero-otitis media).

barotrauma (bar"o-traw'mah) *n.* injury or wound caused by excessive changes in atmospheric pressure as may occur in flying or deep sea diving. The damage may be to the walls of the ear canal or eardrum. Such injury may occur when there is a substantial difference between the pressure in the external auditory canal (atmospheric pressure) and the pressure in the middle ear; *syn*: aero-otitis, barotitis media.

barotrauma, otic. injury to ears resulting from changes in barometric pressure either from flying or diving. It results from the imbalance between the ambient external pressure and that within the middle ear; *syn*: aero-otitis. *adj*: **barotraumatic.**

baryecoia (bar"ĭ-koi'a). (bary-heavy). heavy or hard of hearing; deafness.

barylalia (bar"ĭ-la'le-ah). heavy speech. Difficulty in speaking or speaking with an unusually deep voice.

baseline audiogram. audiogram representative of the hearing of a worker before exposure to noise (or after at least 12 hours of quiet).

basic frequency. the frequency of greatest importance. *syn*: fundamental frequency.

basilar (bas'ĭ-lar) *adj*. **basilary** (bas'ĭ-lar"e) *adj*. of, concerning, or situated at the base.

basilar macula. cluster of cells in the embryonic otic vesicle that develops into the basilar membrane and its associated portions of the inner ear.

basilar membrane. membrane that forms the base of the triangular inner tube of the cochlea. It stretches across the cochlea from the spiral bony lamina to the spiral ligament, and divides the cochlea into two main divisions: the scala vestibuli and the scala tympani. The triangular inner tube is known as the scala media or cochlear duct.

basilar papilla. organ of Corti—the specific receptor organ of hearing.

basis. foundation or base of the cochlea (basis cochleae) adjoining the middle ear at the oval and round window.

basis modioli (mo-di'o-li). base of the modiolus; the part of the modiolus that rests on the bony structure between the oval and round windows.

basis stapedis (stah-pe'dis). base of the stapes; the flat platform fitting into the oval window that supports and is activated by the crura (legs) of the stapes.

bass deafness. deafness to the bass tones.

battery. device for generating electric currents by chemical action. To be technically correct a battery consists of two or more cells, but in common usage a single cell for use in transistorized hearing aids is referred to as a battery. Hearing aid batteries are of various types, depending chiefly upon the material used: *alkaline-manganese.* a larger cell for body aids; voltage 1.5; although more expensive, this has largely replaced the carbon-zinc cell because of its longer life. *carbon-zinc.* penlight size for body aids; initial voltage 1.5, but falls gradually with use. *mercuric-oxide.* can be made quite small; working voltage 1.3; flat discharge. *nickel-cadmium* (*nicad*). working voltage 1.2, this has size limitations and is comparatively expensive, but is rechargeable with care. *silver-oxide.* working voltage 1.4; sizes comparable with mercuric-oxide, but higher voltage for more power. Flat discharge, more constant than mercuric-oxide. *zinc-air.* using air (oxygen) as the cathode, this cell has more room for the anode in the same size cell, so it has a much longer use life. The working voltage is now about 1.35.

battery. a group of subjective and/or objective tests considered together for diagnostic purposes.

battery drain. amount of electric current being drawn from a battery while it is in use. In a hearing aid the drain is determined by the engineering of the circuitry of the aid. In the case of a push-pull circuit the amount of ambient noise will also have an effect on the battery drain; the more sound going through the aid, the greater the drain.

BBA. best binaural average.

BC. bone conduction.

Beasley report. common name for a portion of U.S. Public Health Survey of 1935-36 conducted by Dr. Willis Beasley, which "established a normal hearing reference zero or normal auditory threshold." This became the ASA 1951 audiometric zero and was based on the threshold of hearing of about 1200 normal hearers.

beat *n.* amplitude pulsation resulting from the addition of two or more periodic quantities of the same kind but of slightly different frequencies, i.e., one may hear a pulse or throb of louder sound at intervals when two slightly different tones are sounded together.

beat *v.* to alternate in intensity so as to throb or pulsate.

behavioral audiometry. any audiometric procedure utilizing either a motor or verbal response to auditory stimulation, especially play audiometry; behavioral observation audiometry.

Bekesy audiometer (bek′ĕ-se) (George von Bekesy, Hungarian Physicist, U.S. 1948, 1899-1972). type of semi-automatic audiometer in which the patient controls the intensity of the tone by pushing a button control.

Bekesy audiometry. a type of semi-automatic audiometry. It is diagnostically important from the classification of the results into one of five types based on the comparison of responses to continuous and pulsed tones. The types are described under: audiometry, Bekesy.

bel *n.* unit used to express the ratio of acoustic or electrical power levels named in honor of Alexander Graham Bell. The number of bels is the logarithm of the base 10 of the power ratio. See decibel, one-tenth of a bel, the term commonly used in audiology.

Bell's palsy (Sir Charles Bell, Scottish physician, 1774-1842). facial paralysis caused by a lesion of the VIIth cranial nerve. Hearing impairment may accompany the facial distortion.

Bender gestalt test (Lauretta Bender, New York psychiatrist, 1938). test for personality and possible brain damage among the deaf.

benign (be-nīn′) *adj.* mild, not life-threatening; commonly used to refer to a nonmalignant or noncancerous tumor.

BER. brainstem evoked (or electric) response.

BERA. brainstem evoked (or electric) response audiometry.

Bergmann's cord (Gottlieb H. Bergmann, German neurologist, 1781-1861). stripe of white fibers in the fourth ventricle of the brain involved with the hearing process; acoustic striae.

betacism (ba′tah-sizm) *n.* dialect characteristic or speech defect in which the sounds of b and v lack distinctiveness.

beta wave or rhythm. brainwave pattern of more than ten peaks per second on an electroencephalogram.

Bezold's abscess (ba′zoltz). (Friedrich Bezold, Munich otologist 1842-1908). abscess in the muscle attached to the mastoid process which may cause a running ear.

Bezold's mastoiditis. inflammation of the mastoid process resulting from Bezold's abscess.

Bezold's perforation. perforation of the inner surface of the mastoid, caused by breakthrough of pus from Bezold's abscess.

Bezold's symptom. inflamed fluid-filled swelling at the tip of the mastoid process.

Bezold's triad. diminished perception of the low tones, better bone conduction, and negative Rinne—indicating otosclerosis.

BHI. Better Hearing Institute.

bi- (bi). prefix meaning two.

biaural (bi-aw′ral) *adj.* seldom used variation of the term binaural: using two ears.

biauricular (bi″aw-rik′u-lar) **biauriculate** (-lāt) *adj.* relating to both auricles. Having two auricles—usually refers to different animal hearts rather than external ears.

bibliotherapy (bib″le-o-ther′ah-pe) *n.* the recommendation and use of appropriate readings from books and other literature by the patient so that he will have a better understanding of his problem.

BICROS (bi′cros). bilateral-cros; amplifying system that is a modification of the contralateral routing of signals (CROS); provides a microphone to pick up signals (sound pressure waves) on the side of the greater impaired ear and sends them electrically to the better ear. In this system the better ear also needs amplification, which is provided by another microphone through the same amplifier.

BICROS, open. bicros arrangement that utilizes open earmolds, or tubing alone, to the aidable ear.

BIFROS. binaural frontal routing of signals. A hearing aid amplifier system using microphones set in the front of eyeglass frames to send electrical signals through the bows to each ear. Devised by A. R. Dunlavy.

bifurcate (bi-fur′kat) *v.* to divide into two parts.

bilabial (bi-la′be-al) *adj.* 1. concerning a consonant produced with both lips, e.g., b, p, m. 2. having two lips.

bilateral (bi-lat′er-al) *adj.* pertaining to both ears or both sides of the head.

bilateral contralateral routing of signals. see BICROS.

bilateral fitting. hearing aid with two cords and two receivers with only one amplifier ("Y" cord arrangement).

bilirubin (bil″i-roo′-bin). bile pigment, the product of degenerated hemoglobin, which causes jaundice. Often found deposited in the brain and spinal cord of infants with hearing impairments, cerebral palsy, or both. **kernicterus,** a form of icterus neonatorum (jaundice in the newborn).

bimastoid *adj.* pertaining to or joining the mastoid processes.

bimodal *adj.* concerning the utilization of two methods of brain stimulation, e.g., audition and vision.

bimodal method. combination of manual and oral education of the deaf child; *syn:* simultaneous method.

binaural (bi-naw'ral) *adj.* two-eared; hearing with both ears.

binaural cros. amplifying system that provides a microphone at each ear with a wire leading to an amplifier and receiver at the other ear. It is designed to allow the use of greater binaural power through ear-level hearing aids. *syn:* criss-cros.

binaural diplacusis (dip"lah-ku'sis). the listener believes that the same pure tone presented to the left and right ears alternately is of a different pitch in each ear. *syn:* diplacusis binauralis.

binaural fitting. two complete hearing aids (amplifiers, microphones, and receivers)— one for each ear and ideally at ear level (as opposed to bilateral "Y" or "V" cord).

binaural fusion. single mental impression that results, although there are differences between the sound signals reaching each ear.

binaural loudness balance test. procedure for comparing judgments of loudness. In alternate binaural loudness balance testing, sound is presented first to one ear then to the other; the intensity of the sound presented to one ear is adjusted until the sounds in both ears are judged to be equally loud. This is a commonly used test of loudness recruitment. In simultaneous loudness balancing, the tone is presented to both ears at the same time. The objective is to localize the tone in the midline or center of the head.

binaural summation. cumulative effect of sound reaching both ears, resulting in a threshold lower than that of the better ear alone.

binaural test. test of the ability to integrate and understand speech sounds presented to each ear simultaneously through narrow band-pass filters—high to one ear and low to the other. Only a normally functioning auditory system can get a perfect score.

binauricular (bin"aw-rik'u-lar) *adj.* concerning or having two ears; binaural.

Binet-Simon Scale test (Alfred Binet, French psychologist, 1857-1916). test of intelligence originally designed for children and later extended in range.

Bing test. comparison of the response to a bone vibrator stimulus (or tuning fork) when the ear is left open and then closed; an occlusion test.

binotic *adj.* concerning or having two ears; binaural.

biochemical genetics. study of the effects of chemicals or drugs on genes and heredity.

biofeedback. electronic instruments are used to detect and amplify signals from the body, which the individual is trained to use in modifying specific physiological functions and emotional reactions. One application is in the management of tinnitus.

bisensory *adj.* concerning the use of two senses.

bisyllabic *adj.* concerning a word of two syllables. If the syllables are stressed equally it is called a spondaic word or a spondee.

bithermal caloric test. the use of water or gas of two different temperatures in caloric testing of the vestibular (balance) mechanism.

bi-tonal (bi-tōn'al) *adj.* having two tones; sometimes used as a synonym for diplacusis, the hearing of two tones when only one is presented to the ear.

bitragion diameter. diameter of head at notch above the tragus—the anterior notch.

Blainville ears (Henri Blainville, French zoologist and anthropologist, 1777-1850). unequal appearance in size and shape of external ears.

blast-, blasto- suffix used to designate an immature cell or structure that gives rise to a definitive structure, growth, or sprout.

blast *n.* violent effect of a wave of increased atmospheric pressure followed by a wave of decreased atmospheric pressure resulting from an explosion; may cause acoustic trauma to those nearby.

blastema (blas-te'mah) *pl.* **blastemas, blastemata** *n.* mass of living substance from which cells and tissues are formed. *adj:* **blastematic, blastemic.**

bleb (bleb) *n.* small blister or vesicle.

blennotorrhea (blen"no-toh-re'ah) *n.* discharge of matter from the ear.

blocked electrical impedance. impedance measured at the electrical terminals of an electromechanical transducer when the mechanical system is blocked.

BOA. behavioral observation audiometry (see behavioral audiometry).

body baffle effect. 1. change produced by the presence of a body in the sound field. 2. effect on the response of a box-type or conventional hearing aid when worn on the body, especially under clothing. The greatest attenuation is in frequencies above 1000 Hz.

body hearing aid. hearing aid worn on the body, usually in a pocket or special carrier garment, for those with severe to profound hearing impairments. *syn:* box-type or conventional hearing aids.

Boel's test. noisemaker test developed in Sweden for neonates.

boilermaker's ear, boilermaker's deafness. hearing loss resulting from noise exposure; typified by the high frequency loss of many workers who have spent years repairing or assembling boilers.

bone-air gap. the difference in hearing sensitivity as revealed by comparison of bone conduction and air conduction audiometric test results.

bone conduction. transmission of sound pressure waves through the bones of the skull to the inner ear.

bone conduction, absolute. ABC. 1. test to establish levels of threshold sensitivity in response to the stimulus of a bone oscillator while the ears are occluded (closed). 2. tuning fork test made by comparing the bone conduction of the patient with that of the examiner. The ear canal of the patient is closed by the finger of the examiner and the base of the tuning fork is placed on the mastoid process. If the examiner can still hear the fork in the same manner after the patient has ceased to hear it, this reduced absolute bone conduction usually indicates a sensorineural impairment.

bone conduction hearing aid. hearing aid utilizing a bone conduction receiver to transmit sound.

bone conduction receiver. vibrator or oscillator designed to transmit sound pressure waves through the skull.

bone conduction, relative. test to establish levels of threshold sensitivity in response to the stimulus of a bone oscillator while the ears are open (unoccluded). Compare absolute bone conduction.

bone conduction test. test conducted by placing a bone oscillator on the skull, usually the mastoid process, to determine the threshold of hearing sensitivity when the conductive mechanism of the ear is bypassed. The test is designed to determine how well the balance of the hearing sense is functioning.

bone conduction threshold. level of intensity at which pure tone can just be recognized through a bone oscillator pressed against the skull.

bone conduction vibrator. device for conveying mechanical vibration to the mastoid process (or other parts of the head) in a bone conduction test; bone oscillator.

bone, mastoid (processus mastoideus). rounded hard protrusion at the lower end of the skull behind the external ear. It is honeycombed with air-filled cells.

bone, tympanic (anulus tympanicus). cartilaginous or bony ring that supports the eardrum.

bony cochlea. cavity in the petrous part of the temporal bone that contains the cochlea.

bony endolymphatic canal. canal in the temporal bone through which the membranous tube containing endolymph passes.

bony labyrinth. cavity in the petrous portion of the temporal bone that contains the inner ear.

bony vestibule. cavity in the temporal bone that contains the membranous vestibule of the inner ear.

bougee (boo-zhe') *n.* slender, hollow, flexible instrument that is inserted into a cavity or tube (e.g., eustachian) for diagnosis or treatment.

bowl. portion of the earmold that fits into the bowl (concha) of the ear.

box *n.* blow or slap on the ear.

box *v.* to strike the ears with the hand.

brady- (brad'e). prefix meaning slow or dull.

bradyacousia (brad"e-ah-ku'se-ah) *n.* dull hearing.

bradylalia (brad"e-la'le-ah) *n.* abnormally slow speech.

brainstem audiometry. shortened term for brainstem evoked (electric) response audiometry (BSER, BERA) or auditory brainstem response (ABR) testing.

brainstem response audiometry. BSER. electronic method of making an objective measurement of response to acoustic stimuli. *syn*: auditory brainstem response (ABR).

bridge *n.* 1. electronic instrument containing a circuit for measuring resistance, inductance, capacitance, or impedance of the middle ear mechanism. 2. in reference to earmolds, the portion of the earmold that extends from the canal to the point where the concha rim and helix are joined.

Bright's disease (Richard Bright, English physician, 1789-1858). inflammation of the kidneys, sometimes accompanied by sensorineural hearing loss. *syn*: nephritis.

bristle cells. hair cells of the organ of Corti.

broad-band noise. sound containing a wide range of frequencies.

Broca's area (bro'kahz) (Pierre P. Broca, French physician, 1824-1880). speech center in the cortex of the left hemisphere of the brain.

bruit (brwe, broot) *n.* 1. sound, as of blood moving within the patient's ear, which may be heard by an examiner through an auscultation or ear-to-ear tube. 2. abnormal internal body sound.

brux (bruks) *v.* to grind the teeth, especially while sleeping.

brux *n.* sound of grinding teeth.

BSER. brainstem evoked (electric) audiometry.

BTE. behind the ear. A hearing aid worn behind the ear and coupled to the ear by tubing attached to an earmold; postauricular hearing aid.

BTL. Bell Telephone Laboratories.

buccal cavity (buk'al kav'ĭ-te). the mouth between the teeth and cheeks.

bulla ossea. enlarged section of the bony portion of the external ear canal.

bulla, tympanic. bony cavity which encloses most of the middle ear cavity in some mammals. In the canoids (dogs, bears, raccoons, etc.) it is undivided, while in the feloids (cats, civets, hyenas, etc.) it has a bony divider to form two cavities.

bullous (bul'us) *adj.* containing watery or serous fluid.

bullous myringitis. viral infection of the eardrum that may cause it to split open; myringodermatitis.

bundle, olivacochlear (ol"i-va-kok'le-ar). olive-shaped group of nerve cells which carry impulses from the brain to the cochlea.

bundle of Rasmussen. group of efferent nerve fibers running between the superior olivary complex and the cochlea.

C

C scale. the broadest and flattest scale of a sound level meter. It measures sound pressure levels in decibels relative to .0002 dyne cm^2 and is essentially equally sensitive to all frequencies from 20 to 10,000 Hz. Flat from 100 to 2000 Hz, the C scale has gradual dips which make it 6 dB less sensitive at 21 Hz and at 11,000 Hz.

C tracings. tracings resulting from a continuous tone stimulus used in automatic audiometry.

CA. chronological age.

ca. about.

Cagot ear (ka-go'). external ear having no lobe. *syn:* Aztec ear.

caiculus, aural. impacted wax in the external auditory canal.

calibrate (kal'i-brāt) *v.* to adjust the intensity levels of an audiometer in correlation with its headphones. 2. to adjust a hearing aid to a predetermined response slope of intensity. *n:* **calibration, calibrator.**

California test. answers to questions are analyzed in a personality test used with deaf children.

caloric test. pouring water, either above or below body temperature, into the ear and measuring the involuntary eye response

(nystagmus—eye oscillation) that results. Caloric testing is often done with an electronic measuring device, the electronystagmograph, which records the eye movements by means of a stylus on a moving paper tape. The resulting chart is called an electronystagmogram.

caloric test, Barany. early test of vestibular function devised by Robert Barany, early 20th century otolaryngologist.

canal, auditory. external: the passage from the pinna to the eardrum through which sound waves travel. **internal:** an opening in the petrous portion of the temporal bone through which the auditory and facial nerves and blood vessels pass.

canal, bony endolymphatic. canal in the temporal bone through which the membranous tube containing endolymph passes.

canal, Corti's. spiral canal within the organ of Corti between the outer and inner hair cells. Triangular in shape, it is bounded by the outer and inner pillar cells (the pillars of Corti) and is filled with fluid. *syn:* Corti's tunnel.

canal, fallopian. more common name for the fallopian aqueduct.

canal, horizontal or lateral. one of the semicircular canals—part of the human balance mechanism.

canal, Jacobson's. (Ludwig L. Jacobson, Danish physician, 1783-1843). minute bony tube containing Jacobson's (the tympanic) nerve. It runs from the tympanum to the lower surface of the petrous portion of the temporal bone. *syn:* canaliculus tympanicus, tympanic canal.

canal, lateral or horizontal. one of the semicircular canals—part of the human balance mechanism.

canal-lock. canal earmold that has an additional ridge of plastic fitting into the bowl of the ear to help hold the earmold in place.

canal, Lowenberg's. (Benjamin B. Lowenberg, French physician, 1836-?). cochlear duct, membranous cochlea, or scala media. The middle triangular tube of the cochlea. *syn:* ductus cochlearis, cochlear duct, membranous cochlea, scala media.

canal mold. earmold that uses only a canal section to hold the plastic tube from the ear-level hearing aid.

canal, posterior vertical. one of the semicircular canals—part of the human balance mechanism.

canal, Rosenthal's (Isidor Rosenthal, German physician, 1836-1915). membranous spiral tube of the cochlea, containing the scala media, the scala tympani, and the scala vestibuli. *syn:* canalis spiralis cochleae, spiral cochlear canal.

canal, semicircular. one of three fluid-filled ducts, each describing a little more than half a complete circle, within the labyrinth of the ear. Together with the utricle and the saccule they make up the organ of balance. The three canals, positioned at 90 degree angles to each other, are known as the superior, the posterior vertical, and the lateral or horizontal semicircular canals.

canal, spiral cochlear. commonly known as the spiral canal of the cochlea. A portion of the bony labyrinth of the inner ear about 30 mm long making 2¾ turns about a central bony supporting structure known as the modiolus. Contains the scala tympani, scala vestibuli and cochlear duct. *syn*: Rosenthal's canal.

canal, spiralis modiolus (spi-ral'is mo-di'o-lus). commonly known as the spiral canal of the modiolus. The minute channel within the modiolus where the spiral ganglion of the cochlear nerve lies.

canal, superior. one of the semicircular canals—part of the human balance mechanism; sometimes described as the anterior vertical canal.

canal, tubotympanic. embryonic stage in the development of the eustachian tube and tympanic cavity.

canal, tympanic (canaliculis tympanicus). minute bony tube containing Jacobson's (tympanic) nerve; runs from the tympanum to the lower surface of the petrous portion of the temporal bone.

canaliculis (kan"ah-lik'u-lus) *pl.* **canaliculi** *n.* minute canal, channel, or tube; e.g., auricular, cochlear, tympanic. *adj*: **canalicular.**

canalis *pl.* **canales** *n.* canal, channel or tube: semicircular, etc.

canals, central of cochlea (canales longitudinales modioli). minute channels in the center of the bony structure that supports the cochlea (modiolus) through which pass blood vessels and nerves to the apex.

canals, Siebenmann's (Friedrich Siebenmann, German physician, 1852-1928). tiny blood vessels in the aqueduct of the cochlea.

cannula (or canula) *n.* thin tubular surgical instrument used to drain body cavities.

canthus *pl.* **canthi** *n.* junction of the upper and lower eyelids. *adj*: **canthal.**

canthus, lateral. outside corner of the eye.

canthus, medial. inner corner of the eye.

capacitance *n.* 1. a measure of the ability of two conducting surfaces separated by a nonconductor (or dielectric) to store an electric charge. 2. ability of a circuit to oppose a change in voltage. 3. amount of energy a battery can deliver under controlled conditions. 4. by definition: a capacitor (or condenser) has a capacitance of 1 farad if it can store 1 coulomb of electrical charge when 1 volt is applied.

capacitor *n.* device consisting of two conducting surfaces separated by a nonconductor or dielectric—used to store and control electrical energy. *syn*: condenser.

capacity *n.* amount of electrical energy available from a battery under controlled conditions.

capitis (caput) mallei (kap'ĭ-tus mal'e-i) *pl.* **capita.** the head of the malleus moving with the incus.

capitis stapedis (sta'pe-dis). head of the stapes; knob of the stirrup that connects with the anvil (incus).

capitulum *n.* (kah-pit'u-lum) *pl.* **capitula.** rounded head or knob of a bone.

capitulum malleus. head or large rounded part of the malleus (hammer) which moves with (articulates) the incus (anvil) at the incudo-malleolar joint.

capitulum stapes. small rounded end of the stapes (stirrup) that fits into the lenticular process of the incus (lentiform nodule of Sylvius) and moves with it at the stapedo-incudal joint.

capsule, auditory. cartilaginous capsule in the embryo which becomes the external ear.

capsule, otic. membranous sac that contains the inner ear.

capsulitis of the labyrinth. old term for otosclerosis.

carbon hearing aid. obsolete hearing aid that depended upon carbon granules or carbon shot in the microphone.

carbon microphone. device for converting sound pressure waves into electrical energy which utilized the unique properties of carbon.

carcinoma (kar"si-no'mah) *n.* malignant tumor or cancer arising in the membranous tissue (epithelium) lining the canals, cavities, or ducts of the body.

cardi-, cardia-, cardio- (kar'de). prefix referring to the heart.

cardiac (kar'de-ak) *adj.* relating to the heart.

cardiac evoked response audiometry, CERA. measurements made of changes in heart activity which result from sound stimulation; a type of electrophysiologic audiometry.

cardioid response (kar'de-oid). heart-shaped pattern of sensitivity displayed by directional microphones.

cardiopathy (kar"de-op'ah-the) *n.* heart disease.

Carhart notch. dip in the bone conduction audiogram of 5 dB at 500 and 4000 Hz, 10 dB at 1000 Hz, and 15 dB at 2000 Hz. It results from the inability of the fluids to move freely in the cochlea when the footplate of the stapes is firmly fixed in the oval window.

carrier phrase. phrase preceding the test word in speech audiometry, e.g., "Say the word—". It is used both to instruct the subject and to monitor the speaker's (examiner's) voice.

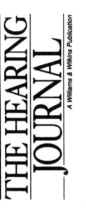

THE HEARING JOURNAL

A Williams & Wilkins Publication

Dictionary of Audiology Survey
August 1993

- What do you think are the Dictionary's strengths and weaknesses? How could we improve it?

- Does the Dictionary look complete to you? Does it look up-to-date?

- Do you have an audiology dictionary, the dictionary?

- Who do you think is the group most likely to use the Dictionary? Audiologists? Students? Manufacturers? Educators? Others?

- How many pages do you think would be necessary? What do you think would be an appropriate price for the Dictionary? Should illustrations be included and if so when?

- Who would be qualified to revise the Dictionary? When you think of prominent audiologists, what names come to mind?

- Would you buy the Dictionary if it were available as you described?

cartilage (kar'tĭ-lij) *n.* tough, light colored, and elastic connective tissue (gristle) that shapes the external ear and lines the eustachian tube as well as the outer one-third of the external ear canal. *adj:* **cartilaginous.**

cartilage, acoustic meatus (me-a'tus). cartilage that forms part of the wall of the external auditory canal.

cartilage, annular. ring composed of cartilage, e.g., the ring that holds the eardrum in place.

cartilage, auditory. cartilage that shapes the external ear (pinna); *syn:* auricular or conchal cartilage.

cartilage, auditory tube (cartilago, tubae auditivae). trough-shaped cartilage that forms part of the wall and roof of the external auditory canal.

cartilage, auricular. cartilage that shapes the external ear; *syn:* conchal cartilage, auditory cartilage.

cartilage, conchal (kong'kal). cartilage of the external ear.

case history. review of the patient's background in regard to the problem involved; information may come from the patient himself or from relatives.

CAT. 1. children's apperception test. 2. computer averaged technique. 3. computerized axial tomogram (scan); *syn:* CT.

catarrh (kah-tahr') *n.* inflammation of any mucous membrane. *adj:* **catarrhal.**

catarrhal deafness. hearing impairment associated with the common cold or allergic blockage of the eustachian tube.

catarrhal otitis media (o-ti'tis me'de-ah). disorder in which the middle ear is filled with thin and watery fluid. More commonly known as serous otitis or middle ear effusion.

catheter (kath'ĕ-ter) *n.* eustachian: tubular device with a gently curved beak to inflate the eustachian tube, or the middle ear through the nasal passage.

cathode (kath'ōd) *n.* negative electrode or element that releases electrons when heated in a vacuum tube. *adj:* **cathodic.**

cathode ray. one of a stream of high-speed electrons projected from the heated cathode of a vacuum tube.

cathode-ray tube. vacuum tube which emits a stream of high speed electrons that are projected on a screen.

cation (kat'i-on) *n.* ion with a positive charge; one that migrates to the cathode.

cauliflower ear. ear thickened and malformed by injury.

causalgia (kaw-zal'je-ah) *n.* burning pain that often follows nerve injuries.

cavity, buccal. the mouth—especially between the teeth and cheeks.

cavum conchae (ka'vum kong'ka). conchal cavity; the lower portion of the concha at the entrance to the external auditory canal below the cymba.

cavum tympani (tim'pan-e). tympanic or middle ear cavity in the temporal bone.

CCC. Certificate of Clinical Competence awarded by ASHA.

CCM. contralateral competing message.

CCS. Crippled Children's Services.

CEC. Council for Exceptional Children.

cecum (se'kum) *n.* narrow space with one outlet.

cecum, cupular (se'kum ku'pu-lar). upper end of the cochlear duct (at the helicotrema).

cecum, vestibular. lower end of the cochlear duct in the vestibule.

cell *n.* 1. metal capsule containing electrodes and an electrolyte for generating electricity by chemical action to provide energy to power hearing aids. 2. unit of a battery. 3. smallest unit of body protoplasm. It is specialized to take part in each of the body functions. *adj:* **celled.**

cell, acoustic. hair cell in the organ of Corti.

cell, Corti's. uncommon name for a hair cell of the organ of Corti.

cell, hair. 1. one of the specific sensory cells of the end organ of hearing (organ of Corti). One end has hair-like projections (cilia) embedded in or in contact with the tectorial membrane. The other end is in close contact with many nerve endings. 2. one of the specific sensory cells of the organ of balance within the vestibule and semicircular canals of the inner ear.

cell, sustentacular (sus"ten-tak'ul-lar). cell that serves as a support for other specialized cells, e.g., Deiter's or Hensen's cells.

cells, bristle. hair cells of the organ of Corti.

cells, Claudius'. supporting cells on the basilar membrane external to the organ of Corti.

cells, Deiter's. supporting cells, like fingers or phalanges, interspersed between the outer hair cells of the organ of corti.

cells of Hensen. outer cells that support the inner structure of the organ of Corti.

cells, mastoid. air-filled cavities in the mastoid process of the temporal bone.

cells, phalangeal (fah-lan'je-al). cells that support the inner hair cells of the organ of Corti.

cells, pillar. cells that support the walls of the inner tunnel of Corti.

cells, tunnel. cells that line the inner tunnel of Corti. *syn:* pillar cells, rods of Corti.

cells, tympanic (tim-pan'ik). small groove-like depressions in the walls of the middle ear that connect with small cavities in the lower wall of the eustachian tube.

cellular (sel'u-lar) *adj.* pertaining to cells or cell-like structures. *n:* **cellularity** (sel"u-lār'ĭ-te).

cellulitis (sel"u-li'tis). inflammation of connective or cellular tissue.

cent. interval between any two sound waves whose frequency ratio is the twelve-hundredth root of two. One hundred cents constitutes an equally tempered semi-tone. Formula:

$$\text{Number of cents} = 1200 \log 2 \frac{f1}{f2}$$

center, epiotic (ep″e-ot′ik). junction joint of the embryonic cartilages that become the mastoid processes.

centimeter-gram-second *adj.* CGS. pertaining to a system of measurement based upon the centimeter as the unit of length, the gram as the unit of mass, and the second as the unit of time.

central *adj.* pertaining to or arising in the central nervous system, e.g., central deafness.

central canals of cochlea (kok′le-ah) (canales longitudinales modioli). minute channels in the center of the structure that supports the cochlea (the modiolus) through which blood vessels and nerves pass to the apex.

central deafness. deafness due to inability of the brain to recognize or understand sounds.

central masking. shift in threshold of the test ear by 5 dB, which results from the effect of masking on the central nervous system. This 5 dB difference should be considered in interpreting the audiogram.

central pathway involvement test. comparison of the speech discrimination results when monosyllables are given to each ear separately, then both together. If the discrimination score fails to improve binaurally, a lesion of the central auditory pathway is indicated.

cephalad (sef′ah-lad) *adv.* toward the head or the front.

cephalic (se-fal′ik) *adj.* pertaining to or near the head.

cephalization (sef″al-i-za′shun). evolutionary tendency for concentration of important nervous functions in the forward part of the brain.

CERA. cardiac evoked response audiometry.

cerebellar vermis. narrow lobe of the brain between the two hemispheres of the cerebellum.

cerebellum *n.* part of the brain, consisting of two hemispheres, located in the back and lower part of the skull.

cerebral (ser′ĕ-bral, sĕ-re′bral) *adj.* concerning the cerebrum of the brain.

cerebral cortex. outer layer of gray matter of the brain.

cerebral deafness. deafness due to damage to the cerebral portion of the brain resulting from illness or accident.

cerebral palsy. ineffective or incomplete muscular (motor) control resulting from brain damage before or during birth. The speech and/or hearing areas of the brain may also be affected.

cerebral vascular accident. CVA. bursting or clotting of a blood vessel in the brain that causes sudden loss or lowering of consciousness and loss of voluntary muscular control. More lasting physical problems and speech and language disorders may follow the initial onset; commonly referred to as a stroke, or less often, apoplexy.

cerebrum (ser′ĕ-brum, sĕ-re′brum) *n.* the largest part of the brain. Divided into two hemispheres, the cerebrum is said to be the site of conscious mental processes.

cerumen (sĕ-roo′men) *n.* yellow or brown wax-like substance of bitter taste (earwax) secreted in the outer one-third of the external ear canal by the ceruminous glands. *adj:* **ceruminal, ceruminous.**

cerumen, inspissated (in-spis′āt-ed). thickened and dried earwax plugging the outer ear canal.

ceruminoma (sĕ-roo″mĭ-no′mah) *n.* benign tumor of ceruminous glands of the external ear canal.

ceruminosis (sĕ-roo″mĭ-no′sis) *n.* excessive formation of earwax.

ceruminospoon. device designed to scrape wax out of the ear canal.

ceruminous deafness (sĕ-roo′mĭ-nus). deafness due to an impacted plug of wax in the outer ear canal.

ceruminous glands. glands within the external auditory canal that secrete cerumen or earwax.

CGS. centimeter-gram-second.

CHAA. certified hearing aid audiologist.

CHABA. Committee on Hearing and Bio-Acoustics.

chain, ossicular. the three small bones (ossicles) in the middle ear that convey the sound waves from the drumhead to the oval window of the inner ear—the malleus (hammer), the incus (anvil), and stapes (stirrup).

chair, Barany. chair designed to allow the patient to be turned in a circular motion to test the effect on equilibrium.

CHAMPUS. Civilian Health and Medication Program of the Uniformed Services.

charge *v.* to store up energy in a battery or cell.

charge *n.* amount of electricity available in a cell or battery.

chemoprophylactic (ke″mo-pro-fī-lak′tik) *adj.* pertaining to chemoprophylaxis—the prevention of infectious disease by the use of chemicals.

chemoprophylaxis (ke″mo-pro-fī-lak′sis) *n.* prevention of disease by the use of chemicals or drugs.

chemotherapy (ke″mo-ther′ăh-pe) *n.* treatment or control of diseases by the use of chemicals.

children's apperception test. CAT. personality test that can be adapted for use with a deaf child.

chip. popular informal term for the integrated circuit used in hearing instruments.

chloral hydrate. sedative drug used for electrophysiologic testing of the hearing of some children.

choana (ko'a-nah) *n.* funnel-like opening into the nasopharynx from the nostrils.

cholesteatoma (ko"le-ste"ah-to'mah) *n.* tumor or cyst that forms in the middle ear or deeper portion of the external auditory canal.

cholesteatosis *n.* progressive middle ear disease resulting from a cholesteatoma.

chondroma (kon-dro'mah) *n.* benign cartilaginous tumor; a possible cause of tinnitus.

chorda tympani (tympanic cord). branch of the facial nerve that passes through the upper part of the middle ear. It conveys taste sensations and during middle ear operations it may be temporarily affected in such a way that food tastes unnatural.

chromatid (kro'mah-tid) *n.* one of the paired complex filaments of a chromosome.

chromatin (kro'mah-tin) *n.* the portion of a cell nucleus that can be stained (the unstainable part is achromatin). *adj:* **chromatinic.**

chromatolysis (kro"mah-tol'ĭ-sis) *n.* disintegration of chromophil material (as chromatin) of a cell, especially of a nerve cell. *adj:* **chromatolytic.**

chromomere (kro'mo-mēr) *n.* one of the filaments of chromatin within the chromosome. *adj:* **chromomeric.**

chromonema (kro"mo-ne'mah) *pl.* **chromonemata** *n.* coiled filament within the chromosome that carries the genes. *adj:* **chromonemal, chromonematic, chromonemic.**

chromophone *n.* a teaching device using gradations of colored lights to show speech sounds and their intensity.

chromosomal (kro"mo-so'mal) *adj.* pertaining to chromosomes.

chromosome (kro'mo-sōm) *n.* portion of the cell nucleus that contains the chromatin and the chromatids. The number of chromosomes is distinct and constant with any one kind of animal or plant. *adj:* **chromosomic.**

chronic. continuing or often recurring.

chronic adhesive otitis media (o-ti'tis me'de-ah). disease in which the middle ear is filled with thick, gummy fluid. In advanced stages, adhesions develop around the eardrum, the windows, and the ossicles. Often called glue ear or mucoid (or mucous) otitis.

chronic eustachian salpingitis (u-sta'ke-an sal"pin-ji'tis). blockade of the eustachian tube, usually as the result of repeated inflammations.

chronic suppurative otitis media (sup'u-ra"tiv). continually running ears as a result of infections.

chronological age. CA. length of time an entity has lived from birth to current date. *syn:* actual age.

cicatrix (sik-a'triks, sik'ah-triks) *pl.* **cicatrices** (sik-ah-tri'sēz), **cicatrixes** (sik-ah-trik'sēz) *n.* contracted scar resulting from a healing wound. *adj:* **cicatrical, cicatrizant.**

cicatrization (sik"ah-trĭ-za'shun) *n.* formation of a scar at the site of a healed wound. *v:* **cicatrize.**

CID. Central Institute for the Deaf.

cilia (sil'e-ah) *n.* (plural of cilium). the hair-like fibers rooted in the hair cells. *syn:* stereocilia.

ciliated cells. cells that have microscopic hair-like structures extending from the body of the cell, e.g., the hair cells of the organ of Corti.

cilium (sil'e-um) *pl.* **cilia** *n.* a hair-like fiber.

cinchonism (sin'ko-nizm) *n.* temporary deafness, ringing in the ears, headaches, etc., caused by the use of cinchona or its alkaloid derivatives (such as quinine).

circuit *n.* combination of electronic components that carries electric current from the microphone through the receiver or earphone.

circuit, integrated. electronic circuit made up of electrical elements combined on one small substrate.

circuit, printed. a circuit printed, etched, or built up with a conductive material to include the necessary wiring, condensers, and resistors for an electronic device such as a hearing aid.

circuitry *n.* the parts that make up an electric circuit.

circular stairways. translation of the Latin word, scala, referring to the three tunnels or canals within the cochlea.

circumambient *adj.* surrounding—usually shortened to ambient.

circumaural *adj.* around the ear; especially refers to headphones that encircle the pinnae rather than resting on the ears (supraaural). There are also circumaural earmuffs for protection from noise.

clang deafness. deafness in which sounds are heard without the ability to recognize small distinctions.

classic cros. basic CROS system that picks up sound from the side with the impaired ear and transmits it to the good ear.

classes of hearing handicap. see Table 2, page 28.

Claudius' cells. (Friedrich M. Claudius, Austrian anatomist, 1822-1869). Supporting cells on the basilar membrane external to the organ of Corti.

cleft palate. congenital lack of lengthwise closure of the roof of the mouth; occasionally extends to a harelip.

click *n.* a quick sharp sound.

click *v.* to make a quick sharp noise.

Table 2. Classes of Hearing Handicap
AAOO Committee on Conservation of Hearing (1965)

Hearing Threshold Level dB (ANSI) ISO	Class	Degree of Handicap	Average Hearing Threshold level for 500, 1000, and 2000 Hz in the Better Ear*		Ability to Understand Speech
			More Than	Not More Than	
25	A	Not Significant		25 dB (ANSI) ISO	No significant difficulty with faint speech
40	B	Slight Handicap	25 dB (ANSI) ISO	40 dB	Difficulty only with faint speech
55	C	Mild Handicap	40 dB	55 dB	Frequent difficulty with normal speech
70	D	Marked Handicap	55 dB	70 dB	Frequent difficulty with loud speech
90	E	Severe Handicap	70 dB	90 dB	Can understand only shouted or amplified speech
	F	Extreme Handicap	90 dB		Usually cannot understand even amplified speech

* Whenever the average for the poorer ear is 25 dB or more greater than that of the better ear in this frequency range, 5 dB are added to the average for the better ear. This adjusted average determines the degree and class of handicap. For example, if a person's average hearing-threshold level for 500, 1000, and 2000 Hz is 37 dB in one ear and 62 dB or more in the other, his adjusted average hearing-threshold level is 42 dB and his handicap is Class C instead of Class B.

click pitch. sharp sound that lasts long enough to give an auditory sensation of tonality.

clicking tinnitus. another name for Leudet's spasmodic head noises or Leudet's tinnitus. *syn*: objective tinnitus.

CLD. central language disorder.

clinical audiologist. one who practices audiology in a clinic or doctor's office.

clinical audiometer. now called a wide-range audiometer.

clip *v.* to control intensity by limiting output of a hearing aid or amplifier.

CLL. comfortable loudness level.

clonus (klo′nus) *n.* muscular spasm characterized by rapid alternation of contraction and relaxation. *adj*: **clonic.**

closure, auditory. recognition of complete words when only parts are spoken or heard.

clothing noise. noise produced in a body-worn hearing aid by clothes rubbing across the microphone.

CM. cochlear microphonics.

CMI. Cornell Medical Index.

CNC. monosyllabic word made up of consonant, nucleus (vowel portion), and consonant.

CNC list. word list including CNC words.

CNE. could not establish.

CNS. central nervous system.

CNT. could not test.

cochlea (kok′le-ah) *n.* winding tubular cavity within the inner ear, shaped like a snail-shell; contains the end-organ of hearing which finally changes the pressure waves of sound into nerve impulses. The central bony support of the cochlea is called the modiolus. A thin bony plate, the spiral lamina, extends from the modiolus and partially divides the cochlea. The division is completed by the fibrous support for the organ of Corti—the basilar membrane. One passageway above the divider begins at the oval window—the scala vestibuli. Another begins at the round window—the scala tympani. They are joined at the apex or helicotrema. Between the two is the scala media, or cochlear duct, which contains the organ of Corti. When extended the cochlea is about 1⅓"(35 mm) long. It has 2¾ turns and is about 5 mm high and 9 mm in diameter. *adj*: **cochlear.**

cochlea, bony. cavity in the petrous part of the temporal bone that contains the cochlea.

cochleagram (kok'le-ah-gram) *n.* graph indicating the levels of acoustic stimuli necessary to evoke a cochlear microphonic response at different frequencies.

cochlear aqueduct. tube or duct that conducts perilymph between the cochlea and the cerebrospinal fluid, which cushions the brain.

cochlear duct (ductus cochlearis). membranous cochlea, or scala media; middle triangular tube of the cochlea; contains endolymph.

cochlear hydrops (hi'drops). accumulation of fluid in the cochlea; a possible cause of tinnitus.

cochlear implant. electronic device designed to stimulate the hearing mechanism. It utilizes a coil of wire embedded under the skin behind the ear with an extension of wire into the fluid of the inner ear (cochlea). It is activated by an amplifier, similar to a body-type hearing aid, carried in a pocket. There is sometimes a side benefit in that tinnitus is reduced.

cochlear microphonic. electrical voltage produced by the hair cells of the cochlea. The electrical response follows the wave form of the acoustic stimulus in a manner similar to the action of a microphone.

cochlear nerve. branch of the eighth cranial (acoustic) nerve that arises in the cochlea and conveys sound stimuli to the brain; the nerve of hearing.

cochlear nucleus *pl.* **nuclei.** the collective terminations of the cochlear nerve fibers in the brain stem from which the central auditory pathways arise.

cochlear otosclerosis. a growth of spongy bone on the cochlear side of the oval window. Stapes fixation may or may not be involved. *syn*: labyrinthine otosclerosis.

cochlear recess. small depression between the oval and round windows that forms the vestibular end of the cochlear duct.

cochlear reflex. more commonly known as acoustic reflex, it is the reflex contraction of the intra-aural muscles (tensor tympani and stapedius) in response to a sound stimulus. *syn*: intra-aural reflex.

cochlear reserve. term that refers to the ability of a hearing-impaired person to understand speech at higher intensity levels. The cochlear reserve is said to be good if understanding improves with increased intensity.

cochlear window. the round window.

cochleitis, cochlitis (kok"le-i'tis, kok-li'tis) *n.* inflammation of the cochlea.

cochleoapical (kok"le-o-āp'ĭ-kal) *adj.* refers to the portion of the inner ear farthest from the middle ear. Considered the site of lesion when low frequencies are lost.

cochleoapical type hearing loss. elevation of threshold sensitivity in the low frequencies.

cochleobasal *adj.* refers to the portion of the inner ear closest to the middle ear. Considered the site of lesion in high-frequency hearing loss.

cochleobasal type hearing loss. steep elevation of threshold sensitivity in the high frequencies.

cochleo-orbicular (kok"le-o-or-bik'u-lar) *adj.* concerning the cochlea and the eye.

cochleo-orbicular reflex. a wink or twitch at the corner (canthus) of the eye as a result of a sudden sound near the ear. *syn*: acousticopalpebral reflex, auropalpebral reflex, cochleopalpebral reflex.

cochleopalpebral (kok"le-o-pal'pĕ-bral) *adj.* concerning the cochlea and the eyelids.

cochleopalpebral reflex. cochleo-orbicular reflex, acousticopalpebral reflex, or auropalpebral reflex.

cochleovestibular *adj.* concerning the inner ear, to include both hearing and balance.

Cockayne's syndrome. complex of associated symptoms including dwarfism, mental retardation, premature aging, and ear and eye malformations.

Cogan's syndrome (D. Cogan, American physician). disease involving connective tissue; characterized by tinnitus, deafness, vertigo, blurred vision, or blindness.

cognition (kog-nish'un) *n.* the sum of all the brain activities that combine into knowledge. *adj*: **cognitive.**

cognitive development. process of acquiring skills in perception, imagination, conception, memory, judgment, and reason, which are the foundation for cognition. This development is often delayed in the child with a hearing impairment whose problem does not receive early attention.

coil, induction. device designed to transform direct electrical current into intermittent higher voltage.

coin click and **watch tick tests.** outdated and inadequate tests of hearing based on the ability to hear the clicking of coins or the ticking of a watch.

cold-running speech. continuous speech delivery on a topic that is informative in content and delivery, rather than emotional. It may be used to establish the speech reception threshold (SRT).

collagen (kol'ah-jen) *n.* usually white, a gelatinous protein contained within the fibers of connective tissue. Its breakdown causes the floppy ears and collapsed canals of the elderly.

collagenous (kol-laj'ĕ-nus) *adj.* relating to tissue containing high concentrations of collagens.

colliculus, inferior. one of a pair of projections on the midbrain containing the integration centers for auditory reflexes.

colliculus, superior. one of a pair of projections on the midbrain containing integration centers for optic reflexes.

color hearing. sense of color that accompanies certain sounds for some people. *syn:* pseudochromesthesia.

columella (kol″u-mel′lah). bony or cartilaginous structure that functions in birds, reptiles, and many amphibians in a similar manner to the ossicular chain in man. *syn:* columella auris.

columella cochleae. the modiolus—the bony structure that furnishes the inner support for the cochlea.

columella effect. result of one type of tympanoplasty in which a skin graft makes contact with the head of the stapes, thus simulating the columella of birds.

column chart. graph that displays statistical distributions by the use of rectangular blocks. For example, scores may be displayed along the abscissa (horizontal axis) and frequencies on the ordinate (vertical axis). *syn:* histogram.

combination tone. tone heard when two tones are presented at the same time. It may be heard differently in either intensity or pitch.

combined method. 1. manual and oral education of the deaf child. 2. use of speech-reading, speech, electronic amplification, and finger spelling; total communication.

combined tone. distinctive sound heard by the ear that results from the combination of two tones produced together. *syn:* combination tone, summation tone.

communication, total. new name for the old simultaneous method, it utilizes signs, finger spelling, electronic amplification (usually hearing aids), speech, and speech-reading. Facial expressions, gestures, and body English are also considered important.

communicologist (kŏ-mu″nĭ-kol′ah-jist) *n.* one who practices communicology; a speech and language pathologist.

communicology *n.* the study of both oral and aural human communication; the study of speech and hearing as functions of language.

competing messages. differing signals or messages presented at the same time. Often used as a test of a hearing aid fitting to demonstrate the advantage of binaural listening.

complete recruitment. sensation of loudness of a tone in the poor ear equals the sensation of loudness in the good ear at maximum intensity levels.

complex noise masking. sound made up of a mixture of frequencies designed to mask the better ear while the poorer ear is being tested. It is usually of the type known as saw-tooth, and is made up of a fundamental frequency of 60 or 120 Hz together with all its harmonics in random phase. It is most effective in masking frequencies below 1000 Hz.

complex tone. sound made up of a number of pure tones.

complex wave pattern. sound made up of several combined pure tones.

compliance (kom-pli′ans) *n.* ease with which the eardrum and the middle ear mechanism moves; opposite of impedance.

compression (kom-presh′un) *n.* 1. decrease of pressure. 2. first half of the cycle of a sine wave. 3. method of controlling the output of a hearing aid changing the gain of the amplifier circuit in response to an input signal.

compression amplification. method of limiting (or compressing) the amplification of loud sounds in comparison to weak sounds. When this type of circuit is used in a hearing aid or other amplifier, the wave form of a loud sound is less modified than when peak-clipping is used.

compression, curvilinear. method of controlling output that takes effect more quickly and progresses upward from lower levels than the usual type of automatic volume control.

compression, linear. method of controlling output that does not take effect until a pre-set level of pressure is reached.

compression, logarithmic. method of controlling output that is said to vary logarithmically with the input.

computer average technique. CAT. method of studying electrical responses of the cerebral cortex by utilizing computers to cause the pattern of response to emerge more clearly from the background of random activity.

concha (kong′kah) *pl.* **conchae** *n.* shell-like cavity of the outer ear in which the entrance to the external ear canal (concha auricula) is located.

concha rim. in reference to earmolds, the portion that outlines the concha just under the rim of the bowl.

conchal cartilage. cartilage of the external ear. *syn:* auditory or auricular cartilage.

conchitis (kong-ki′tis) *n.* inflammation of the concha.

conchoidal (kong-koi′dal) *adj.* resembling a shell, usually as seen from the inside.

condenser. device consisting of two conducting surfaces separated by a nonconductor or dielectric, used to store and control electrical energy; capacitor.

conditioned audio-visual response audiometry. CA-VR. version of play audiometry that utilizes the lighting of a plastic toy to heighten the child's interest. Devised by Rayford C. Reddell and Donald R. Calvert.

conditioned orientation reflex audiometry. CORA. version of play audiometry devised by Tokuro Suzuki and Yoshio Ogiba. It relies on an assessment of the child's localizing ability as lighted toys are coordinated with two loudspeakers.

conditioned response. trained or taught (conditioned) by a reward, shock, or punishment to do something (respond) when a stimulus, such as a sound, is presented.

conductance (kon-duk′tans) *n.* 1. the ability of the ossicular chain to conduct mechanical movement. 2. a measure of the capacity of a material to conduct a current of electricity; opposite of resistance.

conduction *n.* transmission of sound waves from one point to another.

conduction, air. transmission of sound pressure waves through the air to the eardrum, by way of the middle ear mechanism to the inner ear.

conduction, bone. transmission of sound pressure waves through the bones of the skull to the inner ear.

conductive deafness (or conductive loss of hearing). impairment of hearing due to the failure of sound pressure waves to reach the cochlea through the normal air conduction channels. This type of deafness is often responsive to medical or surgical treatment.

conductor. any material that will transmit energy, whether in the form of electricity or sound pressure waves.

condyle (kon′dīl) *n.* knob, knuckle, or rounded end of a bone that moves (articulates) with another at a joint. The condyle of the jawbone (mandible) extends upward into the tissue below the outer ear canal and may affect hearing. It may also cause problems with the earmold, especially in cases of malocclusion (misfitting jaw closure).

cone of light. area on the drumhead, shaped like a triangle, which reflects brighter than the rest of the membrane. Its position to the right or left of the umbo indicates accordingly which ear is being pictured. If the umbo is at 11 o'clock, it is the left ear, if at one o'clock, the picture is of the right ear. *syn*: Politzer's luminous cone.

cone, Politzer's luminous. cone of light.

congenital (kon-jen′ĭ-tal) *adj.* existing at birth; conditions that develop in the uterus and are not necessarily the result of heredity.

congenital atresia. closure, or lack of, external ear from birth.

congenital deafness. deafness that develops in the uterus or during the birth process; not necessarily a result of heredity.

consanguineous (kon″san-gwin′e-us) *adj.* with the same blood or ancestry.

consensual *adj.* concerning an involuntary reaction to a stimulus, e.g., stapedius reflex in one ear when the other ear is stimulated.

consonant *n.* speech sounds higher in frequency than vowel sounds, the consonants are produced by putting a sudden check on the expiration of air or by closure of some part of the mouth or throat.

consonant, vowel, consonant. CVC. monosyllabic word of such form used in speech discrimination tests.

constant stimulus method. procedure for measuring the threshold by which one being measured responds verbally after each discrete stimulus presentation. *syn*: frequency method.

consultant. one who gives advice, or counsel, usually in a specialized field.

contact *n.* 1. connecting point through which electric current passes, as the battery contacts in a hearing aid. 2. device especially made to provide an electrical connection.

continuant. speech sound that may be prolonged without a change in quality, e.g., L, F, or S.

continuous frequency audiometer. one whose output frequency may be changed in steps of one cycle per second throughout its frequency range.

continuous spectrum. spectrum that includes all the pure tones within a given frequency range.

continuous tracings. C tracings. The graph that results when a continuous tone stimulus is used in automatic audiometry.

contours, equal loudness. curved lines that indicate the sound pressures necessary at each frequency to produce sensations of equal loudness for normally hearing listeners.

contralateral (kon″trah-lat′er-al). referring to the opposite side of the body (as opposed to ipsilateral or homolateral).

contralateral masking. the effect on the opposite ear when the masking sound becomes too intense.

contralateral competing message. CCM. speech is introduced through the headphone on the opposite side from the primary message.

contralateral routing of signals. CROS. (contralateral routing of offside signals) amplifying system that provides a microphone to pick up signals (sound pressure waves) on the side of the impaired ear and sends them electrically to the normal ear in cases of unilateral loss; *syn*: across-head fitting.

control. in research, a portion of the group involved which does not receive the treatment being studied.

control, automatic gain. another term for "automatic volume control." In hearing aids, a special circuit designed to prevent sounds from being amplified too much for the impaired ear.

control, frequency. device—usually a dial but sometimes a series of buttons—on an audiometer to provide a means of selecting the frequency of the test tone. *syn*: frequency selector.

control, gain. more commonly known as the volume control, this device enables the user to regulate the output of the amplifier.

control group. group of normals for comparison with the group in the experiment.

control, tone. device designed to allow the user to alter the response of an amplifier by limiting the intensity of a portion of the frequency range.

control, volume. device designed to allow the user to adjust the amount by which the input signal is amplified.

conversion deafness. nonorganic or functional hearing loss sometimes unconsciously developed as a psychic protection under conditions of severe emotional strain. More commonly known as hysterical deafness.

COR. conditioned optical response.

CORA. conditioned orientation reflex audiometry.

cord *n.* 1. small flexible insulated electrical cable used to connect a body-type (or conventional) hearing aid to its receiver, or the earphones to an audiometer. 2. a similar cable used to connect an electrical appliance, such as an audiometer, to a current source.

cord, Bergmann's. stripe of white fibers in the fourth ventricle of the brain, involved with the hearing process; acoustic striae.

cortex *pl.* **cortices, cortexes.** outer layer of gray matter of the brain.

cortex, auditory. portion of the outer layer of the brain that serves as the terminus of nerve impulses from the ear.

Corti, Alfonso. Italian anatomist (1822-1888) who described the sense organ of hearing that bears his name.

Corti, organ of. structure resting on the basilar membrane within the cochlear duct (scala media). It contains the essential sensory elements of hearing, the hair cells, together with their supporting cells.

Corti's arches. meeting points of the inner and outer rods of Corti that form the tunnel of Corti.

Corti's canal. Also called Corti's tunnel, a spiral canal within the organ of Corti between the outer and inner hair cells. Triangular in shape, it is bounded by the outer and inner pillar cells and is filled with fluid.

Corti's cells. uncommon name for the hair cells of the organ of Corti.

Corti's fiber. the structure, made up of the pillars or rods of Corti, that forms Corti's tunnel.

Corti's ganglia. collection of nerve cells from the cochlear branch of the auditory

nerve that pass from the modiolus to the organ of Corti. *syn*: ganglia, spiral cochlea.

Corti's membrane (membrana tectoria ductus cochlearis). the tectorial membrane, the roof membrane into which the cilia of the hair cells project.

Corti's pillar. inner and outer rod cells that line the tunnel of Corti.

Corti's rods. long cells (pillar cells) that rest on the basilar membrane. The cells are joined at the top but spread at the bottom to form arches of the tunnel of Corti.

Corti's teeth. minute toothlike projections along the free margin of the labium vestibulare of the cochlea. *syn*: auditory teeth, Huschke's teeth.

Corti's tunnel. fluid-filled triangular canal within the organ of Corti, formed by the rods or pillars of Corti on two sides and the basilar membrane as the base.

cortical *adj.* concerning or related to the cortex of the brain.

cortical deafness. deafness due to damage to the hearing centers in the cortex of the brain—either from illness or accident.

cortical evoked response audiometry. seldom used term for evoked response audiometry (ERA).

Costen's syndrome (James B. Costen, American physician). earache resulting from loss of (or bad fitting) teeth (malocclusion).

COT. critical off time.

cough, ear. cough which is the reflexive result of irritation of the external ear canal. Hardened wax, for example, may cause a dry hacking cough.

coulomb (koo′lom) *n.* unit of electricity. The amount of electricity furnished by a current of one ampere in one second.

coupler *n.* 1. any device by which one portion of an acoustical system is joined to another, e.g., an earmold coupler. 2. cavity of predetermined shape and size used in measuring the acoustic output of earphones or receivers. A 6 cc coupler is used between the audiometer earphone and the condenser microphone for calibration. A 2 cc coupler is used with hearing aid receivers. (Zwislocki, Kemar, Keller, and Bauer coupling systems have all been designed as possible replacements for the 2 cc coupler.)

covert response. reaction that is invisible to an outside observer.

CP. cleft palate. cerebral palsy.

cps or **c/s.** cycles per second.

CR. conditioned reflex. conditioned response. critical ratio.

cranial (kra′ne-al) *adj.* concerning the head.

cranial nerves. also known as cerebral nerves, 12 major pairs arise in the brain. The two pairs that go through the internal auditory canals are of special audiologic interest. They are the VIIth, known as the facial nerve, and the VIIIth, variously known as the auditory, acoustic, or vestibulocochlear nerve—the nerve of hearing.

craniotympanic *adj.* concerning the skull and the middle ear.

crest, acoustic. thickened section of the lining of the bulbous portion (ampulla) of each semicircular canal. Fibers of the vestibular nerve pass through the crest to the hair cells.

crest of the vestibule (crista vestibuli). ridge on the inner wall of the vestibule of the labyrinth. It contains minute holes through which nerve fibers pass.

cretinism (kre'tin-izm) *n.* congenital or early childhood disorder resulting from severe thyroid deficiency. Hearing impairment may be one of the associated abnormalities.

Crib-O-Gram. device developed by Blair Simmons, MD (Stanford Medical School) to use in screening the hearing of newborn babies. It automatically records the responses to sound stimuli while the baby is in the bassinet in the nursery.

cribrate (krib'rāt). perforated with many tiny holes or pits.

cribrose maculae (krib'ros mak'u-le). rough spots in the walls of the semicircular canals caused by minute holes through which fibers of the vestibular nerve pass.

criss-cros. amplifying system that provides a microphone at each ear leading to an amplifier in the opposite ear; designed to give greater binaural power through ear-level aids. *syn:* binaural CROS, power CROS.

crista ampullaris (kris'ta am-puh-lār'is). crest, acoustic.

crista spiralis (spiral crest) (spi-ral'is). fine-toothed ridge of the bony spiral at the edge of the cochlea. Fibers of the auditory nerve pass through these minute openings.

critical band. narrow range of frequencies that are most effective in masking a particular pure tone.

critical band for loudness. range of frequencies within a narrow band—about ⅓ octave or 100 mels—which sound equally loud when presented together.

critical off time. COT. interval between pulsed tones that has been shortened to a time period that results in the same heightened threshold as a continuous tone.

critically damp distortion. alteration of response in a system resulting from overdamping.

CROS. contralateral routing of signals. An amplifying system that provides a microphone to pick up signals (sound pressure waves) on the side of the impaired ear and send them electrically to the normal ear in cases of unilateral loss. *syn:* across-head fitting.

CROS, binaural. amplifying system that provides a microphone at each ear with a wire leading to an amplifier and receiver at the other ear. It is designed to allow the use of greater binaural power through ear-level hearing aids. *syn:* criss-cros.

CROS, classic. basic CROS system that picks up sound from the side with the impaired ear and transmits it to the good ear.

CROS, focal. CROS or bicros hearing aid arrangement that utilizes a plastic tube to channel sound from the concha of the off-side ear into a microphone placed on that side.

CROS, high. classic CROS hearing aid amplifying system modified to cut the lower frequencies and emphasize the higher frequencies.

CROS, mini- hearing aid system with the microphone on one side and the amplifier and receiver on the other (better) side with a short plastic tube (or none) from the receiver spout to the concha of the ear.

CROS mold. earmold with a minimal frame designed to hold a plastic tube in place in the external ear canal. More properly called an open mold or nonoccluding mold.

CROS, power. amplifying system that provides a microphone at one ear with a wire leading to an amplifier and receiver at the other ear. It is designed to allow the use of greater power through ear-level hearing aids.

cross-hearing. phenomenon that occurs when sound pressure waves presented to one ear are heard in the other ear. This may occur as the waves go around or through the head.

cross-talk. accidental competing messages through auditory training units when two systems are too close together.

CRT. cathode ray tube.

crura (kroo'rah) *sing.* **crus** *n.* 1. the legs of the stapes—or supports of the stirrup. 2. seldom used name for the bulbs at the end of the semicircular canals (the ampulla).

crus (krus) *n.* 1. one of the legs of the stapes, either posterior or anterior. 2. the ridge that divides the bowl of the outer ear into two parts. Also known as the crus helicus, it separates the upper (concha cymba) section from the lower (concha cavum) portion of the ear. 3. Another name for the long leg (long process) of the incus that moves (articulates) with the stapes.

cryosurgery *n.* the use of intense cold to destroy or enervate, e.g., cryosurgery of the labyrinth at the horizontal canal.

crystal, ear. minute crystalline particle of aragonite (a type of calcium carbonate, $CaCo^3$)—also known as otoconia (ear dust) or otolith (ear stone). By pressure upon the hair cells of the semicircular canals, these crystals help activate the sense of balance.

crystal earphone. device for converting electrical energy to acoustical energy by utilizing the distinctive properties of a piezoelectric crystal; e.g., a crystal that responds proportionately to an electric current is connected to a diaphragm, which moves the air to create sound pressure waves.

crystal microphone. device for converting sound pressure waves into electrical energy by utilizing the unique properties of a piezoelectric crystal.

CS. conditioned stimulus; conditioning stimulus.

CSF. cerebrospinal fluid.

CT. computerized tomogram.

cue n. word, phrase, sign, hint, or symbol that serves as a signal to stimulate a response.

cue, acoustic. the portion of a speech sound or formant considered most important in identifying the speech signal.

cued speech. method of using finger signs near the mouth to help in speech-reading when words that look alike on the lips are involved; e.g., men and pen.

cupola (or cupula) cochlear. the little dome at the upper end of the cochlea.

cupola space. space in the middle ear above the ossicles. The tympanic attic.

cupula, of the ampullary crest. gelatinous mass that overlies the hair cells of the semicircular ducts.

cupular cecum (ku'pu-lar se'kum). the upper blind extremity of the cochlear duct.

current. the rate of electron flow through an electric circuit. The unit of measure is the ampere. According to Ohm's law, current is defined as the voltage divided by the resistance.

current, alternating. AC or ac. electric current that flows first in one direction, then in the other. When this reversal occurs sixty times in one second it is called sixty cycle current.

current, direct. DC or dc. electric current that flows continuously in one direction. A current of the type delivered by a battery; sometimes referred to as galvanic current.

current, inducing. primary electrical current that gives rise to the secondary current in an induction coil. syn: primary and secondary current.

curve, articulation. curve that results when an articulation score is plotted on a graph. syn: discrimination curve.

curve, discrimination. curve that results when an articulation score is plotted on a graph. syn: articulation curve.

curve, gradually falling. the audiometric chart of hearing loss falls at about 5 to 10 dB per octave.

curve, gradually rising. the audiometric chart of hearing loss rises at about 5 to 10 dB per octave.

curve, marked falling. the audiometric chart of hearing loss falls at about 15 to 20 dB per octave in the higher frequencies. syn: sharply falling curve.

curve, shadow. false audiogram indicating a threshold of hearing sensitivity in the poorer ear that parallels (at a lower level) that of the better ear. It may occur as the sound waves go around or through the head from the ear under test to the better ear. When this occurs, masking of the better ear is required to avoid a shadow curve; this phenomenon is sometimes called cross hearing.

curve, sharply falling. the audiometric chart of hearing loss falls at about 15 to 20 dB per octave in the higher frequencies. syn: marked falling curve.

cushion, eustachian (u-sta'ke-an). ridge of cartilage above and behind the pharyngeal opening of the eustachian tube.

custom earmold. earmold fabricated from an impression of the ear of a specific individual.

custom hearing aid. one built for a specific individual.

cutaneous (ku-ta'ne-us) adj. pertaining to the outermost layer of skin.

cuticular adj. pertaining to the outermost layer of cells.

cutis n. the layer of skin that lies just below the epidermis. syn: dermis.

CV. cardiovascular. consonant vowel.

CVA. cerebral vascular accident.

CVC. consonant, vowel, consonant. A monosyllabic word of such form used in a list.

cyanosis n. bluish color resulting from a deficiency of oxygen.

cybernetics (si"ber-net'iks) n. science based on the principles of control and communication as they apply both to the operation of complex electronic calculators and the functions of the brain, the human nervous system, and other organisms.

cycle n. one of a recurring series of events (e.g., sound pressure waves) or a recurring period of time.

cycles per second. number of times a wave form or vibration is repeated in a second. The term Hertz (Hz) has replaced cycles per second in audiology.

cymba concha. upper, smaller part of the bowl of the outer ear (concha) above the ridge (crus helicus).

cyst n. sac filled with fluid or other foreign material.

cyt-, cyto- (si'to). combining form referring to a cell.

cytoarchitecture (si"to-ar'ki-tek"tūr) *n.* the study of the physical shape and structure of a cell body.

cytogenetics (si"to-jĕ-net'iks) *n.* branch of genetics dealing with the structure and function of the cell, especially the chromosomes.

cytology (si-tol'o-je) *n.* study of the origin and development of the cell.

cytomegalovirus (si"to-meg"ah-lo-vi'rus) *n.* herpes-type virus that causes enlargement of cells of various glands and organs. An infrequent cause of congenital deafness.

cytoplasmic organelle. specialized portion of a cell outside the nucleus.

D

D scale. dBD. special electronic weighting network included in some sound level meters to measure aircraft noise as it affects listeners in a particular area. The annoyance level of fly-over noise. The weighting scale is based on mirroring the 40 Noy contour to approximate the perceived noise level (PNdB) scale.

D₁ syndrome, or the D₁ trisomy syndrome. variable malformation of infants resulting from irregularities in chromosomes of Group D, no. 13, 14 or 15. Malformed ears appear as one of the signs in all cases. *syn:* trisomy D₁ syndrome or trisomy 13-15 syndrome.

dactyl speech. fingerspelling: the use of the manual alphabet. *syn:* dactylology.

dactylography (dak"ti-log'rah-fe) *n.* the use of a machine to convey speech symbols by touch to blind deaf-mutes.

dactylology (dak"til-ol'o-je) *n.* 1. the use of the manual alphabet. 2. the use of hand or finger-made signs to represent words and phrases.

DAF. delayed auditory feedback. system by which the speaker's own words are returned (feedback) through earphones after a time delay of a few milliseconds. A test of malingering, also known as delayed side tone.

damage risk criteria. delineation of those factors of noise intensity levels, length of time of exposure, and frequency of exposure which may be allowed with minimal risk of hearing impairment.

damped wave train. sequence of cycles of sound pressure in which the amplitude of the successive cycles is diminished progressively.

damping. 1. decreasing the amplitude of successive vibrations by mechanical means. 2. decreasing the amplitude of sound pressure waves through absorption, e.g., with acoustical tiles.

Darwinian ear (Charles R. Darwin, English biologist, 1809-1882). congenitally deformed ear in which the upper border is not rolled over to form the helix, but extends flatly upward.

Darwinian tubercle. small projection from the upper part of the helix. It may appear simply as a thickening of the cartilage.

dB (formerly db). decibel—one-tenth of a bel. The B in the abbreviation is capitalized in honor of Alexander Graham Bell—for whom the bel was named.

DBA. doing business as—

dBA. decibel of sound pressure as measured on the A scale of a sound level meter.

dBB. dB of sound pressure on B scale.

dBC. dB of sound pressure on C scale. ("s" or "f" may be added to indicate slow or fast response circuit).

dBD. dB of sound pressure on D scale.

dc. direct current.

dead room. room with a maximum degree of sound absorption. An anechoic chamber is the ultimate example of a dead room.

deaf *adj.* 1. unable to hear sound. 2. unable to recognize sound or the meaning of sound pressure waves. 3. incapable of developing speech and language through the use of the sense of hearing alone, either unaided or aided. a. congenitally deaf: born deaf. b. adventitiously deaf: born with a normal sense of hearing which became unusable through illness or accident. c. pre-lingual deaf: hearing loss before the development of speech.

deaf-aid. obsolete term for hearing aid.

deaf-and-dumb. seldom used—and unacceptable—term for deaf-mute.

deaf-and-dumb alphabet. unacceptable term for manual alphabet.

deaf-ear crab. West Indian fiddler crab whose extracted juices were believed to cure deafness.

deafen *v.* **deafening.** 1. to numb the sense of hearing. 2. to cause a loss of hearing. *adv:* **deafeningly.**

deafened *n.* one who has lost the use of the sense of hearing after normal speech and language were developed. (The adventitiously deaf become deaf after birth but before normal speech patterns are established.)

35

deafferentation (de-af"er-en-ta'shun) *n.* severance of an afferent nerve. Sometimes tried for relief of tinnitus.

deaf-mute *n.* person who has never learned to speak due to the inability to hear.

deaf-mutism *n.* lack of speech resulting from inability to hear.

deafness *n.* condition of being deaf.

deafness, adventitious (ad"ven-tish'us). deafness resulting from illness or accident after birth but before normal speech patterns have developed.

deafness, bass. inability to hear low frequency tones.

deafness, boilermaker's. deafness in the higher frequencies resulting from exposure to continuous loud noises.

deafness, catarrhal. hearing impairment associated with the common cold or allergic blockage of the eustachian tube.

deafness, central. deafness due to inability of the brain to recognize or understand sounds.

deafness, cerebral. deafness due to damage to the cerebral portion of the brain resulting from illness or accident.

deafness, ceruminous (sĕ-roo'mĭ-nus). deafness due to an impacted plug of wax in the outer ear canal.

deafness, clang. deafness in which sounds are heard without the ability to recognize small distinctions.

deafness, conductive (conduction deafness). impairment of hearing due to the failure of sound pressure waves to reach the cochlea through the normal air conduction channels. This type of deafness is often responsive to medical or surgical treatment.

deafness, congenital. with birth. Condition that develops in the uterus and is not necessarily a result of heredity.

deafness, conversion. nonorganic or functional hearing loss sometimes unconsciously developed as a psychic protection under conditions of severe emotional strain. *syn*: hysterical deafness.

deafness, cortical. deafness due to damage to the hearing centers in the cortex of the brain—either from illness or accident. *syn*: central deafness.

deafness, end-organ. deafness due to a lesion (damage) within the organ of Corti.

deafness, familial. hearing loss that appears among several members of a family but is not apparently hereditary. It may be a result of a blood incompatibility.

deafness, feigned. simulated hearing loss—a loss which has no physical damage as a basis. It is the deafness of a malingerer—one who feigns or pretends deafness for personal advantage to gain industrial-loss compensation or to avoid military service, for example. Children may simulate deafness to explain school deficiencies. *syn*: functional deafness.

deafness, functional. deafness or hearing loss that has no physical damage as a basis. *syn*: nonorganic, psychogenic, simulated, hysterical, conversion, or feigned deafness.

deafness, hereditary. deafness resulting from inherited characteristics (recessive genes).

deafness, hysterical. nonorganic or functional hearing loss sometimes unconsciously developed as a psychic protection under conditions of severe emotional strain. *syn*: conversion deafness.

deafness, industrial. loss of hearing sensitivity as a result of relatively long exposure to industrial noise.

deafness, labyrinthine (lab"ĭ-rin'thĭn). deafness due to damage within the inner ear. The term is sometimes used only when there is an accompanying balance problem.

deafness, luetic (lu-et'ik). hearing loss caused by syphilis.

deafness management quotient. DMQ. formula, including a weighted scale, designed to determine the deaf person's ability to meet the requirements of everyday living.

deafness, mind. 1. cortical deafness. 2. auditory aphasia. 3. functional or nonorganic deafness.

deafness, mixed. hearing loss resulting from malfunction of both the conductive and sensorineural mechanisms.

deafness, music. inability to produce or understand music or musical sounds; musical deafness. *syn*: amusia.

deafness, nerve. obsolete term for sensorineural hearing loss.

deafness, noise-induced. hearing loss which develops gradually from continuous exposure to noise that is above acceptable levels.

deafness, nonorganic. deafness or hearing loss that has no (or little) physical damage as a basis. It may be: 1. a purposeful effort to show a worse than actual hearing loss, as in malingering—feigned or simulated deafness, or 2. a subconscious effort to show a worse than actual hearing loss, as in psychogenic or hysterical deafness. Either type may also be referred to as functional deafness.

deafness, obstructive. older term for conductive deafness.

deafness, occupational. noise-induced hearing loss, from industrial noise.

deafness, paradoxical. paradoxical ability of many who have a conductive hearing loss to hear better in noisy places. paracusia willisiana or Willis' paracusis.

deafness, partial. old term for hearing loss.

deafness, perceptive; deafness, perception. sensorineural hearing loss—one not involving the conductive mechanism. *syn*: nerve deafness.

deafness, peripheral (pĕ-rif′er-al). impaired hearing resulting from a lesion affecting the organ of Corti. *syn*: end-organ deafness.

deafness, postlingual. loss of hearing occurring after the acquisition of speech and language.

deafness, prelingual. hearing impairment occurring before the development of speech and language. May be either adventitious or congenital.

deafness, prevocational. loss of hearing before age 19.

deafness, profound. extreme hearing impairment bordering on total deafness. A degree of loss so severe that hearing aid amplification must be supplemented by speech reading at all times to be effective. Numerically, it is generally considered to be an average of over 90 dB at 500, 1000, and 2000 Hz audiometrically (ANSI 1969).

deafness, psychic. type of deafness in which sounds are heard but not understood. Aphasia.

deafness, psychogenic (si″ko-jen′ik). term used to refer to a deficiency in which hearing loss is psychological rather than organic in nature.

deafness, retrocochlear (ret″ro-kok′le-ar). deafness resulting from a lesion behind (retro) the cochlea. High frequencies are lost first and growth of the sensation of loudness is abnormally slow (decruitment), allowing loud sounds to be well tolerated. The ear with this type of loss usually loses its ability to understand speech or to discriminate. The pure tone loss, however, may be mild or moderate. Surgical intervention in cases of retrocochlear lesions may prove helpful.

deafness, sensorineural. hearing loss that results from damage to the sensory mechanism internal from the oval and round windows. Formerly known as nerve or perceptive deafness.

deafness, severe. hearing loss which is 70 dB or more when the hearing threshold level at 500, 1000, and 2000 Hz in the better ear is averaged.

deafness, simulated. the deafness of a malingerer—one who feigns or pretends deafness for personal advantage, e.g., to gain industrial-loss compensation or to avoid military service. Children may simulate deafness to explain school deficiencies. *syn*: functional deafness.

deafness, speech. auditory aphasia.

deafness, sporadic. hereditary deafness that results from a mutant or recessive gene becoming dominant irregularly among members of a family. Compare familial deafness.

deafness, tone. inability to recognize musical tones or pitch differences. In extreme cases it is known as amusia.

deafness, total. extremely rare case in which there can be no sensation of sound because of damage to—or absence of—some portion of the cochlea or neural pathways.

deafness, toxic. hearing loss resulting from the poisonous and damaging (toxic) effect of drugs such as kanamycin, quinine, etc., on the sensory mechanism.

deafness, word. inability to understand the spoken word although the sound is heard. *syn*: auditory aphasia.

decay rate. speed with which a tone (or other sound pressure level) is fading at a given place and time. The rate may be expressed in decibels per second.

decay, tone. fast adaptation, fast auditory fatigue, or Albrecht effect. This phenomenon is evidenced by the inability of an impaired ear to hear a continuous tone presented at successively higher (5 dB) levels of intensity as the tone appears to the listener to fade out.

deci- (des′i). prefix meaning one-tenth.

decibel. one-tenth of a bel. Commonly noted as dB. A decibel is a unit of measurement used to express logarithmic ratios (to the base 10) of intensity, power, pressure, etc. Its reference base must always be given; e.g., re. input, re. .0002 dynes cm²— or referred to in some manner as SPL (sound pressure level), SL (sensation level) etc. A decibel is approximately equal to a just noticeable difference (jnd) in constant changes of intensity.

decibel meter. an instrument calibrated in decibels designed to measure voltage differences when the line impedance (in ohms) is known.

decibeloscope *n*. a teaching device using lights to show the intensity of speech sounds.

decimal (des′i-mal) *adj*. fraction expressed in relation to one-tenth part of the whole. The prefixes and symbols for decimal multiples and decimal parts of the whole are shown in the table:

Table 3.

Decimal Power	Prefix	Symbol
10^1	deka–	da
10^2	hecto–	h
10^3	kilo–	k
10^6	mega–	M
10^9	giga–	G
10^{12}	tera–	T
10^{-1}	deci–	d
10^{-2}	centi–	c
10^{-3}	milli–	m
10^{-6}	micro–	μ
10^{-9}	nano–	n
10^{-12}	pico–	p
10^{-15}	femto–	f
10^{-18}	atto–	a

decrement (dek're-ment) *n.* gradual decrease or percent of decrease. The opposite of increment.

decruitment (de-krŌŌt'ment) *n.* condition in which the growth of the sensation of loudness is slower than normal. *syn*: de-recruitment.

decussate (de-kus'āt) *v.* to cross, as in the formation of the letter T. Often used to describe nerve fiber crossings between sense organ centers.

decussation (de″kus-sa'shun) *n.* the crossing or interlacing of nerve fibers in their pathways to and from lower centers of the central nervous system.

decussation, Held's. refers to the crossing of some of the acoustic nerve fibers.

deferent (def'er-ent) *adj.* conducting away from; *syn*: efferent.

deflected wave. a wave diverted from its straight path.

degeneration (de-jen″er-a'shun) *n.* 1. a gradual lowering of the ability of an organ, muscle, or nerve to function. 2. feedback that is out of phase with an input by 180 degrees; negative feedback.

Deiter's cells (Otto Deiters, German anatomist, 1834-1863). supporting cells, like fingers (or phalanges) interspersed between the outer hair cells of the organ of Corti. *syn*: phalangeal outer cells.

Deiter's terminal frame. flattened-out ends of Deiter's cells where they meet the Hensen cells to frame the outer tunnel of the organ of Corti.

delayed auditory feedback. DAF. a system by which the speaker's own words are returned (feedback) through earphones after a time delay of a few milliseconds. A test of malingering also known as delayed side tone.

delayed feedback audiometry. DFA. a method of estimating a speech reception threshold by determining the amount of intensity of a delayed speech signal required to cause a change in the voice pattern of the person being tested.

delayed side-tone. delayed auditory feedback.

delayed speech. failure of speech to develop as expected with chronological age. It may be due to hearing impairment or brain injury, as well as slow maturation.

delayed speech feed-back test. delayed auditory feedback test.

delta wave or rhythm. a very slow brainwave pattern on an electroencephalograph during normal sleep. It is abnormal if subject is awake.

demography. *n.* study of a population in regard to distribution, births, marriages, deaths, and other statistics of interest. *adj*: demographic.

demyelinating *adj.* causing the loss or destruction of the myelin sheath that sur-

rounds most nerve cells and speeds up the nerve impulse. *v*: **demyelinate,** *n.* **demyelination.**

dendrite (den'drīt) *n.* filament of a nerve cell at the end of a nerve fiber that reaches toward other nerve cells at a junction point known as a synapse. *adj*: **dendritic, dendritical.**

deoxyribonucleic acid. DNA (de-ok″se-ri″bo-nu-kla'ic). (sometimes desoxyribonucleic). an acid found in the nucleus of cells—a nucleic acid believed to be the carrier of hereditary characteristics.

deprivation (dep-rĭ-va'shun) *n.* lack of auditory stimulus—sensory deprivation.

dermis *n.* any of the layers of skin that line the external auditory canal.

descending method. determining an audiometric threshold of sensitivity by decreasing the intensity of a previously identified stimulus until it is no longer audible. The opposite of the ascending method.

desiccant (des'ĭ-kant) *n.* a drying agent.

desiccate (des'ĭ-kāt) *v.* to dry. *n*: **desiccation.**

desquamated epithelium (des'kwah-ma″ted ep″ĭ-the'le-um). flakes of epithelium (a skin layer) that have broken off.

desquamation (des″kwah-ma'shun) *n.* shedding of flakes of skin or epithelium.

detectability threshold. threshold of sensitivity; that is, the point at which 50% of the presentations of a pure tone can be heard; *syn*: absolute threshold; detection threshold

dextral *adj.* concerning the right side as opposed to: sinistral, the left side of the body.

dextraural (deks-traw'ral) *adj.* concerning one in whom the right ear appears to be dominant.

DFA. delayed feedback audiometry.

diabetes mellitus (di″ah-bē'tēz mel-li'tus). imbalance of blood sugar that may cause inner ear deafness.

diabow microphone. diagonally bowed ceramic substrate microphone.

diacritic (di-ah-krit'ik) *n.* sign or mark used to indicate pronunciation.

diagnosis *n.* identification of a disease or disorder as a result of a study of its symptoms.

diagnostic audiogram. usually includes measurements at the half-octaves of 750 and 1500 Hz as well as lower and higher frequencies.

dialect. localized variation of a language with respect to pronunciation, vocabulary, or grammar. *adj*: **dialectal,** *adv*: **dialectally.**

diapason (di″ah-pa'son) *n.* 1. outburst of sound. 2. tuning fork. 3. standard or pitch expressed in cycles per second.

diaphragm (di'ah-fram) *n.* thin flexible plate that vibrates in response to sound pressure waves (as in a microphone) or vibrates in response to electrical stimuli to create sound pressure waves.

diathesis (di-ath'-ĕ-sis) *n.* inherited weakness or bodily predisposition to certain diseases or disorders.

dichotic, dichotomic, dichotomous (di-kot'ik, di-kot'ahm-ik, di-kot'ahm-us). 1. having two sides, divisions, or attitudes. 2. presentation of a different signal to each ear. *n.* **dichotomy.**

dichotic listening. listening to different signals presented to each ear. Diotic listening involves identical signals at each ear.

dichotic stimulation. stimulation of two sides at the same time.

diction *n.* careful pronunciation, enunciation, and choice of words.

didactic *adj.* designed to teach or instruct.

dielectric (di'ĕ-lek'trik) *n.* material or part that does not conduct.

diencephalic (di"en-se-fal'ik) *adj.* of, pertaining to, or involving the second portion of the brain (the diencephalon).

diencephalon (di"en-sef'ah-lon) *n.* the second from the left subdivision of the brain.

difference limen. (dif'fer-ens li'men). DL. sometimes called just noticeable difference or differential threshold. The smallest change in frequency or intensity which can be recognized.

difference tone. distinctive sound heard by the ear whose pitch represents the difference between the frequencies of two generating tones.

differential threshold. just noticeable difference (jnd) or difference limen (DL). *syn:* difference threshold.

diffraction (dǐ-frak'shun) *n.* scattering or distortion of sound waves around small obstacles.

diffuse sound. results when sound pressure waves are equal in all directions.

digitus auricularis (dij'ǐ-tus aw"rik-u-la'ris). the little finger was at one time called *auricularis* because it was used to scratch the outer ear canal.

dihydrostreptomycin (di-hi"dro-strep"to-mi'sin). antibiotic that may damage hearing.

dilatation (dil"ah-ta'shun) *n.* expansion of an opening with a dilator. e.g., enlarging the opening of an ear canal by inserting successively larger earmolds.

dimenhydrinate (di"men-hi'drǐ-nāt). drug used to control nausea.

din *n.* loud noise made up of a mixture of discordant sounds.

dineuric (di-nu'rik) *adj.* pertaining to a nerve cell having two axons, as found among the acoustic ganglion cells. *syn:* dineuritic.

ding *v.* to produce a ringing sound.

diode (di'od) *n.* 1. a vacuum tube made up of two elements (electrodes) one of which (known as a cathode) emits electrons when heated. The electrons are collected on the other element (known as the plate or anode) which is positively charged. 2. in solid-state circuitry, a semi-conducting crystal with two terminals fulfills the same function; that is, it conducts in one direction only—and only when voltage reaches a certain level.

diotic *adj.* 1. having two ears. Binaural. 2. presenting the same signal to both ears.

diotic listening. listening to an identical signal presented to both ears. Dichotic listening involves differing signals presented to each ear.

diphasic (di-fa'zik) *adj.* having two phases.

diphasicity (di"fa-zis'i-te) *n.* quality of having two phases.

diplacusis (dip"lah-ku'sis) *n.* literally, double-hearing. One tone is heard as two. *syn:* paracusia duplicata.

diplacusis, binaural. the listener believes that the same pure tone presented to left and right ears alternately is of a different pitch in each ear **(diplacusis binauralis).**

diplacusis dysharmonica (dis-har-mon'i-ka). the listener believes the same sound has a different pitch in each ear. *syn:* binaural diplacusis.

diplacusis echoica (e-ko'ik-a). a single sound appears to be repeated in the affected ear.

diplacusis monauralis (mon-aw-ra'lis). one tone appears to have two pitches or to be a noise in the same ear. Sometimes known as diplacusis uniauralis.

diplacusis uniauralis (u"nǐ-aw-ra'lis). more commonly known as displacusis monauralis.

diplopia (dǐ-plo'pe-ah) *n.* double vision. It sometimes occurs as one of the symptoms of syndromes that also affect the ear.

diprosopus (di-pros'o-pus) *n.* having four ears.

direct current. DC or dc. electric current that flows continuously in one direction. A current of the type delivered by a battery; sometimes referred to as galvanic current.

directional hearing aid. a hearing aid designed to utilize a directional microphone. It has greater sensitivity to sounds from the front than from the rear.

directional microphone. a microphone designed for ear-level aids with two openings so there will be greater sensitivity to sounds coming from the front (or direction toward which the head is turned). Sounds from the rear are attenuated in various ways.

directivity factor. effect of the direction from which a sound pressure wave is approaching a microphone.

directivity index. measurement in decibels of the directivity factor.

disarticulate (dis"ar-tik'u-lat) *n.* lack of interconnection of the bones of the ossicular chain. It results in a loss of hearing sensitivity of about 25 dB.

discrete (dis-krēt') *adj.* 1. separate and individually limited to pure tone frequencies—not continuous. 2. electronic circuit made up of separate components rather than utilizing a chip or integrated circuit.

discrete frequency audiometer. audiometer that presents pure tones at preselected intervals—usually octaves and half-octaves.

discrimination *n.* ability to distinguish and understand sounds.

discrimination intensity. more commonly called loudness discrimination, it is: 1. ability to detect changes in intensity. 2. measurement to detect changes in intensity—the difference limen (DL) for intensity.

discrimination loss. the difference, as expressed in percent, between the percentage of PB (phonetically balanced) words heard correctly and 100 per cent.

discrimination score. the score that results when a list of phonetically balanced monosyllabic words are presented and the number of those repeated correctly is expressed as a percentage of 100.

discriminator *n.* an electronic circuit that is designed to pass or reject preselected bands of signals.

disease, Meniere's. condition whose intermittent symptoms include dizziness, nausea, tinnitus, and progressive deafness. It is sometimes referred to as endolymphatic or labyrinthine hydrops, and Meniere's syndrome.

disease, Saint Zachary's. disease characterized by inability to speak, mutism.

disease, Voltolini's. disease of the labyrinth that in young children may lead to deaf-mutism.

disease, von Meyenburg's. type of blood disease that may result in deformity of the cartilages of the ear and nose.

disease, von Recklinghausen's. disease characterized by numerous tumors involving nerve endings; *syn*: neurofibromatosis.

dispense *v.* to prepare and distribute. *n*: **dispenser.**

dissonance (dis'so-nans) *n.* mixture of discordant sounds. *adj*: **dissonant.**

distal (dis'tal) *adj.* at the greatest distance from the center.

distance receptor. sense organ that can respond to a stimulus originating at a distance from the body. e.g., the ear. *syn*: telereceptor.

distorted speech test. same as filtered speech test. Test of speech discrimination in which words are presented at a level that is comfortably loud but filters allow only controlled frequency bands to be heard.

distortion *n.* inexact reproduction of a sound wave pattern. *adj*: **distortional.**

distortion, amplitude. inexact reproduction of a sound wave pattern that results when

the output of an electro-acoustical system is not proportional to the input. *syn*: distortion.

distortion, critically damp. alteration of response in a system resulting from over-damping.

distortion, harmonic. 1. inexact reproduction of the frequencies in a sound wave pattern. 2. new frequencies introduced by amplitude distortion are harmonically related to the original frequency, hence the term.

distortion, intermodular. type of amplitude or nonlinear distortion that results when two or more frequencies transmitted through a system generate a set of new frequencies that have no harmonic relationship.

distortion, nonlinear. inexact reproduction of a sound wave pattern that results when the output of an electro-acoustical system is not proportional to the input. *syn*: amplitude distortion.

distortion, transient. inexact reproduction of a sound wave pattern resulting from sudden changes of voltage or of load.

disyllabic (di"sil-ab'-ik) *adj.* consisting of two syllables.

dizygotic (di"zi-got"ik) *adj.* twins resulting from the fertilization of two ova; fraternal twins.

DL. difference limen.

DLD. difference limen difference.

DLF. dlf. difference limen for frequency.

DLI. dli. difference limen for intensity.

DLST. difference loudness summation test.

DMQ. deafness management quotient.

DNA. 1. did not answer. 2. deoxyribonucleic acid.

DNR. did not respond.

DNT. did not test.

Doerfler-Stewart test. test of functional or nonorganic hearing loss. Based on a comparison of the ability to understand spondaic words in quiet and in noise. The test was designed by Leo G. Doerfler and Kenneth Stewart.

doing business as. DBA.

Doppler effect. (Christian J. Doppler—Austrian mathematician and physicist in America 1803-1853). change in frequency observed (as a change in pitch) when a constant source of sound waves is in rapid motion toward or away from the listener.

Doppler shift. sometimes used in reference to sound to mean the same as Doppler effect. More accurately used to refer to a change in light rays rather than a change in sound frequency as a result of the movement of the source of the rays or waves.

dorsal (dor'sal) *adj.* pertaining to, or toward, the back. *opp*. ventral.

dorsal cochlear nucleus. cochlear nucleus in the back portion of the brain stem.

dorsum (dor′sum) *n.* the upper part and/or the back.

dosimeter (do-sim′ĕ-ter) *n.* instrument used to measure and record an individual's exposure to noise.

double-blind. research design that prevents both the researcher and the subjects from knowing the makeup of the test or control groups during the experiments.

double vibration. one cycle of a sound wave. This older term (dv) was replaced by cycles per second (cps), which has been in turn replaced by Hertz (Hz).

Down's syndrome. (John Langdon Haydon Down, English physician, 1828-1896). monogolism. Mental retardation and hearing impairment as well as physical deformities are characteristic.

DR. dynamic range.

drawl. to lengthen and soften the vowel sounds while speaking slowly.

DRC. damage risk criteria; dynamic range compression.

Drever-Collins Scale. an intelligence test that may be used with the deaf.

DRF. Deafness Research Foundation.

driving frequency. frequency of the generator driving an electrodynamic system.

drop-off *n.* abrupt change in the higher frequencies typical of a "ski-slope," precipitous, or "waterfall" loss of hearing.

drum. shortened term for eardrum.

drumhead. eardrum.

drum membrane. eardrum or tympanic membrane.

drumskin. tympanic membrane.

DS. discrimination score.

D-S. Doerfler-Stewart (test).

DSHL. decibel sum hearing (threshold) levels.

duct, acoustic. external ear canal; *syn:* acoustic meatus.

duct, cochlear (ductus cochlearis). triangular inner tube of the cochlea. It contains endolymph and connects with the sacculus by the ductus reuniens (or duct of Hensen). *syn:* scala media.

duct, endolymphatic. tiny canal that conducts endolymph from the saccule of the inner ear to the endolymphatic sac.

duct of Hensen. short membranous tube passing from the cochlear duct to the saccule of the membranous labyrinth.

duct, semicircular (ductus semicircularis). one of the three membranous tubes in the bony labyrinth of the inner ear that participate in the sense of balance.

dumb *adj.* unable to speak.

dura mater (du′rah ma′ter). outer, tough, fibrous membrane that covers the brain and spinal cord.

dv. double vibrations. Term that preceded cycles per second (cps) and Hertz (Hz).

dynamic earphone. earphone whose diaphragm of an especially thin sheet of metal is activated by an alternating signal current flowing through a connecting wire coil suspended in a magnetic field. The diaphragm thus activated changes (transduces) the electric current into sound pressure waves for introduction directly into the ear canal; *syn:* moving coil magnetic earphone.

dynamic microphone. device for converting sound pressure waves into electrical energy as a thin diaphragm is moved, causing an alternating current to flow through a connecting wire coil suspended in a magnetic field.

dynamic range. DR. the individual dynamic range is found by subtracting the speech reception threshold (SRT) from the threshold of discomfort (TD) (also known as the tolerance level [TL] or uncomfortable level [UCL])—the level at which speech becomes uncomfortably loud.

dynamic range compression. DRC. similar to logarithmic compression, this system operates only in the input stage of the hearing aid circuit.

dyne (din) *n.* measure of energy. The amount of power necessary to accelerate a weight of one gram a distance of one centimeter per second.

dyne/cm^2. dyne per square centimeter.. basic unit of measurement of sound pressure. Also known as a microbar, it represents the amount of energy required to move a mass of one gram a distance of one centimeter in one second.

dys- prefix meaning bad, difficult, ill, or painful. By extension it also means abnormal or impaired.

dysacousia (dis″ah-koo′ze-ah) *n.* **dysacousis** (dis″ah-koo′sis) **dysacusia** (dis″ah-ku′ze-ah) **dysacusis** (dis″ah-ku′sis). 1. literally, bad or difficult hearing. Properly confined to a loss of understanding rather than a loss of hearing sensitivity. 2. pain or discomfort from exposure to noise (seldom used).

dysacusis, paroxysmal (par″ok-siz′mal). hearing impairment as a result of a sudden change in blood circulation to the ear.

dysarthria (dis-ar′thre-ah) *n.* 1. poor articulation of speech due to lack of muscular coordination. 2. stammering.

dysarthria literalis (lit″er-al′is). medical term for stammering.

dysarthria syllabaris spasmodica (sil″la-bar′-is spaz″mod′i-ka). medical term for stuttering.

dysarthric *adj.* relating to problems in speaking (articulating) distinctly.

dysaudia *n.* speech disorders due to deafness.

dyseneia (dis-ē-ne'a) *n.* disturbance of speech (articulation) resulting from impaired hearing.

dysiconia, auditory (dis-ĭ-ko'ne-a). defective ability to formulate auditory images.

dysfunction (dis-funk'shun) *n.* failure to function normally.

dysglossia (dis-glos'se-ah) *n.* disorders of speech (articulation) resulting from structural anomalies of the lips, tongue, jaw, and soft palate.

dyslalia (dis-la'le-ah) *n.* 1. defect of speech (articulation) due to structural abnormalities of the organs of speech. 2. defect of speech due to impaired hearing (dyseneia is preferred term).

dyslexia (dis-lek'-se-ah) *n.* lack of ability to read with understanding that is not caused by aphasia or speech disorders.

dyslogia (dis-lo'je-ah) *n.* defective speech and language resulting from brain lesion or arrested mental development.

dyslogomathia (dis-lo-go-math'e-ah) *n.* difficulty in learning speech and language. (Hallowell Davis, MD)

dysmathia (dis-math'e-ah) *n.* difficulty in learning.

dysosteogenesis (dis-os″te-o-jen'ĕ-sis) *n.* defective or incomplete bone formation; *syn:* dysostosis.

dysostosis (dis″os-to'sis) *n.* defective or incomplete bone formation; *syn:* dysosteogenesis.

dysostosis, otomandibular. incomplete development of the lower jaw, accompanied by malfunctions of the ear; *syn:* : otomandibular syndrome.

dyspepsia, mastoid. nausea symptomatic of mastoiditis.

dysphagia (dis-fa'je-ah) *n.* problems with swallowing.

dysphasia (dis-fa'ze-ah) *n.* **dysphrasia, dysphasic.** broad term covering many forms of aphasia—defective speech and language resulting from brain damage.

dysphemia (dis-fe'-me-ah) *n.* 1. seldom used term (similar to aphemia) covering disorders of hearing that are emotional or nonorganic in origin. 2. obsolete term for stammering. *adj:* **dysphemic.**

dysphonia (dis-fo'ne-ah) *n.* difficulty in speaking. *adj:* **dysphonic.**

dysphrasia (dis-fra'ze-ah) *n.* dysphasia. *adj:* **dysphrasic.**

dysplasia (dis-pla'se-ah) *n.* abnormal growth of cells, (or a tumor) similar to neoplasia (new growth of abnormal tissue).

dyspraxia *n.* painful functioning, as in earache or laryngitis.

dystrophia (dis-tro'fe-ah) *n.* gradual and progressive weakening of a muscle. *syn:* dystrophy. *adj:* **dystrophic.**

dystrophy (dis'tro-fe) *n.* defective metabolism or inability to assimilate food—imperfect nutrition.

dystubal *adj.* concerning the malfunction of the eustachian tube.

E

EA. educational age.

ea. each.

ear (auris). organ of hearing and balance that is divided into:

1. The external ear includes the sound-collecting visible portion (auricle or pinna), the outer ear canal (external auditory meatus), and the outer surface of the eardrum (tympanum).

2. The middle ear includes the inner surface of the eardrum, the ossicular chain (hammer, anvil, and stirrup—or malleus, incus, and stapes), the eustachian tube, and the outer surface of the oval and round windows (fenestrae).

3. The inner ear includes the vestibule, the semi-circular canals, the inner surface of the oval and round windows, and the cochlea.

earache *n.* ear pain. Any ache or pain arising in the ear. Technically it may be called otalgia or otodynia.

ear advantage. the right ear, stimulating the left hemisphere of the brain, is considered the better ear for speech discrimination. The left ear, stimulating the right hemisphere, responds better to environmental sounds and music.

ear, artificial. device using a microphone in a cavity for the measurement of the acoustic output of an earphone. The cavity (6 cc in volume) is designed to present an acoustical impedance to the earphone equal to the impedance of the average human ear.

ear, aviator's. pain resulting from unequal balance of pressure between the middle and outer ear. *syn:* aero-otitis media, barotrauma.

ear, Aztec. outer ear with no lobe. *syn:* Cagot ear.

ear bank—temporal bone bank. primarily a depository that makes research possible on inner ears.

1. Eastern Temporal Bone Bank Center
Johns Hopkins Hospital
605 N. Broadway
Baltimore, MD 21205
2. Midsection Temporal Bone Bank Center
University of Chicago
950 E. 59th St.
Chicago, IL 60637
3. Southern Temporal Bone Bank Center
Baylor College of Medicine
Texas Medical Center
Houston, TX 77025
4. Western Temporal Bone Bank Center
University of Calif. Medical Center
3rd & Parnassus
San Francisco, CA 94122

ear, boilermaker's. sometimes called boilermaker's deafness. Hearing loss resulting from noise exposure. It is typified by the high frequency loss of many workmen who have spent years repairing or assembling boilers.

ear, Cagot (ka-go'). outer ear with no lobe; *syn*: Aztec ear.

ear calculus. ear crystals; *syn*: ear dust, otolite, otolith, otoconia, and otatoconia.

ear canal (external auditory meatus). channel through which sound waves travel to reach the eardrum.

ear, cauliflower. ear thickened and malformed by injury.

ear closure. atresia of the external ear canal.

ear cough. cough that is the reflexive result of irritation of the external ear canal. Hardened wax, for example, may cause a dry, hacking cough.

ear crystal. minute crystalline particle of aragonite (a type of calcium carbonate, $CaCO_3$) also known as otoconia (ear dust) or otolith (ear stone). By pressure upon the hair cells of the semicircular canals, these crystals help activate the sense of balance.

ear, Darwinian. congenitally deformed ear in which the upper border is not rolled over to form the helix, but extends flatly upward.

ear defenders. ear inserts (plugs) or muffs designed to protect the ear from dangerous noise levels.

ear dropsy. seldom used name for Meniere's disease or endolymphatic hydrops.

eardrum *n.* the eardrum (or tympanic membrane) stretches across the inner end of the external ear canal and forms the outer boundary of the middle ear. It reacts to sound waves and starts the ossicular chain moving.

eardrum, artificial. paper or plastic device designed to convey sound vibrations to the oval window, through a reed (also of plastic).

ear dust. another name for ear calculus, ear crystals, ear stones, otoconia or otolith.

ear, far. ear on the other side of the head from the signal source.

ear fungus growth. there are many types and terms including aspergillus, otomycosis, mycomyringitis, and myringomycosis.

ear hypertrophy. abnormally enlarged ears; *syn*: macrotia.

ear impression. pattern of the external ear canal made by inserting a soft plastic-like material which hardens into the shape of the individual ear canal and concha. The resulting impression is used as the matrix for molding the final earpiece to conduct amplified sound waves into the ear from the receiver of the hearing aid. See illustration on page 184.

ear inflammation. may be given any one of a number of names: otitis, otomycosis, myringitis, tympanitis, labyrinthitis.

ear, inner. portion of the ear bounded externally by the oval and round windows and internally by the internal auditory canal. It contains the cochlea and semicircular canals.

earlobe *n.* lower fleshy part of the ear, not reinforced by cartilage. **lobulus auriculae.**

ear, lope. an external ear that projects directly outward from the head.

earminded *adj.* (As contrasted to visual minded). audile.

earmold *n.* plastic piece designed to conduct amplified sound waves into the ear from the receiver (earphone) of a hearing aid. Sometimes called the earpiece.

earmold cotton block. pellet of cotton used to block the impression material in the ear canal. Sometimes a plug made of spongy plastic (polyurethane) is used instead of cotton.

earmold, CROS. earmold with a minimal frame designed to hold a plastic tube in place in the external ear canal. At the same time the ear canal itself is left as open as possible.

earmold, custom. one fabricated from an impression of the ear of a specific individual.

earmold, CFA. continuous flow adapter (CFA) earmold was designed by Norm Schlaegel of San Francisco to facilitate the changing of earmold tubing. It has a constant inside diameter.

earmold, FGM. the frequency gain modifier (FGM) earmold was designed by Harry Bennett of Fresno, CA, to change and control the frequency response of the hearing aid.

earmold, Janssen. an earmold frame designed for "tube only" fittings by Gwen Janssen of Oklahoma City. It directs the tubing toward the eardrum and holds it in place without occluding the canal.

earmold, Killion. Mead C. Killion, PhD, devised and made available to the hearing aid industry a coupling system that included the Killion "Horn" and especially designed acoustically tuned earmolds.

earmold, stock. earmold that is one of several standard sizes used for demonstration or temporary use until a custom earmold can be made.

earmold terms. terms standardized by the National Association of Earmold Laboratories, June, 1971, and in general use today. For descriptions of earmolds, see Appendix VI, page 183.

earmold vent. hole drilled in an earmold to relieve pressure or alter acoustic response. A diagonal vent is a hole drilled from the outside into the sound bore of the mold, and a parallel vent is a hole drilled parallel to the sound bore of the mold. The 1971 standard vent diameter sizes: $\#1 = 3/64''$, $\#2 = 4/64''$, $\#3 = 5/64''$, $\#4 = 7/64''$.

earmuff *n.* covering for the ear used to protect the ear from loud sounds.

ear muffler. device, such as a cotton-filled glass tumbler, formerly used to minimize transient masking noise during hearing tests.

ear, near. the ear on the same side of the head as the signal source.

ear noises. noises originating within the ear itself. Variously known (among other things) as susurrus aurium (ear whispers), tinnitus aurium, tinnitus cerebri, and more commonly simply as tinnitus.

earphone *n.* a device (also known as a receiver) designed to be closely coupled to the ear, for converting electrical energy to acoustical energy. It is an electro-acoustic transducer that is also sometimes referred to as a headphone since it is usually worn on the head and held to the ear by means of a headband. Note: The terms earphone, headphone, and receiver are often used interchangeably. Many authorities, however, reserve the term *receiver* to designate the device that performs the same function in the hearing aid and is much smaller. The telephone receiver is excluded from this definition because of the modifying term *telephone.*

earphone, crystal. a device for converting electrical energy into acoustical energy by utilizing the distinctive properties of a piezoelectric crystal, i.e., a crystal that responds proportionately to an electric current is connected to a diaphragm that moves the air to create sound pressure waves.

earphone, dynamic or moving coil. earphone whose diaphragm (of an especially thin sheet of metal) is activated by an alternating signal current flowing through a connecting wire coil suspended in a magnetic field. The diaphragm thus activated changes (transduces) the electrical current into sound pressure waves for introduction directly into the ear canal.

earphone, magnetic. earphone in which a soft iron diaphragm is activated by changes in electrical signal current flowing through soft iron poles of a permanent magnet to change electrical energy to acoustical energy.

earphone socket. socket within an earmuff designed to hold an earphone to allow communication in extremely noisy surroundings.

earpiece *n.* 1. plastic piece designed to conduct amplified sound waves into the ear from the receiver of a hearing aid. More commonly called the earmold. 2. button of a hearing aid that contains the receiver.

ear plastic surgery. surgery intended to rebuild the ear or to correct defects. Related terms include otoplasty, myringoplasty, and tympanoplasty.

ear plugs. devices intended to be inserted in the external ear canal to protect the ear from loud noise or water.

ear protectors. devices to insert into the ear canal (as an earplug) or to cover the outer ear (as a muff) to lessen the effect of loud noise.

ear resistance. opposition to free movement of various parts of the middle ear as measured by an impedance bridge or meter.

ears, Blainville. unequal appearance in size and shape of external ears.

ear scoop. spoonshaped instrument used for removing ear wax or middle ear granulations.

ear, scroll. outer ear in which the rim appears to be rolled forward and inward.

earshot *n.* distance within which the unaided voice may be heard by a normal ear.

ear specialist. commonly accepted name for a medical ear specialist is otologist. He may also be known as an aural surgeon or aurist. Other medical men especially interested in ears are variously known as otolaryngologists or otorhinolaryngologists— (oto) ear, (rhino) nose, (laryngo) throat specialists.

ear speciality. the medical specialty devoted to the ear is known as otology.

ear speculum. a short, funnel-shaped tube to facilitate inspection of, or operating in, the external or middle ear.

earsplitting *adj.* painfully loud.

ear squeeze. failure to equalize pressure in the middle ear while skin or scuba diving. Bleeding or transudation into the middle ear may result.

ear stone. otolith or calcium compound. Also called ear calculus, ear crystals, ear dust, and otoconia.

ear trumpet. device with a large opening at one end designed to gather sound waves and direct them through a smaller opening into the outer ear canal.

earwax *n.* wax in the external ear canal; *syn:* cerumen.

earwax obstruction. the problem caused by wax obstructing the ear is technically known as ceruminosis.

ECG, EKG *n.* electrocardiogram.

echeosis (ek″e-o′sis) *n.* emotional upset resulting from continued exposure to disturbing noises.

echo *n.* reflected sound waves.

echo *v.* to reflect sound.

echoacousia (ek″o-ah-koo′ze-ah) *n.* abnormal condition of hearing in which a sound seems to be repeated.

echo diplacusis. single sound appears to be repeated in the affected ear.

echoencephalography (ek″o-en-sef″ah-log′rah-fe) *n.* use of ultrasound waves in investigating skull and brain conditions.

echo, flutter. reflections of an original sound wave stimulus that occur in rapid succession. If the reflections are periodic and audible they may be called musical echoes.

echoic *adj.* pertaining to an echo.

echolalia (ek″o-la′le-ah) *n.* involuntary repetition of words or phrases just spoken by someone else. Also known as echologia, echophasia, echophrasia, echo speech, and mimic speech.

echolocation *n.* method of locating distant or invisible objects by means of sound waves reflected back by the objects (as used by bats). A man-made apparatus for the same purpose is known as an echometer or sonar.

echologia (ek″o-loj′e-ah) *n.* involuntary repetition of words or phrases just spoken by someone else. More commonly known as echolalia and sometimes as echophasia, echophrasia, echo speech, or mimic speech.

echometer *n.* apparatus for locating distant or invisible objects by measuring the time involved in transmission and reflection of sound waves; *syn:* sonar.

echo, multiple. reflections of an original sound wave stimulus that occur in separately distinguishable intervals. Echoes that occur more rapidly are called flutter echoes.

echo-opthalmography *n.* use of a sounding device to locate a foreign body in the eye or to aid in differentiation of lesions.

echopathy (ek-op′ah-the) *n.* involuntary imitation of actions or words.

echophasia (ek-o-fa′se-ah) *n.* form of aphasia characterized by involuntary repetition of words or phrases just spoken by someone else (often with rising inflection as in a question). *syn:* echophrasia, echolalia, echo speech, mimic speech.

echophotony (ek″-fot′o-ne) *n.* the sensation of color some people have when they hear certain sounds.

echophrasia (ek″o-fra′se-ah) *n.* involuntary repetition of words or phrases spoken by someone else. *syn:* echophasia, echolalia, echo speech, mimic speech.

echo sounder instrument for measuring depths by timing the transmission and reflection of sound waves.

echo speech. involuntary repetition of words or phrases just spoken by someone else. More commonly referred to as echolalia, less often as echologia, echophasia, echophrasia, and mimic speech.

ECR. electrocardiographic response.

-ectomy (combining form). suffix indicating surgical removal; e.g., stapedectomy, the surgical removal of the stapes.

ectopia, ectopy (ek-to′pe-ah) *n.* congenital misplacement of a body part.

ectopic (ek-top′-ik) *adj.* in an abnormal location or out of place.

EDA. electrodermal audiometry.

edema (ĕ-de′mah) *n.* abnormal accumulation of fluid in body tissues or body cavities. *syn:* hydrops, as in endolymphatic hydrops—Meniere's.

edematous (ĕ-dĕm′ah-tus) *adj.* concerning edema.

EDR, EDRA. electrodermal response audiometry.

educational age. EA. grade standing of an individual as measured by achievement tests scored in age units.

educational audiologist. hearing screening and hearing conservation programs of students are conducted by educational audiologists in public and private school systems.

educational quotient. EQ—a number given to represent the relationship between chronological age and grade standing in school.

EEA. electroencephalic audiometry.

EEG. electroencephalography, electroencephalogram.

EENT. eye, ear, nose and throat.

EER. electroencephalographic response.

effect, Albrecht. also known as fast adaptation, fast auditory fatigue, or tone decay. This phenomenon is evidenced by the inability of an impaired ear to hear a continuous tone presented at successively higher (5dB) levels of intensity as the tone appears to the listener to fade out.

effect, body baffle. 1. change produced by the presence of a body in the sound field. 2. effect on the response of a box-type or conventional hearing aid when it is worn on the body—especially under clothing. The greatest attentuation is in frequencies above 1000 Hz.

effect, Doppler. the apparent change in pitch that results when listener and sound source are moving rapidly away from or toward each other; *syn:* the Doppler phenomenon, Doppler shift.

effect, electrophonic. sensation of hearing that results when an alternating electrical current of suitable frequency and intensity is passed through a person. It is most effective on the head near the inner ear.

effective level. difference between the total energy of a critical band and the threshold energy of a pure tone in the center of the band. It approximates the sensation level of the critical band of noise.

effective masking. 1. noise of sufficient intensity to interfere with the hearing of another sound. White noise may be introduced in the better ear, for example, to mask out the speech that is being tested for threshold of sensitivity (SRT) in the poorer ear. Narrow bands, pink noise, and complex noise may also be used for masking when a pure tone threshold is sought. 2. this term, when used by some audiometer manufacturers, indicates that additional energy is built into the masking level—as indicated on the dial—to compensate for the air conduction shadow curve.

effective sound pressure. sound pressure having sufficient energy to cause a predetermined response.

effector *n.* 1. nerve cell terminal at the transmission end of the nerve fiber. 2. motor (efferent) nerve ending which activates a muscle, gland, or body organ. 3. organ, gland, or muscle that reacts to efferent stimulation.

effect, precedence. when the same sound reaches the ear from two sources at different distances, the precedence effect results in the sound being heard as coming from the nearer source rather than both.

effects, microphonic. unwanted sound generated in a loudspeaker or in an electrical circuit by mechanical movements of normally nonmoving parts.

efferent (ef'er-ent) *adj.* 1. conducting away from—as opposed to afferent (conducting toward). 2. nerve fibers that carry impulses away from the brain.

efferent auditory fibers. nerve fibers that carry impulses from the superior olivary nucleus in the brainstem to the cochlea.

effusions *n.* accumulations of fluid in the middle ear.

eighth (VIIIth) nerve (or eighth cranial nerve). cable of nerve fibers that carry impulses between the inner ear and the brain. It consists of two branches: vestibular (balance) and cochlear (hearing). The nervus vestibulo-cochlearis is sometimes called the nervus acusticus or acoustic (auditory) nerve.

EKG. electrocardiogram.

elasticity *n.* capacity of some materials to return to their original size and shape after being deformed.

ELBA. ear level bilateral attachment.

electret microphone. condenser microphone that has been miniaturized to the point it can be used in hearing aids.

electrical impedance. opposition to the flow of electrical current comparable to friction in a water pipe. It is the ratio of the voltage across two terminals to the electrical current passing through them.

electrical impedance, blocked. impedance measured at the electrical terminals of an electromechanical transducer when the mechanical system is blocked.

electrical potential. amount of electrical pressure (electromotive force measured in volts) potentially available in an electrically charged body.

electric pulse code. system of electrical impulses relayed along the auditory nerve in response to a stimulus that the brain decodes and identifies.

electric response audiometry. ERA—also referred to as evoked response audiometry—it is a form of electrophysiologic audiometry in which an analog computer is included in the circuit to average out ongoing or spontaneous brain-wave activity. A characteristic pattern of response to a sound stimulus may then become evident.

electristor *n.* type of semiconductor that utilizes a tiny layer of a radioisotope to energize the flow of electrons.

electroacoustic *adj.* concerning the relationships of electrical and acoustical forms of energy.

electroacoustic characteristics. qualities (frequency range, efficiency, and distortion, for example) of a device (transducer) designed to change electrical energy into acoustical energy or vice versa.

electroacoustic locator. device designed to locate foreign bodies in tissue by measuring resistance to sound waves.

electroacoustic transducer. device designed to change electrical energy into acoustical energy and vice versa, e.g., hearing aid receivers and microphones.

electroacupuncture. use of electrodes at acupuncture points. It is sometimes used as a treatment for sensorineural hearing impairment.

electrocardiogram *n.* EKG. graphic recording or tracing of heart action produced by an electrocardiograph.

electrocardiograph *n.* instrument for graphically recording heart action as revealed by changes of electrical potential during heartbeat.

electrocardiographic response audiometry. form of electrophysiologic audiometry. Measurements are made of changes in heart activity that result from sound stimulation; *syn*: cardiac evoked response audiometry (CERA).

electrocochleogram *n.* audiogram based on cochleography—the measurement of the electrical activity of the cochlea by means of electrodes placed in the external auditory canal or through the eardrum onto the promontory.

electrocochleography. measurement of the electrical potential of the VIIIth nerve.

electrode *n.* 1. one of the poles of an electrical storage battery. 2. one of the elements in a vacuum tube. Either the source of free electrons (cathode) or the collector of the electrons (anode). 3. device designed to provide contact between a metallic and non-metallic conductor. 4. instrument with a point or surface to be placed on the patient (or into a research animal) to complete an electrical circuit or to measure an electrical potential.

electrode, negative. 1. cathode or element that releases electrons when heated in a vacuum tube. 2. cathode of a hearing aid cell that releases negative ions.

electrode, positive. 1. anode or element that collects the free electrons released by the negative electrode (cathode) in a vacuum tube. 2. anode of a hearing aid cell.

electrodental *adj.* pertaining to the use of a tooth as a transducer (electrophonic effect) or for bone conduction. Sometimes associated with the idea of building a hearing aid in a false tooth (transdental).

electrodermal *adj.* pertaining to the electrical properties of the skin, especially the activities of the sweat glands through the autonomic nervous system. The change in electrical resistance is known as the Fere effect. The change in electrical potential is known as the Tarchanoff effect.

electrodermal audiometry. EDA—method of determining hearing thresholds by measuring changes in skin resistance, associated with a conditioned response to sound (PGSR).

electrodiagnosis *n.* identification and measurement of degree of hearing deficit by means of electronic instruments.

electrodynamics *n.* branch of physics devoted to the study of electric charges in motion. See electrostatics.

electroencephalic *adj.* shorter term for electroencephalographic. Pertaining to the tracings of brain activity made by an electroencephalograph.

electroencephalic audiometry—EEA or electroencephalographic audiometry—EEG. type of eletrophysiologic audiometry. The electroencephalic response (EER) resulting from sound stimulation causes changes in the pattern of the encephalogram (EEG). These changes are measured and quantified.

electroencephalogram (e-lek″tro-en-sef′ah-lo-gram″) *n.* sometimes known as an electrogram. The tracing made by an electroencephalograph. Usually abbreviated EEG.

electroencephalograph *n.* EEG—instrument for recording the electrical current produced by brain activity.

electroencephalographic *adj.* pertaining to the tracing of brain activity by an electroencephalograph.

electrogram. short term sometimes used in place of electroencephalogram.

electrolyte. solution in a battery that conducts ions between the negative and positive poles and is decomposed in the process.

electromagnetic wave. wave produced by periodic variations of intensity of an electric charge; e.g., light waves and radio waves.

electromanometer *n.* electronic instrument designed to measure gas or liquid pressure. It is an important part of the electroacoustic impedance meter.

electromechanical transducer. device designed to change electrical energy into mechanical energy and vice versa, e.g., hearing aid bone vibrator.

electromotive force *n.* abbreviation: EMF, Emf, or emf. pressure causing the flow of electrons in an electric current. It is measured in volts.

electromyography *n.* study of the reflex of the stapedius muscle by means of recordings of the action potential after acoustic stimulation.

electron. one of the subatomic negatively charged particles that surround the positively charged nucleus to form the atom. *adj:* **electronic.**

electron microscope. microscope that can magnify up to 100,000 times by using electron beams with wave lengths thousands of times shorter than visible light in place of light.

electronegative *adj.* state of being charged with negative electricity.

electronics *n.* branch of physics concerned with the study of electrons and the practical application of this knowledge in useful electronic devices.

electronystagmogram (e-lek″tro-nis-tag′mo-gram) *n.* chart resulting from tracings made by an electronystagmograph.

electronystagmograph *n.* electronic measuring instrument used to chart the involuntary eye movements during caloric tests in evaluating vestibular function.

electronystagmography (e-lek″tro-nis″tag-mog′rah-fe) *n.* electronic charting of tracings made by an electronystagmograph.

electrophonic effect. sensation of hearing that results when an alternating electrical current of suitable frequency and intensity is passed through a person. It is most effective on the head near the inner ear.

electrophysiologic audiometry. inclusive term covering many types of so-called objective audiometry designed to measure the individual's response to a sound stimulus without subject cooperation being necessary.

An instrument is used that records changes in brain waves, heart rate, or skin resistance to sound stimuli. The response may be pre-conditioned or reinforced by a mild electric shock that follows the sound stimulus at an interval of about 0.6 second.

ERA—evoked (or electric) response audiometry.

CERA—cardiac evoked response audiometry.

ECR—electrocardiographic response

EDA—electrodermal audiometry.

EEA—electroencephalic audiometry.

electrophysiologist *n.* one who studies both the reaction of living cells and nerves to external electrical stimuli or the generation of electrical currents by living cells and organs of the body.

electrophysiology *n.* study of the electricity generated by the chemical and physical activity of the human body.

electropositive *adj.* state of being charged with positive electricity.

electroscope *n.* electronic device that detects and measures positive and negative electric charges in the body.

electrostatic *adj.* of or pertaining to static electricity.

electrostatics *n.* branch of physics devoted to the study of the behavior of electrical charges at rest.

electrotactile *adj.* concerning electronic devices designed to convert various stimuli (e.g., sound waves) into vibratory signals that can be felt by the deaf.

electrotonus *n.* change in sensitivity of a nerve when a current of electricity passes through. *adj*: **electrotonic.**

electrowriter. an attachment to a telephone that allows both parties to communicate by writing.

elevated threshold. a poorer threshold of sensitivity, indicated by marks at higher numbers on the audiogram; *syn*: higher threshold.

elide (e-līd') *v.* to omit a syllable in pronunciation.

elliptical recess. small cavity in the upper part of the wall of the vestibule in which the utricle is lodged. The utricular fossa.

embol-, emboli-, or embolo- combining form for embolus.

embolus *pl.* **emboli** *n.* a foreign particle (solid, liquid, or gaseous) circulating in a blood vessel.

embolectomy *n.* surgical excision of an embolus.

embolic *adj.* pertaining to or caused by an embolus or embolism.

embolism *n.* sudden obstruction of a blood vessel by a foreign substance. Sometimes considered responsible for a sudden loss of hearing; vascular accident.

embrace, Moro's. a startle reaction of the newborn described by Moro (German pediatrician) as a drawing of the infant's arms across its chest in response to a sudden loud sound. A version of the Moro reflex or response.

-eme. suffix denoting a significantly distinctive unit of language structure; as phoneme.

EMF. electromotive force.

EMG. electromyograph.

-emia, -aemia. a suffix or combining form referring to the blood.

emission *n.* flow of electrons from a cathode.

emphasis *n.* stress given to a syllable or word.

empiric *n.* one who depends on practical experience or observation. *adj*: **empirical.**

empyema *n.* pus in a body cavity.

empyema, mastoid. presence of pus in the air cells of the mastoid process.

EMR. educationally mentally retarded.

enceph-, encephal-, or encephalo- prefix and combining forms denoting the brain.

encephalic *adv.* pertaining to the brain or to the structure within the skull.

encephalitis *n.* brain inflammation.

encephalograph (en-sef'ah-lo-graf″) *n.* term used for either an x-ray of the brain (encephalogram) or as a shortened version of electroencephalograph — an instrument used to make tracings of brain wave activity.

encephalography *n.* x-ray studies of the brain after the cerebrospinal fluid has been replaced by air.

encephalomyelitis (en-sef″ah-lo-mi″ĕ-li'tis) *n.* inflammation of both the brain and spinal cord at the same time. *syn*: myeloencephalitis.

encephalon *n.* the brain.

encyst *v.* to enclose in a cyst. *n*: **encystment, encystation.**

end- or endo- prefix or combining form meaning within, inside, or inner; as endolymph—the fluid within the scala media as compared to perilymph—the fluid that surrounds the scala media in the scala vestibuli and scala tympani.

endaural (end-aw'ral) *adj.* pertaining to the inner surface of the external auditory canal.

endaural incision. surgical cut through the external auditory canal.

endbrain *n.* forward part of the brain.

endemic, endemical (en-dem'ik) *adj.* peculiar or native to a region or locality. *n:* **endemicity, endemism.**

endochondral (en"do-kon'dral) *adj.* concerning the formation of bone as it replaces cartilage.

endocranium *n.* inner surface of the skull.

endocrine glands (en'do-krĭn). ductless glands that produce secretions that have a stimulating or retarding effect on tissues or organs of the body. One effect of endocrine disorders in children may be impaired hearing.

endogenous (en-doj'ĕ-nus) *adj.* originating within the body. *opp:* exogenous.

endolymph (en'do-limf) *n.* fluid contained within the scala media (inner tube of the cochlea) and the semicircular canals. It is secreted by the stria vascularis. *adj:* **endolymphatic.**

endolymphatic duct. a tiny canal that conducts endolymph from the saccule of the inner ear to the endolymphatic sac.

endolymphatic hydrops (hi'drops). Meniere's disease. malfunction of hearing and balance caused by excessive inner ear fluids. *syn:* Meniere's syndrome.

endolymphatic labyrinthitis (lab"y-rin-thi'tis). inflammation of the inner ear: otis interna.

endolymphatic potential (en"do-lim-fat'ik). energy in the form of steady voltage between the endolymph inside the cochlear partition and the perilymph outside.

endolymphatic sac. a pouch embedded in the mastoid—filled with endolymph.

endomastoiditis *n.* inflammation of the lining of the mastoid process. *syn:* intramastoiditis.

end-organ. structure at the end of a nerve fiber or a nervous system that changes a stimulus into nervous activity. The end-organ of hearing is the organ of Corti.

end-organ deafness. deafness due to a lesion (damage) within the organ of Corti.

end-organ of hearing. organ of Corti.

endosalpingitis (en"do-sal"pin-ji'tis) *n.* inflammation of the membrane that lines the eustachian tube.

endoscope *n.* medical instrument used for the inspection of a hollow organ.

endosteum (en-dos'te-um) *n.* membrane lining the marrow cavity of bone.

endothelial *adj.* concerning endothelium.

endothelium *n.* layer of thin cells that lines internal body cavities.

end-plate. structure at the end of a motor nerve that activates a muscle fiber.

energize *v.* 1. to supply electric current to a circuit (as by the battery of a hearing aid). 2. to charge a battery.

energizer *n.* term sometimes applied to a hearing aid battery.

energy *n.* power either in use or available. When in use the unit of measure is the erg. One erg is the amount of energy used up when a force of one dyne acts through a distance of one centimeter.

energy, acoustic. power generated by sound waves.

ENG. electronystagmography.

engorgement *n.* congested with fluid.

enhance *v.* to improve or strengthen.

enhancement *n.* improvement or strengthening of a quality.

ENT. ear-nose-throat.

ent- or ento- combining form. Inner or within.

enucleation (e-nu"kle-a'shun). removal of a tumor without rupturing its capsule.

envelope total distribution of frequencies contained in a sound signal.

envelope frequency. fundamental frequency.

eosinophil granuloma (e"o-sin'o-fil). disease characterized by localized bony lesions—often of the temporal bone.

EP. evoked potential. endocochlear potential.

ephedrine (e-fed'rin). a drug sometimes used to shrink the mucous membranes of the nose, thus allowing better functioning of the eustachian tube.

ep-, epi- combining form. At, on, after, above, besides, near or in addition to.

epicanthal fold (ep"ĭ-kan'thal). heavy layer of skin at the inner angle of the eyes (one of the characteristic features of the Waardenburg syndrome).

epicranial *adj.* located on the bones of the skull.

epidemic parotitis. mumps.

epidermis *n.* outermost layer of skin. *adj:* **epidermal, epidermoid.**

epidermoid cyst. granulation or squamous tissue. A sac filled with discarded skin cells.

epileptiform *adj.* concerning behavior that resembles epileptic symptoms.

epineurium (ep"ĭ-nu're-um) *n.* connective tissue that forms a sheath for a nerve trunk.

epiotic (ep"e-ot'ik) *adj.* near or above the ear.

epiotic center. junction point of the embryonic cartilages that become the mastoid process.

episodic (e-pi-sod'ik) *adj.* intermittent or occurring in cycles; e.g., a characteristic of Meniere's.

epistaxis *n.* severe nose bleed.

epithelial (ep"ĭ-the'le-al) *adj.* concerning the epithelium—the skin, or the lining of the mucous membrane.

epithelial atrophy. degenerative changes within the cochlea, beginning at the base and proceeding toward the apex. Considered a characteristic of presbycusis.

epithelium *n.* cellular tissue that forms the surface layer of the skin and mucous membrane lining of various tubes and cavities of the body.

epithelium, neural. surface layer of cells that contain nerve endings of special sense; e.g., the hair cells of the inner ear.

epitympanic (ep″ĭ-tim-pan′ik) *adj.* above or near the eardrum.

epitympanic recess. attic or upper portion of the middle ear, the epitympanum.

epitympanic recess, inflammation of. atticitis. Inflammation of the attic.

epitympanum *n.* the attic of the middle ear cavity.

EQ. educational quotient.

equal loudness contours. curved lines that indicate the sound pressures necessary at each frequency to produce sensations of equal loudness for normally hearing listeners.

equal loudness contours, monaural. equal loudness contours determined by testing one ear alone.

equation method. procedure for determining thresholds by which the subject varies the intensity of a stimulus to match or barely differ from a reference stimulus. *syn*: method of adjustment.

equilibrium (e″kwĭ-lib′re-um) *n.* state of balance. The ability to control position in space.

equilibrium senses. semicircular canals: esp. the rudimentary balance organs.

equipotentiality in CNS (central nervous system) (e″kwe-po-ten″she-al′ĭ-te). power of one part of the brain to take over the function of another.

equivalent SRT (speech reception threshold). average of the two better (lesser loss) frequencies of 500, 1000, and 2000 Hz. The same as the Fletcher method of estimating the speech loss from the pure tone audiogram.

ERA. evoked (or electric) response audiometry.

eremophobia (er″ĕ-mo-fo′be-ah) *n.* morbid fear of being alone.

ERI. Ear Research Institute. Now House Ear Institute.

erg *n.* unit of measure of energy: the amount of energy required to accelerate a mass of one gram one centimeter per second.

erythroblast (ĕ-rith′ro-blast) *n.* cell found in red bone marrow that is the first stage in the formation of red blood cells. *adj*: **erythroblastic.**

erythroblastic kernicterus. infant jaundice that results from erythroblastosis.

erythroblastosis. abnormal condition characterized by the presence of too many erythroblasts in the blood that causes a breakdown of the red blood cells.

erythroblastosis fetalis. specific type of erythroblastosis in the newborn resulting from RH incompatibility in the parents. Anemia, jaundice, and enlargement of the liver and spleen are characteristic of this disease. *adj*: **erythroblastotic.**

ESN. educationally sub-normal.

esophageal (ĕ-sof″ah-je′al) *adj.* of or concerning the esophagus.

esophageal speech or voice. speech produced by belching swallowed air through the upper narrow portion of the esophagus.

ESP. extrasensory perception.

esophagus (ĕ-sof′ah-gus) *n.* tube in the throat through which food passes to the stomach.

esthesiometer *n.* device for measuring sensory stimulation.

etiologic, etiological *adj.* pertaining to the causes of disease.

etiology *n.* the study of the factors that cause an abnormal condition or disease.

etymotic (ĕ-te-mah′tik) *n.* word coined to express the mathematical difference between the unaided and aided frequency response at the eardrum when a hearing aid is used; *syn*: real ear gain, orthotelephonic gain, insertion gain.

euphony (u′fon-e) *n.* sound of words that are pleasant to the ear.

eurhythmics (u″rith′miks) *n.* harmonizing of body movements with spoken words. Often used in helping the deaf learn the rhythm of speech.

eustachian catheter (u-sta′ke-an kath′ĕ-ter). a tubular device with a gently curved beak to inflate the eustachian tube or the middle ear through the nasal passage.

eustachian cushion. ridge of cartilage above and behind the pharyngeal opening of the eustachian tube. *syn*: torus tubarius.

eustachian salpingitis, acute (sal″pin-ji′tis). closure of the eustachian tube by inflammation.

eustachian salpingitis, chronic. blockade of the eustachian tube (usually as a result of repeated inflammations).

eustachian tonsil. mass of lymphatic tissue in the mucous membrane of the eustachian tube near its opening into the pharynx. Adenoids.

eustachian tube. (Bartolomeo Eustachio, Italian anatomist, 1510-1574). tube about 1½ inches (36 mm) long and ⅛″to ¼″(3 mm to 6 mm) in diameter, leading from the nasopharynx to the middle ear. Normally makes possible equalization of pressure between the middle-ear and outside air. *syn*: auditory tube (tuba auditiva).

eustachitis. inflammation of the eustachian tube; *syn*: salpingitis.

evaginate (e-vaj′ĭ-nat) *v.* to protrude or turn inside out.

evagination *n.* protrusion or outgrowth.

evaluation, hearing aid. HAE. any method of trying to select a suitable hearing aid for an impaired ear. In actual practice, a misnomer, in that it does not refer to a method of judging hearing aids; i.e., evaluation of hearing aid performance.

everyday speech test. a test of speech understanding based on the use of sentences especially prepared at the Central Institute for the Deaf that were designed to represent everyday American speech.

evoked potential—EP. electrical potential generated by brain wave activity in response to a stimulus; e.g., sound.

evoked response audiometry, ERA. a form of electrophysiologic audiometry in which an analog computer is included in the circuit to average out ongoing or spontaneous brain-wave activity. A characteristic pattern of response to a sound stimulus may then become evident. *syn*: electric response audiometry.

Ewing tests. tests of infant hearing designed by the Ewings of England that are based on the quiet presentation of familiar sounds; e.g., cup and spoon.

exacerbate (eg-zas'-er-bāt) *v*. to increase in severity. *n*: **exacerbation.**

exogenous (eks-oj'ě-nus) *adj*. originating outside the body.

exostosis (ek"sos-to'-sis) *pl*. **exostoses** *n*. bony growth within the external auditory canal.

exponent *n*. small number (placed high and to the right of the natural number) that indicates how many times the primary number is to be multiplied by itself or the number of zeros to add to the natural number in the case of logarithms to the base 10 (as in decibels).

exposure-equivalent rule in TTS. if a temporary threshold shift (TTS) already exists from one type of noise exposure, this time can be added to the time of exposure of the new noise.

expressive aphasia. inability to say a word needed to express a thought. *syn*: motor aphasia.

extended high frequency audiometer. audiometer designed to generate pure tone frequencies from 8000 to 20,000 Hz.

external auditory canal, (external auditory meatus). passageway that allows sound waves to reach the eardrum. Its diameter is about 7 mm (¼ to ⅓ inch), length from the tragus is about 40 mm, and from the pore it is about 25 mm (about 1 inch).

external auditory canal pore. outer opening of the external ear canal.

external auditory meatus. outer ear canal. The external auditory canal. *syn*: external acoustic meatus.

external ear. outer ear—the portion of the hearing mechanism made up of the external ear flap (auricle or pinna) and the external auditory canal terminating at the eardrum (tympanic membrane).

external hair cells. hair cells in the organ of Corti that rest on the outer edge of the basilar membrane; i.e., the edge away from the modiolus.

external otitis. inflammation of the walls of the external auditory canal.

exteroceptors. groups of nerve cells (receptors) that respond to stimuli from outside the body; e.g., in the ear.

extirpation (ek"ster-pa'shun) *n*. removal by surgery.

extraneous noise. sounds of the environment; *syn*: ambient noise.

extratympanic manometry. measurement of middle ear muscle reflexes by means of a device that monitors changes in external ear canal pressures in response to acoustic stimuli.

extravasate (eks-trav'a-sāt) *v*. to filter or exude blood, lymph, or serum from a vessel into surrounding tissue. *n*: **extravasation.**

exudate *v*. to exude or ooze through minute openings in tissue.

exudate *n*. fluid, pus, or serum that passes into a cavity such as the middle ear.

exudation (eks"u-da'shun) *n*. oozing of fluid into the middle ear cavity.

exude *v*. to ooze through minute openings or pores in tissue, e.g., into the middle ear or ear canal.

eye blink test. closure or blink of an eye (the auropalpebral reflex) resulting from stimulation of the hearing mechanism by sudden sound at controlled levels.

F

facial canal. more commonly known as fallopian aqueduct or canal.

facial nerve. VIIth cranial nerve. It accompanies the VIIIth nerve through the internal auditory canal. Some of its branches control muscles of the external and middle ear, e.g., chorda tympani.

facial palsy. facial paralysis caused by a lesion of the VIIth cranial nerve. Hearing impairment may accompany the facial distortion; *syn*: Bell's palsy.

FACP. Fellow of the American College of Physicians.

FACS. Fellow of the American College of Surgeons.

factor, recruitment. degree by which an abnormally rapid increase in the sensation of loudness affects the ability of an individual to handle loud or amplified sound.

factor, RH. a protein in most blood types. If the blood of the mother does not contain this protein and the father's does, the incompatibility may result in damage to the newborn. The factor was first described in 1940 and associated with deafness in 1950.

fading-numbers test. almost obsolete group hearing test in which a phonograph record presents pairs of one-digit numbers at successively lower (3 dB) levels of intensity.

faint speech test. test of speech discrimination in which monosyllabic words (PB lists) are presented at 5 to 15 dB above threshold (SL—sensation level).

fallopian aqueduct. bony passage through which the facial nerve traverses the middle ear into the internal auditory canal. *syn*: fallopian canal.

fallopian canal (Gabriele Fallopius, 16th century Italian anatomist). more common name for fallopian aqueduct.

false negative response. lack of reaction to a sound stimulus when it has actually been heard. Most often this term is used if an infant has not responded during a hearing screening test when his hearing is within normal limits as revealed by other tests.

false paracusis. sensation of improvement in hearing when others speak loudly because of noisy surroundings.

false positive response. appearance of a reaction to a sound stimulus when it has not actually been heard. Most often used if an infant has responded during a hearing screening test when his hearing is not within normal limits as revealed by other—more objective—tests.

familial deafness. hearing loss that appears among several members of a family, but is not apparently hereditary. It may be the result of a blood incompatibility.

far ear. ear on the other side of the head from the signal source; *syn*: offside ear.

farad *n.* named for Michael Faraday, English physician and chemist (1791-1867), the farad is the unit of electrical capacity. It is the capacity of a condenser which, charged with 1 coulomb, gives a difference in potential of 1 volt.

farmer's ear. one ear shows loss of sensitivity as a result of exposure to tractor noise—as he looks back over shoulder.

fascia (fash'e-ah) *pl.* **fasciae** *n.* 1. thin tissue that forms a sheath around the body under the skin. It also surrounds muscles separately or in groups. It is sometimes used in eardrum reconstruction. 2. a bandage.

fascia, temporalis. thin tough tissue covering the temporal muscle.

fasciculus (fah-sik'-u-lus) *n.* a bundle of nerve or muscle fibers.

FAST. filtered audiometric speech test.

fast adaptation. also known as fast auditory fatigue, the Albrecht effect, or tone decay. This phenomenon is evidenced by the inability of an impaired ear to hear a continuous tone presented at successively higher (5 dB) levels of intensity as the tone appears to the listener to fade out.

fast auditory fatigue. tone decay or fast adaptation.

fatigue, auditory. also known as temporary threshold shift (TTS). The change in the threshold of hearing that may result from continuous exposure to sound. It is expressed in dB per frequency and related to exposure time.

fatigue, perstimulatory. apparent diminishing of the loudness of a stimulus when presented continuously at an intensity level that is above threshold. A type of tone decay.

FCP. functional communication profile.

febri- prefix referring to fever.

febrile (feb'ril) *adj.* concerning fever.

Fechner's Law (Gustav Theodor Fechner, German physicist, 1801-1887). In 1860 he said that a sensation resulting from a stimulus seems to increase by a constant amount (arithmetically by addition) as the intensity of the stimulus is constantly increased (logarithmically by multiplication). Compare with Weber-Fechner law.

feedback. 1. return of a portion of the output of an amplifier to an input stage. 2. response to a stimulus. 3. efferent nervous system.

feedback, acoustic. high-pitched squeal caused by recirculation and reamplification of sound waves between microphone and speaker or earphone. Occurs when units are too close together, amplification is too high, or there is earmold leakage in the case of hearing aids.

feedback, auditory. hearing and monitoring of one's own vocalizations.

feedback, degenerative. return of an out-of-phase (or inverted) signal of an amplifier from an output stage to an input stage to reduce amplification of harmonic distortion; *syn*: negative, inverse, or out-of-phase feedback.

feedback, delayed auditory. DAF. system by which the speaker's own words are returned (feedback) through earphones after a time delay of a few milliseconds. A test of malingering also known as delayed side tone.

feedback, in-phase. return of a portion of the output signal to be added to an input stage for greater amplification. Also known as positive or regenerative feedback.

feedback, internal. acoustic feedback (squeal) usually resulting from the unshielded proximity of the microphone and receiver in an ear-level hearing aid.

feedback, inverse. negative, out-of-phase, or degenerative feedback.

feedback, mechanical. acoustic feedback (squeal) usually caused by the vibrations of the microphone or receiver against the hearing aid case.

feedback, negative. out-of-phase, degenerative, or inverse feedback.

feedback, out-of-phase. degenerative, inverse, or negative feedback.

feedback, positive. the result, for example, when a portion of the output voltage is returned and added to the input voltage. *syn:* regenerative or in-phase feedback.

feedback, regenerative. in-phase or positive feedback.

feeling, threshold of. the minimum intensity level at which sound pressure produces a sensation of feeling that is distinct from the sensation of hearing. It may also be described as discomfort.

feigned deafness. simulated hearing loss—a loss that has no physical damage as a basis. It is the deafness of a malingerer—one who feigns or pretends deafness for personal advantage to gain industrial loss compensation or to avoid military service, for example. Children may simulate deafness to explain school deficiencies. *syn:* functional deafness.

felix. tactual vocoder developed by Levine and his associates at MIT in the 1950s. Its operation was based on the separation of speech signals into frequency bands with variations in intensity. Later improvements included the separation of coded speech into vibratory signals that varied in intensity, frequency, and vibration placement.

fence, high. upper limit of the hard of hearing range of hearing impairment expressed as an average of 500, 1000, and 2000 Hz; 92 dB ISO (ANSI) or 82 dB ASA. Greater loss is considered deaf.

fence, low. lower limit of hearing impairment expressed as an average of 500, 1000, and 2000 Hz; 27 dB ISO or 16 dB ASA 1951.

fenestra (fĕ-nes′trah) *pl.* **fenestrae** *n.* a window or small opening in a body structure, usually closed by a membrane: e.g., the fenestra ovalis or oval window. *adj:* **fenestral.**

fenestra cochleae. the round window. *syn:* fenestra rotunda.

fenestra novovalis (nov″o-val′is). window or artificial opening created in a semicircular canal to allow transmission of sound pressure waves in the fenestration operation.

fenestra ovalis. the oval window. *syn:* fenestra vestibuli.

fenestra rotunda. the round window; *syn:* fenestra cochleae.

fenestra tympanica. the round window; *syn:* fenestra cochleae; fenestra rotunda.

fenestra vestibuli. the oval window.

fenestrate (fen′es-trāt) *v.* to create a window by surgery.

fenestrated (fen′es-trāt″ed) *adj.* having a window created by surgery.

fenestration (fen″es-tra′shun) *n.* surgical creation of a window in the bony structure of the inner ear to allow passage of sound pressure waves.

Feré effect (fā′rā). change in the electrical resistance of the skin that results from an external stimulus.

Feré method. electrodes are attached to the skin to measure the change in resistance to a minute external electric current that results from a sound stimulus—as in GSR or EDR audiometry.

FET. field effect transistor.

fetal erythroblastosis (ĕ-rith″ro-blas-to′sis). specific type of erythroblastosis in the newborn that results from RH incompatibility in the parents. Anemia, jaundice, and enlargement of the liver and spleen are characteristic of this disease.

FF. free field.

fiber *n.* threadlike cell body, e.g., nerve fiber.

fiber of Corti. the structure, made up of the pillars or rods of Corti, that forms Corti's tunnel.

fibers, afferent. nerve fibers that carry impulses toward the brain or spinal cord.

fibers, efferent. nerve fibers that carry impulses away from the brain or spinal cord.

fibers, internal spiral. nerve fibers in the cochlea that are believed to be terminal to the efferent nervous system; that is, from the brain to the ear.

fibers, Retzius'. fibers in the outer phalangeal or Dieter's cells.

fibril *n.* very small fiber.

fibrin *n.* the whitish protein that is the basis for the clotting of blood.

fibrinogen (fi-brin′o-jen) *n.* the protein occurring in blood that is converted into fibrin to cause blood clots.

fibroareolar tissue (fi″bro-ah-re′o-lar). loose, fibrous connective or interlacing tissue.

fibrosis (fi-bro′sis) *n.* formation of fibrous tissue.

fibrotic (fi-brot′ik) *adj.* concerning fibrosis.

fibrotic drum. drumhead whose motion is inhibited by the formation of fibrous tissue.

field effect transistor. transistor with extremely high input impedance. It is used to lower the impedance of ceramic and electret microphones.

field, free. unbounded area or area in which the boundaries have little effect on sound pressure waves, e.g., an anechoic chamber. In practice, most so-called free field tests are actually done in sound field.

field, sound. area or room in which sound waves originate from a loud speaker system.

fifth (Vth) nerve. the Vth cranial nerve serves part of the head, jaws, and eyes. A branch connects with the tensor tympani; *syn*: trigeminal nerve.

filter *n.* device used to control (or filter) the frequencies allowed to pass through an amplifying system.

filter *v.* to separate by means of a filter.

filter, acoustic. device or material (such as lamb's wool) used to alter the acoustic response of an amplifier.

filter, band-pass. electrical filter that allows a fixed or preselected band of frequencies to pass—to be transmitted. Acoustic signals or frequencies above or below the band-pass filter are rejected—not transmitted or amplified.

filter, electric wave. band-pass filter.

filter, high-pass. band-pass filter that allows only selected higher frequencies to pass.

filter, low-pass. band-pass filter that allows only selected lower frequencies to pass.

filter, passive. electric filter made up only of passive elements, such as resistors or capacitors.

filter, sintered. small cylinders containing tiny stainless steel balls fused in such an exacting manner that the degree of acoustic attenuation can be controlled closely.

filtered audiometric speech test (or filtered speech test). a test of speech discrimination in which words are presented at a level that is comfortably loud, but filters allow only controlled frequency bands to be heard.

filtered speech. speech that has been passed through filters to alter its characteristics.

filtered speech test. filtered audiometric speech test.

finger spelling. finger-made signs (dactylology). The manual alphabet for the deaf.

first arch syndrome. complex of symptoms similar to Treacher-Collins (incomplete development of the lower jaw and cheek bones, low-set ears and misshaped lower eyelids) but more severe with additional malformations.

fishmouth *v.* to enlarge the opening at the inner end of an earmold canal.

fissure *n.* groove or furrow in a bone or tissue.

fissure, petrotympanic. groove between the tympanic and squamous portions of the

temporal bone. It provides space for the chorda tympani nerve.

fissure, sylvian. the deep narrow cleft that separates the frontal, parietal, and temporal lobes of the brain. (Sulcus lateralis cerebri or fissura cerebri lateralis: the lateral cerebral fissure).

fissure, vestibular. narrow groove in the lower part of the first turn of the cochlea.

fistula *n.* an opening, as 1. tracheo-esophageal fistula—opening between the gullet and the windpipe; 2. abnormal opening from a cavity to the surface or to another cavity; 3. blind pocket or tract in front of the pinna that sheds dead skin and may become infected.

fistulation, fistulization *n.* formation of an opening in a part, as in the membranous labyrinth, which might explain prolonged remission and even total subsidence of attack of Meniere's.

FIT. fusion at inferred threshold.

fitting, bilateral. hearing aid with two cords and two receivers, with only one amplifier (Y cord arrangement).

fitting, binaural. two complete hearing aids (amplifiers, microphones, and receivers)—one for each ear and ideally, at ear level (as opposed to bilateral or Y cord).

Fitzgerald key. (Edith Fitzgerald, 1926). method of aiding the development of language by deaf children. Six symbols are used as keys to verbs, adjectives, pronouns, infinitives, present participles, and connectives.

five dB rule. interpretation by US Dept. of Labor concerning noise exposure risk calculation: when duration of a partial exposure is cut in half the intensity of the exposure can be increased 5 dBA without increasing the risk.

fixed hearing aid. old term for individual amplifier or headphone system installed in churches or other meeting places.

flaccid (flak'sid) *adj.* flabby.

flare *v.* to enlarge the opening at the inner end of an earmold canal.

flat audiogram. in this type of audiogram, hearing loss is approximately equal at all frequencies.

flat response. amplification is approximately equal at all frequencies within a stated range.

Fletcher method (Harvey Fletcher, American physicist, 1885-1981). a method of estimating the loss for speech from the pure tone audiogram: The SRT (speech reception threshold) equals the average of the two better (lesser loss) frequencies of 500, 1000, and 2000 Hz.

Fletcher-Munson curves (Harvey Fletcher and W.A. Munson). a series of equal loudness curves (contours); named for the men who did the original research in recording these human judgments of loudness of different frequencies as compared to a 1000 Hz tone.

Fletcher point-eight rule. a seldom used formula to determine a percentage for hearing loss; the average of the hearing levels at 500, 1000, and 2000 Hz is multiplied by 0.8.

flocculent (flok'u-lent) *adj.* containing flaky masses.

fluctuating noise. noise that varies more than plus or minus 5 dB as it continues.

fluid, Scarpa's. endolymph. *syn*: Scarpa's liquor.

fluorometer *n.* an instrument used to adjust fluoroscope shadows to aid in interpretation.

fluoroscope *n.* device used to make the shadows of x-rays visible after they have passed through the body. *adj*: **fluoroscopic.**

flutter *n.* the first feeling of sound pressure waves when the frequency is too low to be heard as a tone, at about 18 Hz. *syn*: flutter threshold.

flutter, auditory. recognition of the discontinuity of an interrupted sound.

flutter echoes. reflections of an original sound wave stimulus that occur in rapid succession. If the reflections are periodic and audible they may be called musical echoes.

flutter fusion, auditory. loss of the recognition of discontinuity of an interrupted sound due to the increased rapidity of the interruption.

flutter threshold. point (about 18 Hz) at which pure frequencies begin to lose tonal quality.

flux. magnetic flux—the lines of force of a magnetic field. It is the leakage of this flux from the telephone that makes the use of the telephone coil in the hearing aid possible. Flux is also used advantageously in induction loop systems in classrooms and schools for the deaf.

FM. frequency modulation.

focal CROS. a CROS or BiCROS hearing aid arrangement that has a plastic tube to channel sound from the concha of the offside ear into a microphone placed on that side.

folds, malleolar. ridges in the eardrum membrane caused by the attachment of the malleus to the inside of the drumhead.

Folius' anterior process. a tiny projection on the malleus to which the ligaments that fasten it to the bone are attached.

follicle (fol'li-k'l) *n.* 1. small depression from which a hair grows. 2. a small sac or gland capable of secreting material.

follicles. minute depressions in the skin at the entrance to the external ear canal from which hairs (tragi) originate.

follicular (fo-lik'u-lar) *adj.* concerning follicles.

footplate *n.* bony base plate that rests in the oval window. The legs (crura of the stapes) are imbedded in the footplate to complete the stirrup. *syn*: vestibulo-stapedial joint or basis stapedis.

foramen (fo-ra'men) *pl.* **foramina** (fo-ram'i-nah). opening (usually small) through a bone. Sometimes used to refer to the auditory canals.

foramen, external auditory. opening to the external auditory canal.

foramen magnum. opening through which the spinal cord passes into the skull to become the medulla oblongata of the brain.

foramen mastoideum. opening in the mastoid that allows passage of blood vessels.

foramen, obturator (ob'tu-ra"tor). the closure for an opening; e.g., the stapes for the oval window.

foramen, stylomastoid. opening in the temporal bone that allows passage of the facial nerve and the stylomastoid artery into the tympanic cavity.

force, electromotive. EMF, Emf, or emf. pressures causing the flow of electrons in an electric current; measured in volts.

force, nerve. ability of nerve fibers to transmit stimuli.

forelock, white. white patch of hair over the forehead. One of the characteristic features of the Waardenburg syndrome—another is defective hearing.

formant (fôr'mant) *n.* portion of a speech sound that is its characteristic peak intensity and resonance.

formant frequencies. frequencies whose resonance form the characteristic quality of a speech sound. More commonly known as a formant.

formula *n.* group of symbols arranged in a manner to express the combination of factors or elements that will solve a problem.

formulation aphasia. type of aphasia characterized by the inability to join words and phrases into connected language.

forward masking. phenomenon by which a sound continues to be masked (not heard) for a brief period after the masking noise is discontinued. *syn*: residual masking, post-stimulatory threshold shift.

fossa *pl.* **fossae** *n.* depression or furrow in a portion of the anatomy, e.g., the triangular fossa of the auricle.

fossa, mastoid. furrow in the mastoid process for blood vessels.

fossa ovalis. depression in which the oval window rests.

fossa, Rosenmüller's (Johann Christian Rosenmüller—German anatomist, 1771-1826). depression in the wall of the pharynx above and behind the eustachian tube. *syn*: pharyngeal recess.

fossa, scaphoid. depression or boat-shaped furrow beneath the ridge of the helix in the upper posterior portion of the external ear.

fossa, utricular. elliptical recess. A small cavity in the upper part of the vestibule in which the utricle is lodged.

4-C hearing test. test of hearing involving the use of the 4-C group audiometer. Two-digit numbers are given progressively softer. The last number heard by each listener indicates his threshold.

Fourier analysis (foor'e-a) (Jean Baptiste Joseph Fourier, French physicist, 1768-1830). mathematical reduction of a complex tone into its component pure tone frequencies.

Fourier series. graphic representation of the result of Fourier analysis to show the average value of the wave form, a fundamental, and its harmonics.

Fourier synthesis. composition of a complex tone from a set of pure tones.

Fowler test. (Edmund Prince Fowler, American physician). test of recruitment involving loudness balancing.

fragilitas ossium (frah-jil'ĭ-tas ah'se-um). disease characterized by fragile bones that fracture easily. May affect the ossicular chain and cause deafness.

frame, Deiter's terminal. flattened-out ends of Deiter's cells where they meet the Hensen cells to frame the outer tunnel of the organ of Corti.

fraternal (twins) *adj.* dizygotic—of twins resulting from the fertilization of two ova.

free field. unbounded area or an area in which the boundaries have little effect on sound pressure waves, e.g., an anechoic chamber. In practice, most so-called free-field tests are actually done in sound field.

free-field room. anechoic chamber, a room especially built so that the sound waves generated within are almost totally absorbed by the material used to cover walls, ceiling, and floor. There must also be a high degree of isolation from external sounds: "dead" room.

free-field test. hearing test involving the use of loudspeakers rather than earphones. More accurately known as a sound field test.

free morpheme. one that is a complete word, e.g., pan, cat, ban.

free progressive wave, free wave. sound pressure wave in a free field, i.e., in a boundary-free area that can only be approximated in practice.

free wave. free progressive wave.

fremitus (frem'ĭ-tus) *n.* vibration felt by placing a hand on the chest during speech.

fremitus, vocal. sound heard when an ear is pressed against a speaker's chest.

Frenzel's glasses. magnifying glasses with internal lighting for observing eye movements during caloric testing.

frequencies, infrasonic or subsonic. frequencies below the lower frequency limit of normal hearing, i.e., frequencies of fewer vibrations than 16 cycles per second. (Subsonic is currently used chiefly to designate speeds slower than the speed of sound—about 760 miles per hour at sea level).

frequencies, inharmonic. frequencies that have no multiple relationship with each other or the fundamental.

frequency. number of double vibrations or cycles per second (cps) of a sound wave train, now referred to as hertz (Hz). For example, 256 Hz has the same pitch as middle C on the piano. Doubling this produces a tone one octave higher; if it is halved the tone will be one octave lower. Pitch is the psychological response to frequency.

frequency, basic. frequency of greatest importance; *syn*: fundamental frequency.

frequency control. a device—usually a dial but sometimes a series of buttons—on an audiometer to provide a means of selecting the frequency of the test tone. *syn*: frequency selector.

frequency curve. line drawn to show a comparison of how something occurs within given periods of time. *syn*: Gaussian curve.

frequency discrimination. ability to distinguish changes in frequency.

frequency distortion. inexact reproduction of the frequencies in a sound wave pattern.

frequency distribution. chart or report of how often events, items, or numbers are repeated within given periods of time.

frequency, driving. frequency of the generator driving an electrodynamic system.

frequency, envelope. fundamental frequency.

frequency, fundamental. lowest frequency of a complex tone.

frequency, harmonic. frequency that is a multiple of the fundamental frequency; e.g., the second harmonic is twice the fundamental in cycles per second.

frequency, high. inexact term that in audiology, generally refers to any frequency above 1000 Hz.

frequency level. frequency level, in octaves, is the logarithm to the base 2 of the ratio of a given frequency to a standard frequency of 16.352 Hz. (The decibel logarithmic ratio is to the base 10.)

frequency, low. inexact term that, in audiology, generally refers to a frequency of 1000 Hz and below.

frequency method. procedure for measuring the threshold of hearing sensitivity by which the one being measured responds after each discrete stimulus presentation; *syn*: method of constant stimuli.

frequency modulation. FM. variation of the frequency of a radio carrier wave in accordance with an audio or other signal.

frequency, natural or **normal.** number of cycles per second at which it is easiest for a mass to vibrate—whether gas, liquid or solid; *syn*: resonant frequency.

frequency response range. the generally accepted Hearing Aid Industry Conference method of expressing the frequency response range of a hearing aid is determined as follows: The HAIC gain is calculated and noted on the 1000 Hz vertical axis. A horizontal line is then drawn 15 dB below that point to intersect the two extremes of the hearing aid curve as plotted on the graph of frequency response. The frequency response range of the hearing aid is then expressed as from the lowest frequency point of intersection to the highest frequency point of intersection.

frequency range. any series of frequencies between specified limits either controlled (as in an audiometer) or natural (as in the response of the human ear).

frequency, resonant (rez'o-nant). natural or normal frequency.

frequency response. expression of the electrical or acoustic reaction of a device in terms of cycles per second and in relation to an input signal.

frequency selector. frequency control.

frequency, subharmonic. frequency that is a submultiple (or an even fraction) of the fundamental.

frequency theory of hearing. the generally discounted belief that pitch discrimination is dependent upon the number of times per second that impulses pass over the auditory nerve.

frequency translator. (Charles I. Berlin, PhD). hearing aid designed to change the energy of low frequency phonemes into ultra-high frequencies (to 18,000-20,000 Hz).

frequency transposer. hearing aid designed to change the energy of high frequency phonemes into low frequency energy.

frequency transposition. system of changing high frequency information into low frequency energy.

fricative (frik'a-tiv) *n.* consonant sound composed of very high frequencies made by escape of air through the tongue and lips, as "f," "th," and "v" (as in fin, thin, then and very).

fricative *adj.* concerning consonant sounds made by the friction of air.

frontal lobe. forward rounded portion of either hemisphere of the brain.

full mold fitting. use of an unvented receiver earmold to accommodate a high-gain hearing aid.

functional *adj.* referring to a disability not related to a physical or organic dysfunction.

functional communication profile. FCP.

functional deafness. deafness or hearing loss that has no physical damage as a basis; *syn*: non-organic, psychogenic, simulated, hysterical, conversion, or feigned deafness.

functional gain. lowered threshold of hearing sensitivity that results from the increase in sound pressure reaching the eardrum when a hearing aid is used.

functional overlay. an inability to operate normally that arises from a mental (psychical) exaggeration of the results of a physical disability.

fundamental *n.* lowest and loudest tone produced by an instrument that determines its pitch.

fundamental frequency. lowest frequency of a complex tone.

fundamental tone. lowest and loudest frequency of a complex tone; *syn*: fundamental frequency.

fundus *n.* part of a body pouch or hollow at the bottom of or farthest from the opening.

fundus, meatus acusticus internus (me-a'tus). lowest part of the internal auditory canal, situated at the base of the modiolus.

fundus, tympani. base or floor of the tympanic cavity.

fungus growth, ear. there are many types and terms including Aspergillus, otomycosis, mycomyringitis, and myringomycosis.

furuncle *n.* abscess, boil, or infection of a hair follicle.

furuncular otitis. abscess in the external auditory canal.

fusion (fu'zhun) *n.* blending of two sounds into one.

fusion at inferred threshold. FIT. (Moe Bergman, EdD). method of estimating the threshold sensitivity of a much poorer ear by noting the intensity level required to cause an apparent change of sound in the better ear when an identical tone is presented at the same time to the poorer ear at increasing levels of intensity.

fusion, binaural. single mental impression that results although there are differences between the sound signals reaching each ear.

fusion, spectral. the blending into one sound in the central cortex of different bands of noise presented simultaneously to each ear.

G

gain *n.* a magnification or increase in intensity of sound; *syn:* amplification.

gain, acoustic. increase in sound output (intensity or volume) resulting from the amplification of the sound entering the microphone; calculated by subtracting the input in dB from the output in dB.

gain control. more commonly known as the volume control, this device allows the user to regulate the output of the amplifier.

gain control, automatic. AGC. automatic volume control; in hearing aids, a special circuit designed to prevent sounds from being amplified too much for the impaired ear.

gain, HAIC. the Hearing Aid Conference in 1961 agreed on a method of expressing hearing aid gain for comparison purposes as follows: Subtract the standard input figure of 60 dB from the maximum output at 500, 1000, and 2000 Hz to arrive at the gain for each of those frequencies. Add the three gain figures together and divide the total by three to determine the HAIC gain.

gain, peak. the highest point on the frequency response curve of the amplifier.

Galton's whistle. (Francis Galton, English scientist 1822-1911). a tubular whistle, usually activated by a bulb, with a screw-adjustable pitch, formerly used to test the frequency range of hearing.

galvanic *adj.* pertaining to a direct current of electricity produced by chemical action.

galvanic audiometry. shortened term for psycholgalvanic or electrodermal response audiometry.

galvanic battery. a grouping of two or more cells that generate electricity by chemical action.

galvanic current. direct current (DC or dc). An electric current that flows continuously in one direction. A current of the type delivered by a battery.

galvanic skin response. GSR. a change in skin resistance (the Fere effect) that results from a stimulus to the nervous system. *syn:* psychogalvanic skin response.

galvano- (Luigi Galvani, 1737-1798, Italian physicist and physician). comb. form used to indicate direct electric current.

galvanometer (gal″vah-nom′ĕ-ter) *n.* device used to measure electric current.

gamma globulin (gam′ah glob′u-lin) *n.* part of the blood serum that contains antibodies (substances that weaken or destroy bacteria or viruses). *syn:* serum globulin.

ganglia, acousticofacial. embryonic nerve cell mass that separates into the acoustic

ganglion of the VIIIth nerve and the geniculate ganglion of the VIIth nerve.

ganglion *pl.* ganglia *n.* group or collection of nerve cells outside the brain or spinal cord.

ganglion, acoustic. embryonic nerve cell mass that separates into the cochlear and vestibular ganglia.

ganglion, auditory. collection of nerve cells that pass from the organ of Corti to the cochlear nerve. *syn:* Corti's ganglion, spiral ganglion.

ganglion, Corti's. elongated collection of nerve cells from the cochlear branch of the auditory nerve that pass from the modiolus to the organ of Corti. *syn:* spiral ganglion, auditory ganglion.

ganglion, geniculate (jĕ-nik′u-lāt). collection of nerve cells that are part of the facial nerve within the fallopian canal of the middle ear.

ganglion, Scarpa's. collection of nerve cells within the internal auditory canal from the semicircular canals; *syn:* vestibular ganglion.

ganglion, spiral. Corti's ganglion; auditory ganglion.

ganglion, tympanic. collection of nerve cells that separate from the glossopharyngeal nerve in the tympanic cavity.

ganglion, vestibular. Scarpa's ganglion.

gap, air-bone, or bone-air. difference in hearing sensitivity as revealed by comparison of bone conduction and air conduction audiometric test results.

gap, tonal. narrow band of frequencies that cannot be heard as well as the frequency bands on either side.

Gault's reflex. seldom used term for the auropalpebral (APR) reflex.

gauss (gows) *n.* (Johann K. F. Gauss, Germany—1777-1855). basic (cgs) unit of measurement of intensity of a magnetic field (flux).

gaussian curve. a line drawn to show a comparison of how often something occurs within given periods of time. More commonly known as a frequency curve.

gaussian noise. white noise—a sound that contains equal amounts of energy in all frequencies.

Gelfoam (jel′fōm) *n.* trade name for a thin sheet of gelatin preparation used for the closure and repair of defects in membranes such as the oval window in the operation known as stapedectomy.

Gelle's test (zhel-āz′). (Marie-Ernst Gelle; French otologist, 1834-1923). a test designed to determine the mobility of the ossicles and especially the stapes. A tuning fork is applied to the mastoid process while a rubber tube with an air bulb is used to compress the air in the ear canal. If the threshold does not change as the air is compressed the problem is considered to be conductive in that the stapes is fixed.

gene *n.* ultramicroscopic, self-reproducing, protein particle in the chromosome that transmits hereditary characteristics.

gene mutation. failure of a gene to transmit an exact hereditary characteristic due to a change in its internal molecular structure.

gene, recessive. mutant gene whose failure to transmit a normal hereditary characteristic is masked by the dominant gene of a pair.

genetic (jĕ-net'ik) *adj.* concerning hereditary characteristics transmitted by genes.

genetic deafness. deafness transmitted by faulty genes. The trisomy syndromes exemplify the abnormal genetic transmissions that result in hearing impairments.

genetics *n.* science that deals with hereditary characteristics transmitted by genes.

genetics, biochemical. study of the effects of chemicals or drugs on genes and heredity.

geniculate body. one of the centers in the upper nerve pathways where nerve impulses pass between neurons (synapses) on the way to the brain.

geniculate ganglion. the collection of nerve cells that are part of the facial nerve within the fallopian canal of the middle ear.

geniculate otalgia. earache resulting from problems associated with the facial nerve.

geniculum, canalis facialis. the knee-like bend in the facial canal as it turns past the tympanic cavity. It contains the facial nerve portion known as the nervi facialis geniculum.

genotype *n.* the typical hereditary characteristics of an individual transmitted by genes.

geratic (jĕ-rat'ik) *adj.* concerning old age.

geriatric (jer"e-at'rik) *adj.* concerning the aged or the aging process.

geriatrician (jer"e-ah-trish'an) *n.* a specialist in the problems of the aged *syn:* gerontologist.

geriatrics *n.* the science devoted to the study of old age or the aging process. *syn:* gerontology.

germanium (jer-ma'ne-um). a grayish white metallic element used in transistors or semiconductors.

German measles. rubella, an acute contagious disease that is especially damaging to the developing fetus during the first trimester. It often causes hearing problems among other possible defects.

gerontal (or gerontic) (jer-on'tal) *adj.* concerning the physical and mental deterioration associated with the aging process.

gerontological (jer-on"to-loj'ik-al) *adj.* concerning gerontology—the study of problems of aging.

gerontologist. specialist in the problems of the aged and aging. *syn:* geriatrician.

gerontology. the science devoted to the study of old age and the aging process. *syn:* geriatrics.

gestalt (ges-tawlt') *n.* the theory that views the person, action, or object of mind as a whole rather than the sum of its parts.

giga- (jig'ah). (10⁹). prefix indicating one billion. abbreviated G.

gigacycle (jig'-ah-si"k'l) *n.* one billion cycles per second. *syn:* gigahertz, GHz.

gigahertz, GHz (jig'-ah-hertz") *n.* one billion cycles per second. *syn:* gigacycles, kilomegacycles, kilomegahertz.

gigo. "Garbage in, garbage out." Computer language indicating that if worthless or erroneous information is entered into the computer, worthless information will be displayed.

glands, ceruminous (sĕ-roo'mĭ-nus). glands within the external auditory canal that secrete cerumen or ear wax.

glands, endocrine. ductless glands that produce secretions that have a stimulating or retarding effect on tissues or organs of the body. One effect of endocrine disorders in childhood may be impaired hearing or dysacusis.

glasses, Frenzel's. magnifying glasses with internal lighting for observing eye movements during caloric testing.

glioblastoma (gli"o-blas-to'mah) *pl.* **glioblastomas, glioblastomata** *n.* a tumor of the brain that grows rapidly in the supporting tissue.

glioma (gli-o'mah) *n.* an uncontrolled new growth of tissue (neoplasm or tumor) within the brain tissue (parenchyma). *syn:* neuroglioma, gliomatosis.

globulin, gamma. part of the blood serum that contains antibodies (substances that weaken or destroy bacteria or viruses).

globulin, serum. gamma globulin.

glomus (glo'mus) *n.* a small bulblike body that may form a communicative link between arteries and veins.

glomus jugular tumor. a painful tumor that may occur in the middle ear. It tends to be more painful with each pulsation of blood and may be involved in objective tinnitus; *syn:* glomus tympanicum.

glomus tympanicum. glomus jugular tumor.

glossal (glos'al) *adj.* regarding the tongue.

glue ear. common name for a form of adhesive otitis media—chronic disease in which the middle ear is filled with thick gummy fluid. In advanced stages adhesions develop around the eardrum, the windows, and the ossicles. *syn:* mucoid or mucous otitis media.

goatee hairs ("goat's beard"). hairs at entrance to external ear canal. Tragi (singular: tragus). Another name for barbula hirci.

gobo (go'bo) *pl.* **gobos, goboes** *n.* a contrivance to deflect unwanted sound from a microphone.

Go game. a test of hearing in which the child is conditioned to respond to the word "Go" given at various levels of intensity. It is also used in auditory training.

Gradenigo's syndrome (Giuseppe Gradenigo, Italian physician, 1859-1926). a group of symptoms including earache (otalgia), ear discharge (suppurative otitis media), double vision (diplopia), and abscess of the temporal bone associated with localized meningitis involving the fifth and sixth cranial nerves.

gradually falling curve. the audiometric chart of hearing loss falls at about 5 to 10 dB per octave.

gradually rising curve. the audiometric chart of hearing loss rises at about 5 to 10 dB per octave.

gram *n.* the basic unit of weight and mass in the metric system. One gram is equal to a little less that 1/30 of an ounce. One gram is the weight of one cubic centimeter of water.

granuloma *n.* a lump filled with grainy tissue that resembles a skin tumor.

grid. the small wire mesh used in a vacuum tube to control electron flow.

grommet tube (grom'et). a plastic tube inserted through the eardrum to provide pressure equalization when the eustachian tube does not open properly or is blocked. *syn:* indwelling ventilating tube.

groove, tympanic. a shallow trench in the bottom of the inner bony portion of the outer ear canal into which the thickened ring (annulus) of the eardrum fits. *syn:* sulcus tympanicus.

group audiometer. audiometer with a number of head-sets designed to check the hearing of several people at the same time. One type uses live voice or a phonograph record giving numbers progressively softer. The last number heard by the listener indicates his threshold.

group hearing aid. an auditory training or teaching system that consists of a microphone, an amplifier, and a number of head-set receivers to accommodate several students at the same time.

group Massachusetts test. a number of children are screened simultaneously by having them indicate on a scoring sheet whether or not a pure tone is heard as it may or may not have been presented during a series of six bursts.

group pulse-tone test. the binaural group test.

group screening test. test designed to be administered to several people at the same time that will indicate any who may need further attention.

group speech test, Meyerson. a number of children are screened simultaneously by having them point to the appropriate picture in response to the word.

group test, binaural. a screening test of hearing for several persons at the same time. Pure tones are presented in varying numbers of pulses to either ear. The testee indicates the number of pulses heard in both ears at each presentation series. This system is utilized in both the Reger-Newby and Glorig automatic group screening audiometers.

group test, fading numbers. an almost obsolete group hearing test in which a phonograph record presents pairs of one-digit numbers at successively lower (3 dB) levels of intensity.

group test, Johnston. several children are screened simultaneously by having them keep their eyes closed and raise their hands as they hear pure tones that are presented randomly to various parts of the group at the same time.

GSR. glavanic skin response. (variant of PGSR).

gurgle *v. or n.* infant vocalization—usually simple vowel sounds and blowing of air bubbles. Absence of this stage of development may indicate a hearing impairment.

gyrus, Heschl's (ji'rus). the auditory receptor center in the brain; a twisted ridge of gray matter deep in the lateral fissure of Sylvius. *syn:* transverse temporal gyrus (temporalis transversus).

H

H. international hearing aid symbol for high frequency emphasis tone control position.

habilitation (ha-bil"-i-ta'-shun) *n.* education of the deaf or hearing-impaired to function better in society.

habituation *n.* becoming accustomed to a sound or noise to the degree that it is ignored.

HAE. hearing aid evaluation.

HAF. Hearing Aid Foundation; successor to Hearing Aid Industry Foundation.

HAIC. Hearing Aid Industry Conference; successor: Hearing Industries Association, HIA.

HAIC gain. the Hearing Aid Industry Conference in 1961 agreed on a method of expressing hearing aid gain for comparison purposes as follows: Subtract the standard input figure of 60 dB from the maximum output at 500, 1000, and 2000 Hz to arrive at the gain for each of those frequencies. Add the three gain figures together and divide the total by three to determine the HAIC gain; *syn*: average gain.

HAIC ouput. the HAIC has agreed that this term should apply to the average of the three saturation output pressures at 500, 1000, and 2000 Hz. Commonly referred to as the output of the hearing aid.

HAIF. Hearing Aid Industry Foundation. now known as HAF—Hearing Aid Foundation.

hair cell. 1. one of the specific sensory cells of the organ of hearing (organ of Corti). One end has hairlike projections (cilia) that are imbedded in or in contact with the tectorial membrane. The other end is in close contact with many nerve endings. There are about 400 hair cells per millimeter and about 80 cilia per cell. 2. one of the specific sensory cells of the organ of balance within the vestibule and semicircular canals of the inner ear.

hair cells, external. the hair cells in the organ of Corti that rest in the outer edge of the basilar membrane, i.e., the edge away from the modiolus.

hair cells, internal. the hair cells in the organ of Corti that rest in the inner edge of the basilar membrane, i.e., the edge nearest the modiolus.

hairs, auditory. a seldom used name for the cilia of the cochlear hair cells.

half-shell, earmold. a tubing-type mold consisting of a canal and thin shell with bowl extending only halfway to the helix.

hallucination, auditory. sensation of hearing something when there is no external auditory stimulus.

hallucinosis (hah-lu″sĭ-no′sis) *n.* the condition of having auditory hallucinations.

hammer *n.* common name for the malleus—the first ossicle, attached to the eardrum.

handicapped (person). to be unable to compete on equal terms with a peer group because of a defect in the hearing process.

hand language *n.* manualism; communication by signs and the manual alphabet.

hangover tinnitus. as the name suggests, tinnitus that results from the intake of too much alcohol.

hard-of-hearing *adj.* concerning the inability to distinguish sounds at normal levels of intensity. More acceptable term: hearing impaired.

hard peak clipping. the type of peak clipping that occurs in a hearing aid as the maximum acoustic capacity of the system is reached.

hardwire system. an auditory training system that requires the teacher's microphone to be directly connected to the student's headsets through desk-type amplifiers.

harmonic. a multiple of the fundamental tone produced simultaneously. *syn*: overtone; upper partial.

harmonic content. the ratio of the power in all the overtones to the power in the fundamental tone.

harmonic distortion. the new frequencies introduced by amplitude distortion are harmonically related to the original frequency.

harmonic frequency. a frequency that is a multiple of the fundamental frequency, e.g., the second harmonic is twice the fundamental in cycles per second.

harmonics *n.* the overtones of a complex tone that are natural arithmetic multiples of the lowest frequency or fundamental.

harmonics, aural. a type of distortion generated within the ear itself. Increasing the intensity may cause pitches to be heard that are harmonics of the stimulating frequency.

harmonic, second. the (first) overtone that is twice the frequency of the fundamental or lowest tone.

harmonic, third. the overtone that is three times the fundamental or lowest tone.

H.D. hearing distance when in caps.

h.d. hora decubitus (bedtime) when in lower case letters.

HDN. hemolytic disease of the newborn, or hyperbilirubinemia.

head noises. tinnitus, especially when considered an auditory hallucination. *syn*: acousma.

headphone *n.* more commonly called earphone, it is a device (electroacoustic transducer) for converting electrical energy to acoustical energy designed to be held to the ear by a headband.

head shadow effect. the difference in reception at each ear created by the interposition of the head especially when sound waves come from the side. (Six to seven dB in the most important speech frequencies—even more in the higher frequencies.)

health maintenance organization. HMO. A program of public health care initiated by the Department of Health, Education, and Welfare.

hear *v.* to observe through the sense of hearing or to recognize and interpret sound pressure waves.

hearing *n.* one of the five senses—the one that responds to sound pressure waves.

hearing, after. sensation of sound that may continue after the stimulus has ceased. Also known as sound perseveration—it is similar to the afterimage in vision.

hearing age. the ability of a congenitally hearing impaired child to understand speech when compared with the chronological age of a child hearing normally from birth. It is governed by the period of time the congenitally impaired child has had adequate personal amplification and audio therapy.

hearing aid. an electronic amplifying device to make sounds audible to the individual with a hearing loss. Sound pressure waves are converted into electricity by a microphone. The electric impulses are then amplified through controlled electronic circuitry. The amplified electric impulses are then reconverted by a receiver to pressure waves at a much more intense level to be presented to the impaired ear.

hearing aid acoustician. European term corresponding to hearing aid consultant in the United States.

hearing aid, air-conduction. hearing aid designed to present amplified sound pressure waves directly through the ear canal to the eardrum.

hearing aid audiologist. hearing aid specialist who has completed a correspondence course, passed an examination, and agreed to follow a code of ethics governing the fitting and sale of hearing aids prepared by the National Hearing Aid Society.

hearing aid, body. a hearing aid worn on the body—usually in a pocket or special carrier garment—for those with severe to profound hearing impairments; *syn*: box-type or conventional hearing aid.

hearing aid, bone-conduction. hearing aid designed to present amplified sound pressure waves to the inner ear through a bone receiver (bone oscillator or bone vibrator) held against the bone behind the ear (mastoid process).

hearing aid, BTE. hearing aid worn behind the ear and coupled to the ear by tubing attached to an earmold; *syn*: postauricle or over-ear hearing aid.

hearing aid, carbon. an obsolete hearing aid that depended upon carbon granules in the microphone.

hearing aid, CROS & BICROS. fittings designed for severely asymmetrical hearing sensitivity conditions. See CROS.

hearing aid, custom. one built for a specific individual.

hearing aid, directional. hearing aid designed to utilize a directional microphone. It has greater sensitivity to sounds from the front than from the rear.

hearing aid, duopack. old style hearing aid that had one case for the microphone and amplifier and one case for the batteries.

hearing aid evaluation. (HAE). any method of selecting a suitable hearing aid for an impaired ear. In actual practice a misnomer, in that it does not refer to a method of judging hearing aids: Evaluation of hearing aid performance.

Hearing Aid Foundation. HAF.

hearing aid, group. an auditory training or teaching system that consists of a microphone, an amplifier, and a number of head-set receivers to accommodate several students at the same time.

Hearing Aid Industry Conference. HAIC. successor: Hearing Industries Association. HIA. An organization of firms that manufacture or distribute hearing health care products or their component parts.

hearing aid, ITE. in the ear. A hearing aid with all components encased in the earmold or in a case designed to fit entirely in the ear.

hearing aid, loop-induction. hearing aid specifically designed to be used in connection with a magnetic loop in classes for the hard of hearing or deaf. Usually, however, conventional hearing aids equipped with telephone coils are used by the pupils.

hearing aid, mechanical. a device designed to intensify sound waves by concentration rather than electrical amplification. An ear trumpet.

hearing aid, Medresco. free hearing aid distributed by the National Health Service of Great Britain. Designed by the MEDical REsearch COuncil from which its name is taken.

hearing aid, monopack. early name for hearing aid that had only one case for the microphone, amplifier and batteries.

hearing aid, monaural. a hearing aid designed to present amplified sound to only one ear.

hearing aid, postauricle. hearing aid, BTE—behind the ear.

hearing aid, pressure. a hearing aid using a so-called nondirectional microphone. It is said to be sensitive only to the sound pressure at the location of the microphone opening.

hearing aid, pseudobinaural. a hearing aid that separates the amplified sound to present it to both ears. A body aid with a Y or V cord, for example. *syn*: Y cord hearing aid.

hearing aid, transistor. one designed to utilize transistors in its amplifying circuit.

hearing aid, vacuum. one designed to use vacuum tubes—now obsolete.

hearing, color. the sensation of color that accompanies certain sounds for some people. Pseudochromesthesia.

hearing conservation. minimizing or prevention of damage to the hearing mechanism by means of a program of noise control or ear protection.

hearing, cross. a phenomenon that occurs when sound pressure waves presented to one ear are heard in the other ear. This may occur as the waves go around or through the head.

hearing, frequency theory of. the generally discounted belief that pitch discrimination is dependent upon the number of times per second that impulses pass over the auditory nerve.

hearing hallucinations. hallucinosis—the sensation of hearing something when there is no external auditory stimulus.

hearing handicap (classes of). see classes of hearing handicap, Table 2, page 28.

hearing impairment. a loss or lack of hearing sensitivity.

hearing level. HL. the number of decibels above audiometric zero.

hearing loss. see also under "deafness" headings, as congenital deafness or sensorineural deafness.

hearing loss, abrupt or high-tone. steep elevation of threshold sensitivity above 1000 Hz.

hearing loss, adventitious. hearing impairment resulting from illness or accident after birth.

hearing loss, bass. inability to recognize low frequency tones.

hearing loss, boilermaker's. deafness in the higher frequencies resulting from exposure to continuous loud noises.

hearing loss, catarrhal. hearing impairment associated with the common cold or allergic blockage of the eustachian tube.

hearing loss, central. deafness due to inability of the brain to recognize or understand sounds.

hearing loss, cerebral. deafness due to damage of the cerebral portion of the brain resulting from illness or accident.

hearing loss, ceruminous (sĕ-roo'mĭ-nus). deafness due to an impacted plug of wax (cerumen) in the ear canal.

hearing loss, clang. deafness in which sounds are heard without the ability to recognize small distinctions.

hearing loss, cochleoapical. elevation of threshold sensitivity in the low frequencies.

hearing loss, cochleobasal type. steep elevation of threshold sensitivity in the high frequencies.

hearing loss, conductive. impairment of hearing due to the failure of sound pressure waves to reach the cochlea through the normal air conduction channels. This type of deafness is often responsive to medical or surgical treatment.

hearing loss, congenital. literally, with birth. Conditions that develop in the uterus and are not the result of heredity.

hearing loss, conversion. nonorganic or functional deafness sometimes unconsciously developed as a psychic protection under conditions of stress or severe emo-

tional strain. More commonly called hysterical deafness.

hearing loss, cortical. deafness due to damage to the hearing centers in the cortex of the brain—either from illness or accident.

hearing loss, discrimination. the difference (as expressed in percent) between the percentage of PB (phonetically balanced) words heard correctly and 100%.

hearing loss, end-organ. deafness due to a lesion (damage) within the organ of Corti.

hearing loss, familial. deafness that appears among several members of a family, but is not apparently hereditary. It may be a result of a blood incompatibility.

hearing loss, feigned. deafness or hearing loss that has no physical damage as a basis; e.g., the loss of a malingerer—one who feigns or pretends deafness for personal advantage to gain industrial loss compensation or to avoid military service. Children may simulate deafness to explain school deficiencies. *syn*: functional deafness.

hearing loss, functional. deafness that has no physical damage as a basis. *syn*: nonorganic psychogenic, simulated, hysterical, conversion, or feigned deafness.

hearing loss, genetic. deafness transmitted by faulty genes. The trisomy syndromes exemplify such abnormal transmissions that result in hearing impairments.

hearing loss, hereditary. deafness resulting from inherited characteristics (recessive genes).

hearing loss, high frequency. elevated threshold of sensitivity in the frequencies above 1000 Hz.

hearing loss, hysterical. conversion deafness.

hearing loss, industrial. loss of hearing sensitivity as a result of relatively long exposure to industrial noise.

hearing loss, labyrinthine. (lab"ĭ-rin'thĭn). hearing impairment due to damage within the inner ear. The term is sometimes used only when there is an accompanying balance problem.

hearing loss, luetic. deafness caused by syphilis.

hearing loss, mind. 1. cortical deafness. 2. auditory aphasia. 3. functional or nonorganic deafness.

hearing loss, mixed. deafness resulting from malfunction of both the conductive and sensorineural mechanisms.

hearing loss, music. inability to produce or understand music or musical sounds. Musical deafness.

hearing loss, nerve. obsolete term for sensorineural hearing loss.

hearing loss, noise-induced. NIHL. hearing loss that develops gradually from continuous exposure to noise above acceptable levels.

hearing loss, nonorganic. hearing loss that has little or no physical damage as a basis. It may be 1. a purposeful effort to show a worse than actual hearing loss, as in malingering—feigned or simulated deafness. 2. a subconscious effort to show a worse than actual hearing loss, as in psychogenic or hysterical deafness. Either type may also be referred to as functional hearing loss.

hearing loss, nuclear. hearing loss resulting from a lesion within the dorsal and ventral cochlear nuclei. It is said to be a result of RH incompatibility.

hearing loss, obstructive. older term for conductive hearing loss, referring to the cause. An obstruction in the normal pathway of sound pressure waves to the inner ear.

hearing loss, occupational. more commonly known as noise-induced hearing loss from industrial noise.

hearing loss, pancochlear. a hearing loss typified by an elevated threshold of sensitivity at all frequencies.

hearing loss, paradoxical. the ability of many who have conductive hearing loss to hear better in noisy places. Paracusia Willisana or Willis' paracusis.

hearing loss (percentage of impairment). AAOO method of calculation (1959): monaurally, compute the average air conduction threshold at 500, 1000, 2000 Hz; subtract 26 dB and multiply the remainder by 1½%. Binaurally, multiply the percentage of impairment of better ear by 5 and add the percentage for poorer ear—then divide the result by 6. AMA method (1947): now largely replaced by AAOO method, calculation was made from weighted values assigned as follows—500 Hz, 15%; 1000 Hz, 30%; 2000 Hz, 40%; 4000 Hz, 15%. The AAO Committee on Hearing and Equilibrium revised the formula in 1979 to produce Table 4. (The complete report is in Appendix II, Page 168)

hearing loss, perception or **perceptive.** sensorineural hearing loss—one not involving the conductive mechanism. *syn*: nerve deaf.

hearing loss, peripheral. impaired hearing resulting from a lesion affecting the organ of Corti; *syn*: end-organ deafness.

hearing loss, profound. extreme hearing impairment bordering on total deafness. A degree of loss so severe that hearing aid amplification must be supplemented by speechreading at all times to be effective. Numerically it is generally considered to be an average of over 90 dB to 500, 1000, and 2000 Hz audiometrically (ANSI).

hearing loss, psychic. a type of loss in which sounds are heard but not understood. Aphasia.

hearing loss, psychogenic. all-inclusive term used to refer to a deficiency in which

Table 4. Monaural Hearing Impairment*

DSHL†	%	DSHL†	%
100	0.0	240	52.5
105	1.9	245	54.4
110	3.8	250	56.2
115	5.6	255	58.1
120	7.5	260	60.0
125	9.4	265	61.9
130	11.2	270	63.8
135	13.1	275	65.6
140	15.0	280	67.5
145	16.9	285	69.3
150	18.8	290	71.2
155	20.6	295	73.1
160	22.5	300	75.0
165	24.4	305	76.9
170	26.2	310	78.8
175	28.1	315	80.6
180	30.0	320	82.5
185	31.9	325	84.4
190	33.8	330	86.2
195	35.6	335	88.1
200	37.5	340	90.0
205	39.4	345	90.9
210	41.2	350	93.8
215	43.1	355	95.6
220	45.0	360	97.5
225	46.9	365	99.4
230	48.9	370	100.0
235	50.6	(or greater)	

*1. From the audiogram or numerical record of the audiometric test, find the decibel sum of the hearing threshold levels (DSHL) of 500, 1000, 2000, and 3000 Hz. Example:

500	20
1000	25
2000	35
3000	40

Total 120 DSHL

2. Under the DSHL heading 120 DSHL (column 1, line 5) equals 7.5%.

3. Computation of percent of hearing handicap. If the monaural percent figure is the same for both ears, that figure expresses the percent hearing handicap. If the percent monaural hearing impairments are not the same, apply the formula:

$$\frac{(5 \times \%[\text{better ear}]) + (1 \times \%[\text{poorer ear}])}{6} =$$

% hearing handicap

Audiometers are calibrated to ANSI 1969 standard reference levels.

†Decibel sum of hearing threshold levels at 500, 1000, 2000, and 3000 Hz.

hearing loss is psychological rather than organic in nature.

hearing loss, retrocochlear (ret″ro-kok′le-ar). deafness resulting from a lesion behind (retro) the cochlea. High frequencies are lost first and growth of the sensation of loudness is abnormally slow (decruitment), allowing loud sounds to be well tolerated. The ear with this type of loss usually loses its ability to understand speech or discriminate. The pure tone loss, however, may be mild or moderate. Surgical intervention in cases of retrocochlear lesions may prove helpful.

hearing loss, retrolabyrinthine. hearing impairment resulting from damage behind (retro) the labyrinth. More commonly referred to as retrocochlear.

hearing loss, sensorineural. SNHL. deafness that results from damage to the sensory mechanism internal to the oval and round windows; formerly known as nerve or perceptive deafness.

hearing loss, severe. a hearing loss between 70 and 90 dB when the hearing threshold level at 500, 1000, and 2000 Hz in the better ear is averaged.

hearing loss, simulated. deafness of the malingerer; e.g., one who feigns or pretends for personal advantage to gain industrial loss compensation or to avoid military service. Children may simulate deafness to explain school deficiencies. *syn*: functional hearing loss.

hearing loss, "ski-slope". abrupt elevation of threshold sensitivity above 1000 Hz.

hearing loss, speech. auditory aphasia.

hearing loss, sporadic. type of hereditary deafness that results from a mutant or recessive gene becoming dominant irregularly among members of a family. Compare familial hearing loss.

hearing loss, syphilitic. hearing loss caused by syphilis. *syn*: luetic deafness.

hearing loss, temporary. a reversible elevation in the threshold of hearing that may result from continuous exposure to loud sound; *syn*: auditory fatigue; temporary threshold shift.

hearing loss, tone. inability to recognize musical tones or pitch differences. In extreme cases it is known as amusia.

hearing loss, total. the extremely rare case in which there can be no sensation of sound because of the damage to (or absence of) some portion of the hearing mechanism.

hearing loss, toxic. deafness resulting from the poisonous and damaging (toxic) effect of drugs such as kanamycin, quinine, etc., on the sensory mechanism.

hearing loss, transient. temporary loss of hearing sensitivity usually considered more severe than a temporary threshold shift.

hearing loss, "waterfall". a very steep loss in the higher frequencies; "ski-slope" loss.

hearing loss, word. inability to understand the spoken word, although the sound is heard. *syn*: auditory aphasia, aphemesthesia.

hearing mutism. delay in development of speech resulting from hearing impairment; *syn*: atelolalia—delayed speech.

hearing, place theory of. the belief that pitch discrimination is dependent on the response to the stimulation of localized areas along the basilar membrane within the cochlea. The theory is often considered to extend to places within the brain.

hearing, residual. range of hearing between the threshold of sensitivity and the threshold of discomfort.

hearing, stereophonic. three-dimensional hearing made possible by the use of both ears (binaural).

hearing, telephone theory. an oversimplified explanation of the hearing process that says the ear is like a microphone and the auditory nerve a transmission line to the brain.

Rutherford in 1886 advanced the theory that the basilar membrane vibrated as a whole—like a telephone plate. The resulting nerve impulses or electrical charges would travel up the nerve at the same rate of frequency as the tone presented.

hearing test, 4C. test of hearing involving the use of the 4-C group audiometer. Two-digit numbers are given progressively more softly. The last number heard by each listener indicates his threshold.

hearing tests, objective. a measurement of hearing sensitivity that does not depend on a voluntary response from the testee.

hearing threshold. minimum level of intensity at which sound pressure will produce the sensation of hearing.

hearing threshold level. HTL. the degree of intensity, re audiometric zero, at which a sound can first be heard.

hearing, traveling wave theory of. movement of the footplate of the stapes causes a fluid wave to move along the basilar membrane with a rise and fall of amplitude. The point where the wave reaches its maximum amplitude is the point where the frequency of the sound is detected. Frequencies are highest toward the oval window and lowest toward the apex of the cochlea. Georg von Bekesy received the Nobel prize in 1961 for his discovery of the traveling wave phenomenon that resulted in this theory.

hearing, unmasked. modifications of hearing aid response by the use of special receivers or changes in circuitry, to reproduce only the frequencies above 1000 Hz. The purpose is to limit the tendency of the lower-pitched vowel elements to mask out and

suppress the higher-pitched consonants.
hearing, visual. old term for lip-reading.
hearing, volley theory of. the belief that pitch discrimination in the lower frequencies is dependent on nerve impulses firing in volleys, and in the higher frequencies it is dependent on the response to the stimulation of localized areas along the basilar membrane in the cochlea.
Held's decussation (de″kus-sa′shun). (Hans Held, German anatomist, 1866.) the crossing from one side of the head to the other of some of the acoustic nerve fibers (neurons) at the site of the first junction (olivary complex) between the cochlea and the brain.
helicotrema (hel″ĭ-ko-tre′mah) *n.* the opening at the apex of the cochlea that allows a wave to be transmitted through the perilymph of the scala vestibuli to the scala tympani.
helix *pl.* **helixes, helices** *n.* the incurved ridge at the edge of the external ear.
helmet *n.* a device designed to protect against extremely loud noise by covering the head as well as ears.
Helmholtz' resonance theory. (Hermann von Helmholtz, German physician and physicist, 1821-1894). the theory that the hair cells within the organ of Corti act as resonators—each with its own natural period of vibration and each responding only to one tone of one particular frequency.
hem- hemo- haem- haemo- combining form meaning blood.
hemal *adj.* concerning the blood or blood vessels; *syn:* hemic.
hemangioma (hĕ-man″je-o′mah) *n.* a nonmalignant (usually congenital) tumor made up of newly formed blood vessels.
hemangiotympanum (hĕ-man″je-o″tim′pah-num) *n.* a benign bloody tumor on the drumhead.
hematoma (hem″ah-to′mah) *n.* accumulation of blood in tissue surrounding a ruptured blood vessel. If it occurs in the pinna, it is often called a cauliflower ear.
hematoma auris (aw′ris). bloody tumor of the ear sometimes found in the insane; *syn:* asylum ear, othematoma.
hemolysin (he-mol′ĭ-sin) *n.* the substance resulting from the reaction between an antigen and an antibody that frees hemoglobin and destroys red blood cells.
hemolysis (he-mol′ĭ-sis) *n.* destruction of red blood cells through a reaction between an antigen and an antibody that results in the release of hemoglobin—as in RH incompatibility.
hemostasis (he″mo-sta′sis) *n.* the stopping of bleeding.
hemotympanum *n.* an accumulation of blood in the middle ear. Usually the result of a blow to the head.

henry *n.* (Joseph Henry, US physicist, 1797-1878). unit of measurement of electrical inductance.
Hensen's cells. outer cells that support the inner structure of the organ of Corti.
heparin (hep′ah-rin) *n.* a drug used to prevent clotting.
heparinization (hep″er-ĭ-nīz″a′shun) *n.* the prevention of blood clotting by the use of heparin.
hereditary *adj.* genetic influences (characteristic traits) transmitted through generations.
hereditary deafness. deafness resulting from inherited characteristics (recessive genes).
heredodegenerative hypacusia. hereditary deafness resulting from degeneration or atrophy of the organ of Corti during early infancy.
heredopathia atactica polyneuritiformis. Refsum's syndrome. A complex of hereditary defects that includes progressive deafness.
herpes, otitic. a rash in and around the ear that may result in deafness from the spread of the virus infection that caused the rash.
herpes simplex. a communicable virus infection that may affect the lips, nose, and genital area. It is believed responsible for congenital deafness and other severe handicaps when the herpes virus is present in the genital tract during birth.
herpes zoster. shingles. A communicable virus infection that may affect the spiral ganglion and cause perceptive deafness.
hertz, Hz (hertz). the new term for cycles per second—named in honor of the German physicist, Heinrich Hertz, 1857-1894.
hertzian waves. electromagnetic or radio waves; similar to light waves but longer.
Herxheimer reaction (Karl Herxheimer, German dermatologist, 1861-?). syphilitic deafness resulting from insufficient doses of a specific remedy.
Heschl's gyrus (ji′rus) (Richard L. Heschl, Austrian physician, 1824-1881). the auditory receptor center in the brain; a twisted ridge of gray matter deep in the lateral fissure of Sylvius. *syn:* transverse temporal gyrus.
heter-, hetero- combining form meaning different than usual.
heterochromia. differing in color—as the eyes in the Waardenburg syndrome.
heterochromia iridium. different colored eyes. A characteristic feature of the Waardenburg syndrome.
heterophasic. (het″er-o-fa′zik) *adj.* the presentation of differing signals or noises to each ear. *opp:* homophasic.
heterozygosis (het″er-o-zi-go′sis) *n.* formation of a zygote by the union of dissimilar genes.

heterozygote (het″er-o-zi′gōt) *n.* a mixture of genes that do not follow a pure hereditary pattern. Such a cell is said to be the carrier of a deafness gene. *adj*: **heterozygotic, heterozygous.**

HEW. Health, Education, and Welfare.

HIA. Hearing Industries Association. Successor to Hearing Aid Industries Conference (HAIC).

high CROS. a classic CROS hearing aid amplifying system modified to cut the low frequencies and emphasize high frequencies.

high fence. the upper limit of the hard of hearing range or hearing impairment expressed as an average of 500, 1000, and 2000 Hz: 92 dB ISO (ANSI) or 82 dB ASA. Greater loss is considered deaf.

high fidelity *n.* the reproduction or amplification of sound waves with a minimum of distortion.

high frequency. an inexact term which, in audiology, generally refers to any frequency above 1000 Hz.

high frequency earmold. a tubing-type mold that allows the maximum volume of air between the receiver nub, or tubing connection, and the tympanic membrane.

high frequency loss. a deficit in hearing acuity at 1001 Hz and above.

high frequency speech sounds. speech sounds whose greatest intensity occurs above 1000 Hz, e.g., most of the consonants.

higher threshold. a poorer threshold of sensitivity. This is indicated by marks at higher numbers on the audiogram. *syn*: elevated threshold.

high-pass filter. a band-pass filter that allows only selected higher frequencies to pass.

high risk register. 1. broadly speaking, a roll or record of the names of newborns who may possibly have auditory handicaps as the result of birth hazards, e.g., anoxia, hyperoxia, or parental blood incompatibilities. 2. a list of the diseases, syndromes, and defects that may cause auditory handicaps in the newborn.

Hiskey test. a test of hearing or understanding of verbal directions that is said to also indicate levels of intelligence. *syn*: Hiskey-Nebraska test of learning aptitude.

histochemistry *n.* science devoted to a study of the chemical makeup of cells and tissues. *adj*: **histochemical.**

histogram. graph that uses rectangles to display a statistical distribution; e.g., scores may be displayed along the abscissa (horizontal axis) and the frequencies on the ordinate (vertical axis); *syn*: column chart.

histology *n.* the branch of biology that deals with the microscopic structure of tissue.

histopathology *n.* the study of microscopic changes in diseased tissues.

histophysiology *n.* the branch of biology dealing with the microscopic study of tissues.

history, case. a review of the patient's background in regard to the problem involved. The information may come from the patient or from relatives.

Hitzelberger's sign. a test of facial (VIIth) nerve response.

HL. hearing level (re: audiometric zero). Formerly referred to as hearing loss.

HMO. health maintenance organization.

homo- prefix meaning similar, like, or the same.

homograft transplant. a replacement of tissue or bones of the ear with natural tissue or bones.

homolateral *adj.* concerning the same side; also called ipsilateral—as opposed to contralateral, the opposite side.

homonym (hah′mo-nim) *n.* a word that sounds like another but is spelled differently; *syn*: homophone.

homophasic (ho″mo-fa′zik) *adj.* the presentation of signals that are alike in time and phase to each ear.

homophenes (hah′mŏ-fēns) *n.* words that look alike on the lips.

homophenous words (ho-mah′fe-nus). words that look alike on the lips.

homophones (hom′mo-fons) *n.* words that sound alike but are spelled differently, e.g., know, no. *syn*: homonyms. *adj*: **homophonic, homophonous.**

homozygosis (ho″mo-zi-go′sis) *n.* the formation of a zygote by the union of similar genes.

homozygote (ho″mo-zi′gōt) *n.* a mixture of similar genes that follow a pure hereditary pattern. *adj*: **homozygotic, homozygous.**

Horace speech. speech that is defective in the consonant sounds.

horizontal or lateral canal. one of the semicircular canals—part of the human balance mechanism.

horn effect. increased high frequency output of the hearing aid response that results from a progressive increase in the diameter of the coupling system. Term suggested by Mead C. Killion, PhD.

horn, Killion. a progressively stepped larger internal diameter earmold coupler designed by Mead C. Killion, PhD. It provides more high frequencies and a smoother response.

horn, Libby. (E. Robert Libby). smoothly-tapered (small at hearing aid hook, large at earmold) one-piece sound tube adaptation of the Killion acoustic horn principle.

house-tree-person test. H-T-P. a personality test sometimes used with the hearing handicapped.

HPI. hearing performance inventory.

Hr factor. a material found in the blood related to the Rh factor (sometimes considered in the Rh classification) and similar in its reaction.

HSMHA. Health Services and Mental Health Administration.

HTHA. Hearing and Tinnitus Help Association.

HTL. hearing threshold level.

H-T-P. house-tree-person test.

Huschke's auditory teeth. (Emil Huschke, German physician, 1797-1858.) minute projections along the free margin of the labium vestibulare of the cochlea resembling teeth. *syn*: auditory teeth.

Hutchinson's triad. (Sir Jonathon Hutchinson, Eng. physician, 1828-1913.) eighth nerve deafness, notched teeth, and chronic corneal inflammation. A syndrome associated with hereditary or prenatal syphilis.

hyalinization *n.* degeneration of connective tissue—because of disease—into a clear, gluelike substance (hyalin). This may further degenerate into a white chalky material on the eardrum (tympanosclerosis).

hydr-, hydro- combining forms for fluid.

hydramnion, hydramnios (hi-dram'ne-on) *n.* excessive amniotic fluid.

hydrocephalic *n.* person afflicted with hydrocephalus.

hydrocephalus, hydrocephaly *n.* enlarged head and diminished brain resulting from an abnormal accumulation of cerebrospinal fluid within the skull. *adj*: **hydrocephalic, hydrocephalous.**

hydrolabyrinth *n.* accumulation of endolymph in the inner ear.

hydrophone *n.* device used for listening to sound waves transmitted through water.

hydrops (hi'drops) *n.* accumulation of fluid in the body tissues. Sometimes referred to as edema or dropsy.

hydrops, cochlear. accumulation of fluid in the cochlea.

hydrops, endolymphatic. Meniere's disease. Malfunction of hearing and balance caused by excessive inner ear fluids. *syn*: Meniere's syndrome.

hydrops, labyrinthine. endolymphatic hydrops. *syn*: hydrolabyrinth.

hydrotis *n.* accumulation of fluid in any portion of the ear.

hygroscopic (hi''gro-skop'ik) *adj.* pertaining to water absorption; e.g., the properties of earwax that may cause a plug of wax to swell up and block the external canal completely when water enters the ear. *n.* **hygroscopicity.**

hyomandibular bone. an evolutionary forerunner of the stapes.

hypacousia, hypacusia, hypacusis *n.* lessened hearing sensitivity. *syn*: hypoacusia.

hyper- combining form meaning greater than normal.

hyperactive *adj.* abnormally active.

hyperacusia, hyperacusis *n.* 1. unusually sensitive to sound. 2. better than normal hearing. *syn*: paracusis acris; auditory hyperesthesia.

hyperacusia, dolorosa. painfully oversensitive to sound.

hyperbilirubinemia (hi''per-bil''ĭ-roo''bĭ-ne' me-ah) *n.* HDN. neonatal hemolytic disease. abnormal amount of bile pigment (bilirubin) in the blood. A cause of sensorineural deafness. In infants it may be called hemolytic disease of the newborn.

hypercoagulation *n.* the process of clotting too easily—may cause sudden deafness.

hyperemia *n.* an ear infection characterized by blood clots under the lining of the ear canal.

hyperesthesia, hyperaesthesia *n.* abnormal sensitivity of any one of the five senses.

hyperesthesia, acoustic or auditory. abnormal sensitivity of the sense of sound. *syn*: hyperacusia. *adj*: **hyperesthetic.**

hyperexcitability. abnormally excitable. Sometimes used instead of hyperactive.

hyperlipidemia. excessive amounts of lipids (fat-like particles) in the blood. Some authorities believe there may be a relationship between hyperlipidemia and high frequency hearing loss.

hyperostosis *pl.* **hyperostoses** *n.* abnormal growth of bony tissue. *syn*: exostosis.

hyperparathyroidism *n.* the result of excessive secretion from the parathyroids. An end result may be stapedial fixation.

hyperplasia (hi''per-pla'ze-ah) *n.* overdevelopment of a part, organ, or tissue. *adj*: **hyperplastic.**

hyperpyrexia *n.* abnormally high fever that may cause hearing loss.

hyper-recruitment *n.* the sensation of loudness of a tone in the poor ear exceeds the sensation of loudness in the good ear at higher intensity levels. It is also known as over-recruitment.

hypersensitive *adj.* abnormally sensitive—as in pollen allergy. *n*: **hypersensitiveness, hypersensitivity.**

hypertrophy *n.* abnormal enlargement of a part or organ not involving a tumor, e.g., ear hypertrophy or macrotia. *adj*: **hypertrophic.**

hypn-, hypno- combining form for sleep.

hypnoanalysis *n.* the treatment of psychosomatic illness by hypnosis and psychoanalysis.

hypnoid, hypnoidal *adj.* concerning a condition resembling sleep, as in hypnosis.

hypnosis *n.* an artificially induced sleeplike condition characterized by ready acceptance of suggestions by the subject.

hypnotherapy *n.* the treatment of disease by hypnotic methods or prolonged sleep.

hypoacusis (hi″po-ah-ku′sis) *n.* lessened ability to hear. Hard of hearing. *syn:* hypacusis.

hyp-, hypo- combining form indicating less than normal.

hypochondria, hypochondriasis (hi″po-kon′dre-ah) *n.* an exaggerated concern about ill-health. It is usually accompanied by many imaginary symptoms of physical ailments.

hypochondriac *n.* 1. a person suffering from hypochondria. 2. concerning the area beneath the ribs.

hypoemia (hi″po-e′me-ah) *n.* a lowered amount of blood in a tissue or organ. *syn:* ischemia.

hypofunction *n.* lowered function.

hypoglycemic *adj.* concerning the condition in which there is less than the normal amount of glucose in the blood.

hypoplasia (hi″po-pla′ze-ah) *n.* incomplete development of a part, organ, or tissue, e.g., an unusually small external ear. *adj:* **hypoplastic.**

hypothesis *pl.* **hypotheses** *n.* an assumption, idea, or supposition concerning the result of an action that has not been tested by experiment.

hypothesize *v.* to prepare or present a hypothesis.

hypothetical *adj.* suppositional.

hypothyroidism *n.* subnormal thyroid function. It may affect hearing adversely. *syn:* hypothyroidea, hypothyrea, hypothyrosis.

hypotrophy (hi-pot′ro-fe) *n.* early loss of vitality or degeneration of tissue. *syn:* abiotrophy.

hypotympanum (hi″po-tim′pah-num) *n.* the lower portion of the middle ear. *adj:* **hypotympanic.**

hypoxia (hi-pok′se-ah) *n.* lack of oxygen that is less damaging to the body tissues than anoxia. *adj:* **hypoxic.**

hypoxia, natal. hypoxia that occurs during the birth process.

hysterical deafness. nonorganic or functional hearing loss sometimes unconsciously developed as a psychic protection under conditions of severe emotional strain. *syn:* conversion deafness.

hysterical mutism. a type of hysterical deafness in which one can only express himself through writing or gestures.

hysterogenic (his″ter-o-jen′ik) **hysterogenous** (his″ter-oj′en-ous) *adj.* causing hysterical behavior.

Hz. abbreviation for hertz—the internationally accepted symbol for cycles per second.

I

I. international hearing aid symbol for on. ("In" operation as opposed to "O": "Out" of operation.)

I tracing. the graphic result of the presentation of pulsed tones in automatic audiometry. Interrupted tracings.

iatrogenic (i-at″ro-jen′ik) *adj.* accidentally caused during the course of treatment.

iatrogenic trauma. damage unexpectedly occurring during the course of treatment.

iatrogeny (i-ă-trah′jě-ne) *n.* abnormality unexpectedly caused by treatment.

IC. integrated circuit.

ICM. ipsilateral competing message.

icterus neonatorum. disease characterized by deposit of bile pigment in the blood (jaundice) of the newborn. *syn:* kernicterus.

ictus *n.* the beats in a series of sounds.

ictus cordis. heartbeat.

ID. inside diameter. Identification.

identification audiometry. technique involving checking large groups of people rapidly against a preestablished limit of normalcy concerning hearing. *syn:* screening audiometry.

idio- prefix or combining form indicating individual, distinct, personal, or separate.

idiocy, sensorial. extreme mental retardation resulting from the congenital absence, or loss in infancy, of one of the senses.

idiom (id′-e-om) *n.* 1. dialect. 2. expression or phrase unique to a people or community that has a meaning distinct from its elements, e.g., "talking through his hat"—making up a story.

idiomatic *adj.* pertaining to idiom or dialect.

idiopathic *adj.* diseased condition arising from an unknown or undiagnosed cause.

idiopathy *n.* disease or abnormality resulting from an unknown cause.

IHC. inner hair cell.

IEC. International Electrotechnical Commission.

IEEE. Institute of Electrical and Electronics Engineers.

IFROS. ipsilateral frontal routing of signals. Type of eyeglass hearing aid.

IL. intensity level.

ILA. induction loop amplification.
IMC. Instructional Materials Center Network (of Office of Education).
impact noise. impulse noise.
impaction (im-pak'shun) *n.* firmly lodged—as an accumulation of wax in the external ear canal.
impairment *n.* damage or decrease of ability to function.
impairment, hearing. loss or lack of hearing sensitivity.
impairment, sensory. inability of a sense to function normally.
impedance (im-pēd'ans) *n.* the opposition to the free flow of sound pressure waves through the middle ear.
impedance, acoustic. resistance to the flow of sound pressure waves through a medium.
impedance audiometry. not fully accepted, this term is used by some authorities to cover the measurements made through the use of an electroacoustic bridge: tympanometry, acoustic impedance, and acoustic reflex threshold.
impedance, blocked electrical. the impedance measured at the electrical terminals of an electromechanical transducer when the mechanical system is blocked.
impedance bridge. device designed to measure the resistance of the mechanism of the ear to acoustic stimuli.
impedance, electrical. the opposition to the flow of electrical current comparable to friction in a water pipe. The ratio of the voltage across two terminals to the electrical current passing through them.
impedance meter. an electro-acoustic device designed to measure: 1. acoustic impedance at the drumhead—the ability of the eardrum and ossicular chain to transmit sound pressure waves. 2. the stapedius muscle reflex. 3. the compliance of the tympanic membrane.
impedance, middle ear. resistance of the drumhead, the oval window, and the ossicular chain to acoustic stimuli.
impede *v.* to resist movement or flow.
implant, cochlear. an electronic device designed to stimulate the hearing mechanism. It utilizes a coil of wire embedded under the skin behind the ear with an extension of wire into the fluid of the inner ear (cochlea). It is activated by an amplifier (similar to a body-type hearing aid) carried in a pocket. There is sometimes a side benefit in that tinnitus is reduced.
impression *n.* a cast made of the contours within the external ear from which the earmold is made.
impulse noise. transient noise with a sharp rise and fall time around a peak of high intensity, e.g., gunfire and explosions. *syn:* impact noise.

impulsive sounds. momentary or explosive sounds.
inaudible sound. sound that is above the range of the human ear in frequency (e.g., dog whistle) or below the range of the individual ear in intensity.
inches per second. ips.
incident wave. a sound pressure wave moving away from the source. The opposite of a reflected wave.
incision of drum. surgical opening of the drumhead. *syn:* myringotomy, paracentesis tympani.
incomplete recruitment. the sensation of loudness of a tone in the poor ear approaches, but does not equal, the sensation of loudness in the good ear at high intensity levels.
increment *n.* addition or increase. The opposite of decrement.
incudal *adj.* concerning the incus or anvil.
incudectomy *n.* removal of the incus by surgery.
incudomalleal (ing"ku-do-mal'e-al) *adj.* concerning the incus (anvil) and malleus (hammer) as they relate to one another.
incudostapedial joint (ing"ku-do-sta-pe'de-al). point of articulation (movement) between the incus and the stapes.
incudus (in-koo'dus) *n.* the laxator tympani ligament.
incus (ing'kus) *n.* the middle bone in the ossicular chain. The body of the incus is moved by the malleus while the lenticular process of the incus moves the head of the stapes. The incus is about 7 mm long. *syn:* anvil.
incus, long process of. the arm of the incus (anvil) that articulates (moves) the stapes.
incus, necrosis of. death or mortification of the incus.
incus replacement prosthesis. IRP. device made of plastic or other material to replace the incus.
index *pl.* **indexes, indices** *n.* a number or numbering system used to denote relationships.
index, articulation. AI. a number that represents the ability to understand speech in the presence of noise; based on measurements made with 20 controlled noise frequency bands.
index of response irregularity. IRI. a method of comparing hearing aid response curves devised by James Jerger, PhD. Parallel lines are drawn at intervals on the response chart of a given hearing aid. The number of times the response curve tracing crosses the parallel horizontal lines is counted to give the IRI.
index vocalis (vocal index). an obsolete attempt to standardize whispered and voiced tests of hearing by setting up a distance ratio between the two.

indicator, volume-level. device used to monitor voice or music intensity levels. More commonly known as a VU (volume unit) meter.

induce *v.* to produce an electric current by induction.

inducing current. the primary electrical current that gives rise to the secondary current in an induction coil. Also known as primary and secondary current.

inductance *n.* the peculiar trait of electricity by which an electromotive force is generated in an electric circuit by a change of current.

induction *n.* the natural phenomenon that causes an electrical conductor to become electrified when near an electrically charged body.

induction coil. device designed to transform direct electrical current into intermittent higher voltage.

induction loop. a continuous wire carrying electrical energy from an amplifier. The flux or magnetic field thus created when such a loop surrounds a room makes auditory training systems that utilize wearable hearing aids possible.

inductive *adj.* concerning inductance or electrical induction.

inductive reactance. measure of the resistance to electrical current flow in an induction coil.

inductor *n.* a coil or part of an electrical device that acts upon another or itself is acted upon by induction.

industrial audiogram. industrial audiograms commonly include measurements of thresholds at 500, 1000, 2000, 3000, 4000, 6000 Hz.

industrial audiometry. audiometry concerned with monitoring or periodically checking the effects of industrial noise exposure.

industrial deafness. loss of hearing sensitivity as a result of relatively long exposure to industrial noise. *syn:* noise-induced hearing loss or industrial hearing loss.

inertance *n.* acoustic inertance. The resistance to the movement of sound pressure waves in a tube—especially one with a closed end.

infarct, infarction *n.* an organ or portion of tissue that has died as the result of a blood clot.

inferior (in-fēr' e-or) *adj.* below. Lesser.

inferior colliculus. one of a pair of projections on the midbrain containing integration centers for auditory reflexes.

inflammation of the brain. encephalitis.

inflammation of epitympanic recess. atticitus. Inflammation of the attic.

inflammation of inner ear. otitis interna or endolymphatic labyrinthitis.

inflammation of membrane lining eustachian tube. endosalpingitis.

inflect *v.* to modify the sound of a word by changing accent, emphasis, or pitch.

inflection *n.* change in loudness for accent or emphasis. *adj.* **inflectional, inflective.**

infra- prefix meaning within or below.

infra-audible sound. more commonly known as infrasonic sound.

infrasonic *adj.* below the normal hearing range in frequency. *syn:* infra-audible sound, subsonic.

infundibulum (in″fun-dib′u-lum) *n.* canal that connects the nasal cavity with the upper end of the cochlear canal in the cupola.

inharmonic frequencies. frequencies that have no multiple relationship with each other or the fundamental.

initial teaching alphabet. ITA. an alphabet in which each symbol represents only one sound. It is designed to stimulate early reading skills.

inner ear. portion of the ear bounded externally by the oval and round windows and internally by the internal auditory canal. It contains the cochlea and semicircular canals.

inner hair cells. internal hair cells. There are about 3500 in the organ of Corti.

inner rod of Corti. inner leg of cartilaginous structure resting on the basilar membrane (closest to the modiolus) that supports a single row of inner hair cells.

innervate (in′er-vāt) *v.* to stimulate a nerve.

innervation *n.* activation of a part through a system of nerves.

innervation, spiral. the nerve system within the spiral of the cochlea.

in phase. two tones of the same frequency and intensity are said to be in phase when their cycles of compression and rarefaction are identical. The resulting tone will be twice the amplitude of either one. *syn:* pressure phase.

in-phase feedback. the return of a portion of the output signal to be added to an input stage for greater amplification. *syn:* positive or regenerative feedback.

input *n.* sound pressure picked up by the microphone.

insert *n.* a device designed to plug the ear canal as a protection.

insertion (in-ser′shun) *n.* the point of attachment of the stapedius muscle to the stapes.

insertion gain. the additional sound pressure reaching the eardrum when a hearing aid is used. (Compared to the sound pressure reaching the eardrum unaided). *syn:* real ear, etymotic, or orthotelephonic gain.

insertion loss. the lessening of sound pressure reaching the eardrum when the external ear canal is occluded (closed) by an earmold.

71

in situ (Latin) (in si'tu). in place, in position.

inspissate (in"spis'āt) v. to thicken by evaporation or the removal of fluid.

inspissated cerumen (in-spis'āt-ed sĕ-roo'men). thickened and dried earwax plugging the outer ear canal.

inspissation n. thickening of fluid that causes the condition in the middle ear known as glue ear.

insufflate (in"suf'lāt) v. to blow air into a cavity. n: **insufflation**.

integrated circuit. an electronic circuit made up of electrical elements combined on one small substrate.

integration. 1. the unification or meshing of auditory signals from both ears into a single whole. 2. the inclusion of deaf and hearing impaired children in programs with normally hearing children. A program known as mainstreaming.

integument (in-teg'u-ment) n. a covering, e.g., the skin.

intelligence quotient. IQ. the number resulting from dividing the score of a test designed to determine the relative mental capacity of a person by his chronological age and multiplying by 100.

intelligibility. understandability of speech, i.e., a measure of how well speech sounds can be recognized and repeated. It is usually expressed as the percentage of a phonetically balanced word list that is repeated correctly.

intelligibility, threshold of. obsolete term for speech reception threshold—the intensity level at which 50 percent of the words presented can be repeated.

intensity n. range of acoustic energy that gives the sensation of loudness. Sound intensity is defined as a ratio between the sound being measured and a reference level of intensity. This ratio is expressed in logarithmic units called decibels.

intensity discrimination. more commonly called loudness discrimination, it is: 1. the ability to detect changes in intensity. 2. the measurement of the ability to detect changes in intensity—the difference limen (DL) for intensity.

intensity level. IL. the ratio of a sound pressure to a base reference intensity.

inter- prefex meaning between or among.

interaural adj. involving the interaction of the ears.

interaural attenuation. the lessening of intensity that occurs as a sound stimulus passes through the head from one ear to the other.

interaural difference. the different sensations that may be noticed at each ear in reaction to the same stimulus.

interauricular (in"ter-aw-rik'u-lar) adj. located between the outer ears (auricles).

interface n. 1. the surface that forms the boundary between two bodies or masses. 2. mechanical or electronic parts that work together or interconnect. 3. sometimes used as a term of comparison.

interface v. to connect devices.

interference n. the interaction of two series of sound waves that results in increased intensity at some points and zero intensity at others.

interference patterns. the intricate pressure wave systems resulting from the introduction of sounds of the same frequency from two or more sources.

interferometer, acoustic. an instrument designed to utilize lights and mirrors in the measurement of sound wavelengths and velocities.

intermittent adj. operating or not operating at irregular intervals.

intermittent current. electric current that flows at intervals but does not reverse itself as in alternating current.

intermodulary distortion. the type of amplitude or nonlinear distortion that results when two or more frequencies transmitted through a system generate a set of new frequencies that have no harmonic relationship.

intermodulation (in"ter-mod-u-la'shun) n. change in a complex wave as a result of the effects of various component waves on each other.

internal acoustic (auditory) meatus (me-a'tus). the internal auditory canal through which the VIIIth and VIIth nerves pass on their way to the brain.

internal auditory artery. artery that supplies blood to the inner ear.

internal auditory canal. sheath through which the auditory nerve and facial nerve pass on their way to the brain. syn: internal auditory meatus, internal acoustic meatus.

internal auditory canal pore. the hole where the internal auditory canal opens into the brain cavity.

internal ear. inner ear—auris interna, labyrinth.

internal feedback. acoustic feedback (squeal) usually resulting from the unshielded proximity of the microphone and receiver in an ear-level hearing aid.

internal hair cells. the hair cells in the organ of Corti that rest on the inner edge of the basilar membrane, i.e., the edge nearest the modiolus.

internal otitis. inflammation of the inner ear—endolymphatic labyrinthitis.

internal spiral fibers. nerve fibers in the cochlea believed to be terminal to the efferent nervous system, i.e., from the brain to the ear.

internalization. the sensation that a sound is within the head when presented externally.

international phonetic alphabet. IPA. system of symbols for speech sounds adopted by the International Phonetic Association. Each speech sound is represented by a distinctive symbol.

International Standards Association. ISO. popular name for the International Organization for Standardization. An international association of national voluntary associations organized to write standards for industry.

interneuron (in″ter-nu′ron) *n.* a nerve cell (neuron) between two other nerve cells. *adj*: **interneuronal.**

interneurosensory (in″ter-nu″ro-sen′so-re) *adj.* concerning the interaction of more than one nerve and sense modality, e.g., the eyes and ears for balance.

internuncial (in″ter-nun′she-al) *adj.* 1. acting as a link between motor and sensory nerve cells. 2. indicating a nerve cell between two other nerve cells.

interoceptor (in″ter-o-sep′tor) *n.* a group of cells (receptors) responding to stimuli from within the body—viscera.

interposition *n.* an operative technique used in the treatment of otosclerosis.

interrupted tracings. I tracings. tracings that result when pulsed tones are used in automatic audiometry.

interrupter *n.* the switch that interrupts (or presents) the pure tones of an audiometer. *syn*: interrupter switch.

interrupter, mechanical. a mechanical device to automatically interrupt a continuous tone at intervals.

interstitial (in″ter-stish′al) *adj.* concerning the spaces between cells.

intertone *n.* the tone of in-between pitch heard as the average of two primary frequencies sounded simultaneously.

interval *n.* the ratio of the difference in pitch between two tones or notes.

intima (in′tĭ-mah) *n.* the inner coating of an organ or blood vessel. *adj*: **intimal.**

intonation *n.* change of voice pitch in speech; inflection. *adj*: **intonational.**

intone *v.* to speak without change in pitch—monotonously. *n*: **intoner.**

intra- prefix meaning within or between.

intra-aural muscles. muscles within the middle ear; the tensor tympani and the stapedius.

intra-aural reflex. the reflex contraction of the intra-aural muscles (tensor tympani and stapedius) in response to sound. *syn*: acoustic reflex.

intracellular potential. the negative internal polarizations of cells in relation to adjacent tissue fluids. Within the cochlea, intracellular potentials are from -20 to -80 millivolts in relation to the perilymph.

intractable tinnitus. tinnitus that is resistant to any type of relief or treatment.

intracutaneous test. a test of sensitivity by injection into the skin of a substance that may cause an allergic reaction.

intradermal, intradermic *adj.* between the layers of skin.

intraganglionic bundle (in″trah-gang″gle-on′ik). the collection of efferent nerve fibers within the cochlea.

intramastoiditis (in″trah-mas″toi-di′tis) *n.* inflammation of the lining of the mastoid process. *syn*: endomastoiditis.

intraneurosensory (in″tra-nu″ro-sen′so-re) *adj.* concerning stimulation within one sense modality. *syn*: unisensory.

intrinsic, intrinsical *adj.* located entirely within an organ or part.

intubate (in′tu-bāt) *v.* 1. to open the eustachian tube—as with a catheter. 2. to ventilate the middle ear by means of a tube in the eardrum.

intubation (in″tu-ba′shun) *n.* insertion of a hollow cylinder into the eustachian tube to open it.

intumesce (in-tu-mes′) *v.* to swell or enlarge.

intumescence (in-tu-mes′ens) *n.* a swelling or enlargement.

invaginate *v.* to fold in, grow inward, or turn outside in.

invagination *n.* in embryology, the process of growing inward.

inverse feedback. the return of an out-of phase (or inverted) signal of an amplifier from an output stage to an input stage to reduce amplification or harmonic distortion. *syn*: negative, out-of-phase, or degenerative feedback.

inverse-square law. the intensity of a sound lessens inversely with the square of the distance from the source.

ion *n.* an atom that has lost or gained electrons and therefore has a positive or negative electric charge.

IOP. Institute of Physics.

iophendylate (i″o-fen′dĭ-lāt) *n.* ethyl iodophenylundecylate. A type of dye that makes x-rays more definitive by causing a contrast in body cavities and the spinal cord.

IPA. international phonetic alphabet. International Phonetic Association.

ips. inches per second.

ipsilateral, ipsilateral *adj.* on the same side. *opp*: contralateral.

ipsilateral competing message. ICM.

ipsilateral routing of signals. IROS. use of a CROS mold—from an ear-level hearing aid into the ear on the same side.

IQ. intelligence quotient.

IRI. index of response irregularity.

IROS. ipsilateral routing of signals.

IRP. incus replacement prosthesis.

irradiation *n.* application of radium locally or by x-ray in radiotherapy.

irreminiscence, auditory (ir"rem-in-ĭ'sens). loss of ability to recall auditory memories.

iridium, heterochromia. different colored eyes. A characteristic feature of the Waardenburg syndrome.

irrigation (ir"ĭ-ga'shun) *n.* washing with water as in cleaning wax from the ear canal.

ischemia (is-ke'me-ah) *n.* locally lowered amount of blood as a result of an obstruction.

ischemia, labyrinthine. lowered amount of blood in the labyrinth as a result of an obstruction.

island, tonal. a narrow band of frequencies that can be heard better than the frequency band on either side.

ISO. International Organization for Standardization, more commonly known as International Standards Organization.

ISO reference zero levels. see audiometric zero.

ITA. initial teaching alphabet.

ITE. in the ear. A hearing aid with all components encased in the earmold.

-itis (i'tis). suffix indicating inflammation or disease of.

ITPA. Illinois Test of Psycholinguistic Abilities.

ivory mastoid. a mastoid process that has no air cells.

to the mold that does not occlude the ear.

jaundice, neonatal. icterus neonatorum or hemolytic disease of the newborn (HDN). It results from an abnormal amount of bile pigment (bilirubin) in the blood. A cause of sensorineural deafness.

Jena. Karl Brauckmann of Jena, Germany, (hence the name) devised a method of teaching speechreading that concentrates on drill work in the rhythm patterns of speech.

jnd. just noticeable difference.

Johnston group test (Philip W. Johnston). several children are screened simultaneously by having them keep their eyes closed and raise their hands as they hear pure tones presented randomly to various parts of the group at the same time.

joint, incudostapedial (ing"ku-do-sta-pe'deal). point of articulation (movement) between the incus and the stapes.

joint, vestibulostapedial. point of articulation (movement) of the footplate of the stapes—in the oval window.

jumper *n.* one who jumps at a loud sound as the result of a nervous disorder.

Justinian's code. code of laws prepared by Byzantine emperor Justinian in the sixth century. It excluded the "deaf and dumb" from the rights and obligations of citizenship.

just noticeable difference. jnd. also known as difference limen (DL) or differential threshold. The smallest change in frequency or intensity that can be recognized. As the smallest recognizable change in intensity, it approximates the decibel.

J

Jacobson's canal (canaliculus tympanicus). (Ludwic L. Jacobson, Danish physician, 1783-1843.) a minute bony tube containing Jacobson's (the tympanic) nerve. It runs from the tympanum to the lower surface of the petrous portion of the temporal bone.

Jacobson's nerve. the tympanic nerve—an afferent nerve that serves the eardrum and the middle ear.

Janssen earmold (Gwen V. Janssen, Oklahoma City). a formed canal in soft materials with exact I.D. and O.D. of the size tubing needed. The tubing does not go in the canal; it is inserted in a valve about ⅛ inch and joins the hook of the hearing aid

K

kanamycin (kan"ah-mi'sin) *n.* antibiotic drug that is ototoxic—it damages the hair cells.

kc. kilocycle. one thousand cycles per second.

K-complex. a wave form that appears on an electroencephalogram as a result of a sound or other stimulus.

Keller coupler. a conical coupler with 1.5 cc volume designed as a possible replacement for the standard 2 cc coupler—for the measurement of hearing aid performance.

keloid. type of scar tissue. It may create problems in the external ear. More common among blacks.

KEMAR. Knowles Electronics Manikin for Acoustic Research.

keratosis obturans. a hard plug of wax and dry skin sometimes found in the external and auditory canal.

kernicterus (ker-nik'ter-us) *n.* form of icterus neonatorum. Nuclear jaundice. Often associated with deafness, cerebral palsy, or both.

kernicterus, erythroblastic. infant jaundice that results from erythroblastosis.

keyboard send and receive. KSR. a teletypewriter portion of a communications device for the deaf that can be operated only by typing.

Killion earmold. Mead C. Killion, PhD, devised and made available to the hearing aid industry a coupling system that included the Killion horn and especially designed acoustically tuned earmolds.

Killion horn. a progressively stepped larger internal diameter earmold coupler designed by Mead C. Killion, PhD. It provides more high frequencies and a smoother response.

kilo- (kil'o). prefix indicating one thousand.

kilocycle *n.* Kc. one thousand cycles per second.

kilomegacycle (kil"o-meg'ah-si-kl) *n.* one thousand million or one billion cycles per second.

kilomegahertz (kil"o-meg'ah-hertz) *n.* one thousand million or one billion cycles per second.

kinesthesia, kinaesthesia (kin"es-the'ze-ah) *n.* the sense of position, motion, weight, and resistance. It is activated by nerve endings in muscles, tendons, and joints; *syn:* kinesthesis.

kinesthesis *n.* kinesthesia. *adj:* **kinesthetic.**

kinesthetic cues. bodily sensations that aid a deaf person in controlling speech, e.g., jaw and lip positions and nasal vibrations.

Kinzie. Cora Elsie and Rose Kinzie devised a system of teaching speechreading that combined the best features of the Mueller-Walle (analytic) and Nitchie (synthetic) methods.

Kisch's reflex (Bruno Kisch, German physician, b: 1890.) the auriculopalpebral reflex. Closure or blink of an eye resulting from stimulation by sudden sound, heat, or some irritant touching the external ear canal.

Klippel-Feil syndrome (Maurice Klippel, French physician, 1858-1942. Andre Feil, French physician, b: 1884). a complex of symptoms that in addition to deafness, includes a short neck, fused vertebrae, and abnormalities of the brain stem and cerebellum.

klystron (kli'stron) *n.* an electron tube used in the generation and amplification of ultra-high-frequency current.

knee. the point where compression takes over in the output of an amplifier, especially as shown on a chart of such an output increase.

kophemia (ko-fe'-me-ah) *n.* an obsolete term for word deafness.

KRS. keyboard send and receive.

KSU speech discrimination test. a test of speech understanding prepared by Kenneth W. Berger, PhD, of Kent (Ohio) State University. It is based on multiple-choice words in sentences.

kymograph (ki'mo-graf) *n.* a device that makes a record of sound vibrations by means of a stylus activated by a tuning fork as a rotating cylinder passes beneath it.

L

L. international hearing aid symbol for low-frequency emphasis tone-control position.

labial (la'be-al) *adj.* concerning the lips.

labyrinth (lab'ĭ-rinth) *n.* the inner ear consisting of the cochlea, vestibule, and the semicircular canals. *adj:* **labyrinthal, labyrinthian, labyrinthic, labyrinthical, labyrinthine.**

labyrinth, bony (labyrinthus osseus). the cavity in the petrous portion of the temporal bone that contains the inner ear.

labyrinth, capsulitis of. old term for otosclerosis.

labyrinthectomy *n.* surgical removal of the labyrinth.

labyrinthine artery. the internal auditory artery that supplies blood to the inner ear.

labyrinthine deafness (lab"ĭ-rin'thĭn). deafness due to damage within the inner ear. The term is sometimes used only when there is an accompanying balance problem.

labyrinthine hydrops (lab"ĭ-rin'thĭn hi'drops). endolymphatic hydrops; *syn:* hydrolabyrinth.

labyrinthine otitis. disease involving the labyrinth.

labyrinthine otosclerosis. growth of bony tissue within the inner ear.

labyrinthine sense. the sense of balance.

labyrinthine windows. the oval and round windows.

labyrinthitis (lab″ĭ-rin-thi′tis) *n.* inflammation of the labyrinth.

labyrinthitis, endolymphatic. inflammation of the inner ear. Otitis interna.

labyrinth, membranous. the membrane that lines the bony labyrinth of the inner ear.

labyrinth, osseous. the bony labyrinth—the cavity in the petrous portion of the temporal bone that contains the inner ear.

labyrinthotomy *n.* surgical destruction of the membranous labyrinth.

lacuna (lah-ku′nah) *n.* a pit or tiny cavity in a bone.

lacuna pharyngis. a small depression or pit at the pharyngeal end of the eustachian tube.

laddergram *n.* a graph, resembling a ladder, prepared to show the results of a loudness balance test of recruitment.

LAFO. Los Angeles Foundation of Otology.

lagena (lah-je′nah) *n.* evolutionary forerunner of the cochlea.

lalognosis *n.* the understanding of speech, especially defective speech.

lalorrhea (lal″o-re′ah) *n.* abnormal flow of speech.

lamina (lam′i-nah) *n.* a thin plate or flat layer, as of bone or tissue.

lamina, basilar cochlear. the basilar membrane. It extends from the bony spiral lamina to the spiral ligament and provides a base for the cochlear duct and organ of Corti.

lamina, bony spiral. the bony plate that extends outward from the modiolus. It is part of the structure that divides the cochlea into sections.

laminagraphy (sometimes laminography). x-ray pictures at different layers of tissue.

lamina theory. an obsolete idea that portions of the bony lamina resonate in response to stimuli of different frequencies.

landmark *n.* distinctive feature of the eardrum revealed by otoscopic examination.

language *n.* the communication of ideas by symbols—vocal or nonvocal.

language age. the ability of a congenitally hearing-impaired child to understand and communicate ideas by gestures or signs when compared with the chronological age of a child hearing normally from birth. The innate intelligence of an infant may obscure a hearing impairment when this language alone is considered.

lapillus (lah-pil′us) *n.* an otolith—"little stone"—on the hair cells in the vestibule of the inner ear.

laryng- prefix referring to the larynx—the Adam's apple.

laryngeal (lah-rin′je-al) *adj.* concerning the larynx.

laryngeal tone. basic tone as air is expired by the lungs between the vocal cords. Fundamental in men is between 120 and 150 Hz and in women between 210 and 240 Hz.

laryngectomy (lar″in-jek′to-me) *n.* surgical removal of the larynx.

laryngoscope (lah-ring′go-skōp) *n.* device for examining the interior of the larynx.

larynx (lar′inks) *n.* the voice box, Adam's apple, containing the vocal chords. *adj*: **laryngitic.**

latency (la′ten-se) *n.* the delay between the stimulus pulse or click and the response; *syn*: response latency.

lateral (lat′er-al) *adj.* to the side.

lateral or horizontal canal. one of the semicircular canals—part of the human balance mechanism.

lateral canthus. outside corner of the eye.

lateral process of malleus. a prominence on the malleus where the handle becomes part of the body. It appears as a bright spot on the drumhead at the upper end of the malleolar stripe.

laterality *n.* the dominance of either side or hemisphere of the brain in speech and hearing.

lateralization *n.* the sensation of hearing a sound in one ear more than the other when a stimulus is presented through a bone oscillator placed in the middle of the forehead; or through the opposite ear when the stimulus is presented to one ear. The sound is said to be referred to or to lateralize to the other ear.

lateralization test. the Weber test. A bone oscillator or tuning fork is placed in the middle of the forehead and the difference in response between the ears (lateralization) is noted. If the tone is heard in the poorer ear, a conductive loss is indicated. If the loss is sensorineural, the tone will be heard in the better ear.

Laurence-Biedl or **Laurence-Moon-Biedl syndrome.** a complex of hereditary and congenital defects including the eyes and ears.

law, inverse-square. the intensity of a sound lessens inversely with the square of the distance from the source.

law, Ohm's. 1. the human ear perceives the components of a complex wave stimulus separately and not as a single sound. 2. the intensity of an electric current (in amperes) is equal to the electromotive force (emf—in volts) divided by the resistance.

law, power. equation to relate loudness to intensity. Loudness is proportional to the 0.3 power of the intensity (energy flux density).

law, Toynbee's. when brain disease is due to otitis media, the cerebrum is involved in case of inflammation of the tympanic attic;

the cerebellum and lateral sinus are involved in case of mastoiditis.

law, Weber-Fechner. named for Ernest Heinrich Weber and Gustav Theodor Fechner, this generalization in neuropsychology states that the just noticeable difference (jnd) in sensation resulting from a stimulus varies (arithmetically) in proportion to the intensity of the stimulus (logarithmic increase) by multiplication.

laxator tympani (lak-sa'tor tim'pa-ne). one of the ligaments attached to the malleus.

laxator tympani major. the ligament attached to the neck of the malleus.

laxator tympani minor. the ligament attached to the handle of the malleus.

LDC. logarithmic or linear dynamic compression.

LDL. loudness discomfort level; *syn:* threshold of discomfort.

learning difficulty. dysmathia.

LED. light emitting diode.

left ear. auris sinistra, (AS).

left side of the body. sinistral.

leg of the stapes. crus (*pl.* crura) or support of the stirrup.

leipoeneia (li"po-ĕ-na'ah). omission of voiceless consonants in the speech of a hard of hearing child (because the surds have not been heard).

lemniscus *pl.* **lemnisci** *n.* bundle of nerve fibers in the auditory pathways.

Lempert horn (Julius Lempert, U.S. physician). type of ear trumpet used to assist in communicating with a patient.

lengthened off time. LOT. a test for malingering that requires the subject to track his threshold by automatic audiometry while the interrupted signal has a lengthened off-time.

lenticular (len-tik'u-lar) *adj.* having the shape of a lens or a magnifying glass.

lenticular aphasia. aphasia due to a lesion within the lenticular nucleus of the brain.

lenticular process. a knob on the tip of the incus (anvil) into which the head of the stapes fits.

lesion (le'zhun) *n.* a wound or damage resulting from disease.

lesion, retrocochlear. damage behind the cochlea (including the auditory nerve and the brain).

Leudet's tinnitus (Theodore E. Leudet, French physician, 1825-1887). spasmodic clicking head noises arising from muscular spasms near the eustachian tube *syn:* objective tinnitus.

level *n.* a reference value expressed as a number; e.g., sound pressure level (SPL) referred to .0002 dynes per centimeter squared.

level, frequency. frequency level, in octaves, is the logarithm to the base 2 of the ratio of

a given frequency to a standard frequency of 16.352 Hz. (The decibel logarithmic ratio is to the base 10).

level, hearing. HL. the number of decibels above audiometric zero.

level, loudness. the loudness level of a sound is determined by comparison for equal loudness with a 1000 Hz tone re .0002 dyne c/m² when heard binaurally in sound field. The unit of loudness level is known as the phon. It is numerically equal to the SPL of the 1000 Hz tone, but varies with frequency.

level, pitch. pitch level varies with intensity and is numerically equal to the frequency of a 40-phon pure tone whose pitch is judged equal to that of the sound in question. The unit of this subjective measurement of differences in pitch is the mel.

level, sensation. The level of a tone, in decibels, above the individual threshold of sensitivity.

level, sound. shortened phrase for sound pressure level as used in sound level meter.

level, sound pressure. SPL. sound pressure level, stated in decibels, is a logarithmic ratio of the measured sound pressure and a reference sound pressure. As commonly used, SPL indicates the decibels mentioned are referred to .0002 dynes/cm². That is, .0002 dynes/cm² is used as the reference pressure in the formula that is stated as: The sound pressure level of a sound is 20 times the logarithm to the base 10 of the ratio of the sound to the reference pressure.

$$SPL = 20 \log_{10} \frac{P(\text{measured sound pressure})}{P_0(\text{reference sound pressure})}$$

$$SPL \ (re \ .0002 \ dyne/cm^2) = 20 \log_{10} \frac{P}{.0002 \ dyne/cm^2}$$

lexicographer (leks"ĭ-kog'ră-fer) *n.* one who compiles a dictionary or lexicon.

Libby horn (E. Robert Libby). a smoothly-tapered (small at hearing aid hook, large at earmold) one-piece sound tube adaptation of the Killion acoustic horn principle.

ligament (lig'ah-ment) *n.* a tough band of tissue connecting or supporting various body structures.

ligament, annular. the ring-like tendon that holds the footplate of the stapes in the oval window. Ligamenta anulare stapedis.

ligament, Rivinus'. a small, thin, triangular portion of the eardrum. It is in the upper part of the membrane. Since it is not as tense as the rest of the eardrum it is also called the flaccid part, pars flaccida. *syn:* Shrapnell's membrane.

ligaments, auricular. the ligaments that attach the external ear to the temporal bone. *syn:* Valsalva's ligaments.

ligament, (spiral) of cochlea. the thickened portion of the lining of the bony cochlea that forms the outer wall of the cochlear duct.

ligaments, Valsalva's. the auricular ligaments.

light emitting diode. LED. a portion of a telecommunications device for the deaf that provides for readout of single characters as they move across the screen when typed.

light reflex. a triangular bright area on the eardrum. Also known as the cone of light, its base is on the lower edge of the tympanic membrane with the apex pointing toward the center. (Its position to the right or left of the umbo indicates accordingly which eardrum is being pictured.)

limbus (lim′bus) *n.* a border, especially the border of the spiral lamina; *syn:* spiral limbus.

limen (li′men) *n.* the point at which a change in sensation begins to be noticeable.

limen, difference. DL. just noticeable difference (jnd) or differential threshold. The smallest change in frequency or intensity that can be recognized.

limen, terminal. the lowest intensity of sound pressure that, when increased, will cause no further increase in the sensation of loudness; *syn:* terminal threshold.

liminal (lim′ī-nal) *adj.* pertaining to the lowest level that will cause a change in sensation.

limited frequency screening test. screening test limited to 1, 2, or 3 frequencies at preset levels of intensity. It is sometimes referred to as reduced screening.

limited range audiometer. one designed to test by air conduction limited ranges of frequency and sound pressure level. Pure tone frequencies of 500, 1000, 2000, 3000, and 4000 Hz are usually included. Sometimes 6000 Hz is added. Sound pressures may be limited to 0 to 70 dB re standard audiometric zero.

line spectrum. a graphic representation in a series of vertical lines of the frequency components of a complex sound wave.

lingual *adj.* 1. pertaining to the tongue. 2. referring to speech, especially speech sounds involving the tongue.

lip-read *v.* to understand by close observation of the speaker's lips. It is now more commonly known as speechreading, since facial expression and gestures enter into communication. *n:* **lipreading.**

listen *v.* to hear, pay attention, or try to understand what is said or heard.

live room. a room in which sounds tend to echo. A reverberant room.

live voice, monitored. the presentation of speech test materials by a vocal speaker who controls (monitors) the level of his voice through observation of a VU Meter.

LL. loudness level.

lobe *n.* 1. the lower, noncartilaginous portion of the external ear appendage. 2. a portion of the brain.

lobectomy *n.* removal by surgery of a lobe.

lobule *n.* the ear lobe. Lobulus auriculae.

localization *n.* determination of the source of a sound made possible partly by the difference in loudness and partly by the difference in time of reception by the two ears.

localization, median-plane. the sensation that the sound is heard in the middle of the head or equally between the two ears.

locator, electroacoustic. a device designed to locate foreign bodies in tissue by measuring resistance to sound waves.

log-, logo- prefix referring to word, speech, or thought.

log. abbreviation for logarithm.

logamnesia *n.* a form of aphasia characterized by inability to recognize spoken or written words.

logarithm (log′a-rithm) *n.* a smaller number (called an exponent) put higher and to the right of a base number, indicates that the base number must be raised to that power in order to produce a given number. This exponent is called a logarithm and the given numbers are found through the use of tables of logarithms. In audiology, the decibel is a unit of measurement used to express a logarithmic ration to the base 10 (usually written log₁₀).

logarithmic amplification. logarithmic compression. Less often used in reference to automatic gain control (AGC).

logarithmic compression. a method of controlling output that varies proportionately with the input. It utilizes a field effect transistor (FET) in the input stage.

logatome (lo′ga-tōm) *n.* syllable that has no meaning. Nonsense syllable. Also spelled logotome.

logokophosia (log″o-ko-fo′se-ah) *n.* inability to understand the spoken word.

logon (lo′gon) *n.* a 1.5 cycle burst of tone.

logopedia (log-o-pe′de-ah) *n.* logopedics; a branch of science dealing with the physiology of speech and the correction of defective speech.

logopedist *n.* speech pathologist.

logotome *n.* a syllable with no meaning. A nonsense syllable—also spelled logatome.

Lombard test. test for malingering in which the patient is asked to read aloud while wearing headphones. As he reads, continuous sound (usually white noise) is presented to the "deafened" ear or ears. Since the normally-hearing person unconsciously tries to talk above the background noise level (the Lombard effect), the malingerer will usually react in the same way; i.e., raise his voice while reading aloud. *syn*: Lombard voice-reflex test.

long process. a comparatively long projection of bone—that is, long compared to other projections of the same bone, e.g., long process of the malleus.

long process of the incus. the arm of the incus (anvil) that articulates (moves) the stapes.

loop, induction. a continuous wire carrying electrical energy from an amplifier. The flux or magnetic field thus created when such a loop surrounds a room makes auditory training systems that utilize wearable hearing aids possible.

loop induction hearing aid. a hearing aid specifically designed to be used in connection with a magnetic loop in classes for the hard of hearing or deaf. Usually, however, conventional hearing aids equipped with telephone coils are used by the pupils.

loop, magnetic. seldom used term for induction loop.

lope ear. an external ear that projects directly outward from the head.

LOT. lengthened off time.

loud *adj.* marked by great amplitude or intensity.

loudness *n.* subjective sensation of the effect of amplitude or intensity. It is determined partly by the number of auditory nerve fibers activated by the sound wave and partly by the number of impulses carried by each fiber. The unit of measurement of subjective loudness is the sone.

loudness balance test. test for recruitment, by comparing judgments of loudness, performed either binaurally or monaurally.

loudness balance test, binaural. test for recruitment by comparing judgments of loudness between ears. In alternate binaural loudness balance testing, a pure tone is presented first to one normal (or nearly normal) ear—then the intensity adjusted in the other ear until the tones in both ears are judged to be equally loud. The values are plotted at increasing levels of intensity to see if the differences decrease with the changes.

loudness balance test, monaural. test for recruitment by comparing judgments of loudness between frequencies in the same ear. A pure tone of a better (lower, preferably normal or nearly normal) frequency is presented at successively increasing levels above its threshold. A pure tone of a higher frequency is adjusted each time until the tones are judged to be equally loud. The

values are plotted at the increasing levels of intensity to see if the differences decrease with the changes.

loudness contours, equal. curved lines that indicate the sound pressures necessary at each frequency to produce sensations of equal loudness for normally hearing listeners.

loudness contours, monaural. equal loudness contours determined by testing one ear alone.

loudness discomfort level. LDL.

loudness level. LL. the loudness level of a sound is determined by comparison for equal loudness with a 1000 Hz tone re .0002 dyne c/m² when heard binaurally in sound field. The unit of loudness level is known as the phon. It is numerically equal to the SPL of the 1000 Hz tone, but varies with frequency.

loudness recruitment. abnormal growth of the sensation of loudness. See recruitment.

loudness unit. sone. The unit of a subjective loudness scale based on average human judgments of comparative loudness. One sone is the loudness heard by an average normal listener when presented with a 1000 Hz tone at an intensity of 40 dB re .0002 dynes/cm² (or 40 phons). While two sones express the sensation of a sound being twice as loud as one sone, the intensity change required will vary but will represent an increase in phons of about 9 dB.

loudspeaker *n.* a speaker. A device (electroacoustic transducer) that amplifies and radiates sound through the air.

loudspeaker, moving coil. loudspeaker whose diaphragm is activated by a moving coil in a fixed magnetic field.

Lowenberg's canal (ductus cochlearis) (Benjamin B. Lowenberg, French physician, b: 1836). the cochlear duct, membranous cochlea, or scala media. The middle triangular tube of the cochlea.

lowered threshold. a better threshold of sensitivity, e.g., one reflecting lower numbers on an audiogram.

low fence. the lower limit of hearing impairment expressed as an average of 500, 1000, and 2000 Hz: 27 dB ISO or 16 dB ASA 1951.

low frequency. an inexact term that generally refers to a frequency of 1000 Hz and below.

low-pass filter. a band-pass filter that allows only selected lower frequencies to pass.

low-pass filtered signal. LPFS.

low-redundancy speech test. test to determine the ability to understand speech when most of the repetitive factors have been removed by the use of filters.

LPFS. low-pass filtered signal.

lues (loo'ez) *n.* syphilis

luetic deafness (loo-et'ik). deafness caused by syphilis.

lumen (loo'men) *n.* space within the eustachian tube. *adj*: **luminal, lumenal.**

lupus pernio. nodular lesions of the skin and mucous membranes which may involve the ears. Sarcoidosis of Besnier.

Luscher-Zwislocki test (E. Luscher, Jozef Zwislocki). a test of the difference limen (DL) for intensity. A tone is presented which varies in intensity but centers around a sensation level (SL) of 40 dB. The variation in intensity (which the patient hears as beats) is gradually reduced until the beats seem to disappear. This point is the patient's DL for intensity (or jnd for loudness).

lymphoid (tissue). tissue characteristic of the lymph glands. The adenoids, which surround the nasopharyngeal opening of the eustachian tube, are made up of lymphoid tissue.

lymphoidectomy *n.* removal of lymphoid tissue by surgery, e.g., adenoidectomy or tonsillectomy.

-lysis. suffix indicating a dissolution or a decomposition.

lysis (li'sis) *n.* 1. gradual improvement of a disease. 2. decomposition of cells. 3. destruction of bacteria and other microorganisms. *adj*: **lytic.**

M

μ. The Greek letter Mu in its lower case form μ is used as a prefix and abbreviation for micro; as in μbar—microbar.

M. international hearing aid symbol for microphone input selector.

MA. mental age. Master of Arts.

MAC. minimum auditory capabilities battery.

macerated. wrinkled, as by long exposure to water.

Macewen's triangle (mak-u'enz) (Sir William Macewen—Scottish surgeon, 1848-1924). triangular indentation above and in back of the bony portion of the external ear canal. It is one of the landmarks in a

mastoid operation. *syn*: suprameatal triangle.

macro- (mak'ro). prefix meaning large.

macroscopic (mak"ro-skop'ik) *adj.* large enough to be seen without a microscope.

macrosonics. study of ultrasonics as used in high intensities.

macrostructure (mak"ro-struk'tūr) *n.* physical makeup of a body part, the hair cells, as determined by visual study with little or no magnification.

macrotia (mak-ro'she-ah) *n.* ear hypertrophy or abnormally enlarged ears.

macula, basilar. cluster of cells in the embryonic otic vesicle which develop into the basilar membrane and its associated portion of the inner ear.

macula, saccular. raised spot on the wall of the saccule where a portion of the vestibular nerve terminates.

maculae, acoustic. rough spots in the walls of the saccule and utricle caused by the terminations of the vestibular nerve.

maculae, cribrose. rough spots in the walls of the semicircular canals caused by minute holes through which fibers of the vestibular nerve pass.

MAF. minimum audible field.

magnetic earphone. earphone in which a soft iron diaphragm is activated by changes in electrical signal current flowing through soft iron poles of a permanent magnet to change electrical energy to acoustical energy.

magnetic loop. induction loop. A loop of wire that encircles a room and through which amplified electrical impulses are transmitted from a microphone. Usually used in classrooms for the deaf and hard of hearing. Any pupil can pick up the teacher's words through an induction coil in his own aid, and is thus free to move about.

magnetic recorder. device that utilizes an electromagnetic transducer to record electrical signals on ferromagnetic recording tape.

magnum foramen (fo-ra'men) *n.* opening through which the spinal cord passes into the skull to become the medulla oblongata of the brain.

mainstream. to place children with impairments in schools and classes with children having no handicaps.

maladaptive response. avoidance conditioning response, i.e., one where the reward is the lack (or avoidance) of a disagreeable stimulus.

malignant (mah-lig'nant) *adj.* life-threatening. Commonly used to refer to a cancerous tumor—as opposed to one that is benign.

malinger (mah-ling'er) *v.* to feign deafness or a degree of deafness more severe than actually exists.

malingerer *n.* one who malingers, i.e., feigns a hearing loss.

malingering test. any one of a number of tests to determine if one is feigning a handicap.

malleolar folds (mal-e′o-lar). ridges in the eardrum membrane caused by the attachment of the malleus to the inside of the drumhead.

malleolar stripe (stria). indication of the handle of the malleus as it appears attached to the drumhead.

malleus (mal′e-us) *pl.* **mallei** *n.* also called the hammer, the malleus is the first and largest of the ossicles. The handle is attached to the eardrum, while the head is attached to the roof of the tympanic cavity by the superior malleolar ligament, and moves (articulates) with the incus (anvil). It is about 8 mm long.

malleus, capitis or caput. the head of the malleus moving with the incus.

malleus fixation. adherence of the malleus to the wall of the tympanic cavity.

malleus, handle of. portion of the malleus attached to the eardrum. It appears through the drumhead as the malleolar stria or stripe. The manubrium.

malleus, lateral process of. prominence on the malleus where the handle becomes part of the body. It appears as a bright spot on the drumhead at the upper end of the malleolar stripe.

malocclusion *n.* imperfect jaw closure. It may result in earmold problems and, in extreme cases, adversely affect hearing or cause earaches.

malodorous (mal-o′dor-us) *adj.* bad smelling.

mandible (man′dĭ-b′l) *n.* large bone in the lower jaw.

mandibular (man-dib′u-lar) *adj.* concerning the lower jaw.

manometer (mah-nom′ĕ-ter) *n.* instrument designed to measure liquid or gas pressure.

manometric flame. early device that utilized an acetylene gas flame to measure frequency.

manometry *n.* study of the impedance of the middle ear structure by means of a pressure-measuring device. The use of a manometer for this purpose has been superseded, first by the mechanical acoustic measuring bridge and later by the electroacoustic impedance meter, which incorporates an electromanometer.

manual alphabet. orderly arrangement of finger positions and hand movements to represent the various letters of the alphabet.

manualism *n.* communication by hand signals, either by gestures, finger-spelling, or sign-language.

manubrium *n.* the handle of the malleus. *adj:* **manubrial.**

MAO. maximum acoustic output. (Same as MDP).

MAP. minimum audible pressure.

MAPS. Make a Picture Story. A personality test sometimes used with the deaf.

Marfan's syndrome. (B.J.A. Marfan, French physician, 1858-1942.) a complex of symptoms including ear, eye, skull, and finger defects.

marked falling curve audiogram. loss increases about 15 or 20 dB per octave at higher frequencies. *syn:* sharply falling curve.

mask *v.* to introduce a controlled sound into one ear to prevent the hearing by that ear of a tone or sound presented to the other ear.

maskability (mask″a-bil′ĭ-te) *n.* capable of being masked. Most often used to refer to the possibility of masking out annoying tinnitus.

masked threshold. point at which a listener can first determine that a sound is audible in the presence of another or masking sound.

masker, tinnitus. amplifying instrument shaped like a hearing aid but engineered to generate a band of white noise designed to mask out an individual's tinnitus. Sometimes used to help a stutterer attain fluency.

masking *n.* interference with a wanted sound caused by an unwanted sound or noise.

masking audiogram. graphical representation, in the form of a laddergram, of the masking effect of a lower frequency on a higher frequency at increasing levels of intensity. It is a seldom-used technique for differential diagnosis of sensorineural and conductive lesions.

masking, backward. louder noise is introduced within 100 milliseconds after a short pure test tone is presented. The louder noise masks out (makes inaudible) the pure tone even though the louder sound is presented after the test tone.

masking, central. the shift in the threshold of the test ear by 5 dB, which results from the effect of masking on the central nervous system. For this reason 5 dB should be subtracted from the threshold obtained when the opposite ear is masked.

masking, complex noise. sound made up of a mixture of frequencies designed to mask the better ear while the poorer ear is being tested.

masking, contralateral. the noxious effect on the opposite ear when the masking sound becomes too intense.

masking, effective. 1. noise of sufficient intensity to interfere with the hearing of another sound; e.g., white noise may be introduced in the better ear to mask out the speech when a speech reception threshold (SRT) is being sought in the poorer ear. Narrow bands, pink noise, and complex noise may also be used for masking when a pure tone threshold is sought. 2. term used by some audiometer manufacturers to indicate that additional energy is built into the masking level to compensate for the air conduction shadow curve.

masking, forward. phenomenon by which a sound continues to be masked (not heard) for a brief period after the masking noise is discontinued. *syn*: residual masking or poststimulatory threshold shift.

masking, narrow band. the use of filtered bands of white noise for masking purposes. Special circuits designed to present a mixture of tones centering around each test frequency may also be used.

masking noise. 1. a mixture of frequencies made up in various ranges—narrow, broad, white, or complex—introduced into one ear to prevent the hearing by that ear of a tone or sound presented to the other ear. 2. any unwanted sound that interferes with the ability to hear the wanted sound.

masking, precedent. backward masking.

masking, residual. forward masking.

masking, saw-tooth. a sound made up of a fundamental frequency of about 60 or 120 Hz together with all its harmonics to 10,000 Hz in random phase.

masking, upward. phenomenon by which higher frequency sounds are made inaudible by the presence of lower frequency noises.

masking, white noise. masking by means of a broad band of noise that contains equal amounts of energy at all frequencies included.

mass, acoustic. resistance to the movement of sound pressure waves in a tube. *syn*: acoustic inertance, inertance.

Massachusetts group test. a number of children screened simultaneously by having them indicate on a scoring sheet whether or not a pure tone is heard as it may or may not have been presented during a series of six bursts.

mastoid *n.* raised portion of the temporal bone behind the external ear: the mastoid process. *adj*: **mastoid.**

mastoidal or **mastoideal otitis.** inflammation of the mastoid.

mastoid antrim. space in the posterior part of the temporal bone connecting with the middle ear.

mastoid bone. rounded hard protrusion at the lower end of the skull behind the external ear. It is honeycombed with air-filled cells.

mastoid cells. air-filled cavities in the mastoid process of the temporal bone.

mastoid dyspepsia. nausea symtomatic of mastoiditis.

mastoidectomy *n.* removal of diseased mastoid cells by surgery.

mastoidectomy, radical. surgical removal of the middle ear structures in addition to the removal of diseased mastoid cells.

mastoid empyema. presence of pus in the air cells of the mastoid process.

mastoideum *n.* space in temporal bone posterior to the tympanic cavity. *syn*: antrum mastoid or mastoid antrum.

mastoid foramen (fo-ra′men). opening in the mastoid that allows passage of blood vessels.

mastoid fossa. furrow in the mastoid process for blood vessels.

mastoiditis *n.* inflammation within the air cells of the mastoid.

mastoiditis, Bezold's. inflammation of the mastoid process resulting from Bezold's abscess.

mastoid, ivory. mastoid process that has no air cells.

mastoid operation. mastoidotomy—an incision for outward drainage of mastoid cells.

mastoidotomy *n.* surgical opening of the mastoid process to allow drainage from the mastoid cells.

mastoid process. rounded bony structure behind the outer ear usually honeycombed by air cells.

mastoid scoop. instrument used during mastoidectomy to scoop out mastoid air cells.

maternal rubella. German measles during pregnancy. If the mother contracts this viral disease during the first three months of pregnancy, the fetus may be adversely affected. Congenitally impaired hearing is a common result.

mating pattern, assortative. tendency of deaf persons to marry deaf persons.

maximum acoustic output. the greatest sound intensity an amplifying system can produce. *syn*: saturation output, maximum deliverable pressure.

maximum deliverable pressure. MDP. the greatest sound pressure an amplifying system can produce. *syn*: maximum acoustic output; saturation output.

maximum power output. in hearing aids this term is usually used to express the average of the saturation output pressures at 500, 1000, and 2000 Hz. It is more often referred to as the output of the hearing aid. *syn*: maximum deliverable pressure.

maximum sound pressure. the greatest degree of intensity of any single wave or designated range of waves.

maximum tolerable pressure. MTP. the greatest sound intensity an individual can tolerate. *syn*: threshold of discomfort; loudness discomfort level.

MCL. most comfortable loudness.

MCLR, MCR. most comfortable loudness range.

MCU. message control unit.

MDP. maximum deliverable pressure.

mean *n.* statistically, when used without qualification, "mean" usually refers to the arithmetic mean; i.e., the mean of a series of numbers is equal to the sum of the numbers divided by the number of numbers in the series.

mean-square. the sum of a series of numbers squared divided by the number of squared numbers in the series.

measles *n.* childhood infectious fever. When hearing impairment results it is either conductive from otitis media or bilaterally sensorineural due to toxic effects of the virus.

measles, German. rubella. A viral disease that, during the first three months of pregnancy adversely affects the developing embryo. Congenitally impaired hearing is a common result.

meatal cartilage (me-a'tal). cartilaginous (gristly) portion of the external auditory canal.

meato-antrotomy. the cutting into the wall of the external ear canal.

meatus (me-a'tus) *n.* short term sometimes used for either the external or internal auditory canal. *syn*: auditory meatus, meatus auditorius.

meatus acusticus externus. external auditory meatus or porus. Ear canal from earflap to eardrum.

meatus acusticus internus. internal auditory meatus or porus. Auditory canal through which the auditory and facial nerves pass on their way to the brain.

meatus, external auditory. the outer ear canal that allows sound waves to reach the eardrum.

meatus, internal auditory. sheath through which the auditory nerve and facial nerve pass on their way to the brain.

mechanical feedback. acoustic feedback (squeal) usually caused by the vibration of the microphone or receiver against the hearing aid case.

mechanical hearing aid. device designed to intensify sound waves by concentration rather than electrical amplification; e.g., an ear trumpet.

mechanical interrupter. mechanical device to automatically interrupt a continuous tone at intervals.

mechanical ohm. the unit of mechanical impedance; equal to the force of 1 dyne divided by a velocity of 1 centimeter per second.

mechanical trauma. damage to the hearing mechanism as a result of a blow to the head; e.g., a break in the ossicular chain.

mechanoreceptors. the hair cells of the ear.

media (me'de-ah) *n.* middle.

media, barotitis (bar"o-ti'tis). (bar: weight or pressure). damage to the middle ear caused by changes in barometric pressure. *syn*: aero-otitis media, barotrauma.

medial *adj.* toward the middle.

medial canthus. inner corner of the eye.

medial geniculate body. the last of the nuclei in the auditory nervous system before the neurons enter Heschl's gyrus (auditory reception center of the brain).

median *n.* 1. midline. 2. in statistics, the number in the middle of a series or the arithmetic mean of the two numbers in the middle.

median-plane localization. the sensation that the sound is heard in the middle of the head or equally between the two ears.

medium, sound. any material through which sound pressure waves may pass.

MEDRESCO. from Medical Research Council—used as the name of the hearing aid distributed by the Department of Health and Social Security in England.

medulla oblongata. enlargement of the spinal cord as it becomes the lower part of the brain.

medullary sheath. layer of myelin that surrounds some nerve fibers.

medulloblastoma. type of malignant brain tumor that occurs most often in children and has a tendency to spread in the meninges.

mega- (meg'ah). 1. prefix meaning huge. 2. prefix meaning one million, 10^6.

megacephalic, macrocephalous, megalocephalic *adj.* having an unusually large head. *n.* **megacephaly.**

megadyne. one million dynes.

MEK. methyl ethyl ketone.

mel *n.* subjective unit describing tone-pitch relationships. It is equal to about 1/1000 of the pitch of a tone of 1000 Hz at 40 dB above threshold; that is, 1000 mels represents the pitch of a tone of 1000 Hz at 40 dB SL (sensation level, above threshold).
One mel is also about one jnd (just noticeable difference) at any frequency.

melanin *n.* a pigment—lack of which seems to be coincidental with some types of deafness and mental deficiency.

MEM. minimum effective masking.

membrane *n.* thin layer of organic tissue. *adj*: membraned.

membrane, basilar. membrane that forms the base of the triangular inner tube of the cochlea. It stretches across the cochlea from the spiral bony lamina to the spiral ligament, and divides the cochlea into two main divisions: the scala vestibuli and the scala tympani.

membrane, Corti's (membrana tectoria ductus cochlearis). the tectorial membrane—the roof membrane into which the cilia of the hair cells project.

membrane, drum. the eardrum. Also called tympanic membrane or the drumskin.

membrane, mucous. thin layer of tissue, containing fluid-secreting cells, which lines passages or cavities connecting with the air.

membrane, Reissner's. membrane within the cochlea that separates the scala vestibuli from the scala media. *syn:* vestibular membrane.

membrane, Scarpa's. thin layer of tissue that covers the round window. Sometimes called the secondary tympanic membrane: membrana tympani secundaria of the fenestra rotunda.

membrane, secondary tympanic. thin tissue that covers the round window.

membrane, Shrapnell's. flaccid portion of the eardrum. The pars flaccida filling the notch of Rivinus.

membrane, tectorial. common name for Corti's membrane. Gelatinous membrane, attached to bony spiral lamina, which overlies the hair cells within the cochlea of the inner ear.

membrane, tympanic. the eardrum. It stretches across the inner end of the external ear canal and forms the outer boundary of the middle ear. It reacts to sound waves and starts the ossicular chain moving. *syn:* drum membrane, drumskin.

membrane, vestibular. *syn:* Reissner's membrane.

membranous *adj.* pertaining to membrane.

membranous, labyrinth. membrane that lines the bony labyrinth of the inner ear.

Meniere's disease, Meniere's syndrome (men"e-arz'). (Prosper Meniere, French physician, 1799-1862). endolymphatic hydrops—the malfunction of hearing and balance caused by excessive inner ear fluids. A condition whose intermittent symptoms include dizziness, nausea, tinnitus, and progressive deafness. *syn:* labyrinthine hydrops.

meninges (mĕ-nin'jēz) *n.* the three membranes, known as the dura mater, pia mater, and arachnoid mater, which cover the brain and its appendages as well as the spinal cord.

meningioma (mĕ-nin"je-o'mah) *n.* a tumor within the meninges.

meningitis (men"in-ji'tis) *n.* infectious fever of the covering of the brain, the meninges, which may result in severe hearing impairment—either from the toxic effects of the virus or from the drugs used in its control.

meninx *pl.* **meninges** *n.* any one of the three membranes that envelop the brain and spinal cord.

meniscus *n.* line that may be visible through the tympanic membrane when the middle ear cavity is partially filled with fluid.

mental age. MA. numerical expression of individual intellectual age when compared with the norm for the same chronological age.

mentally retarded. MR. below chronological age in mental development.

mes-, meso-. prefix meaning in the middle.

mesencephalic (mez-en"sĕ-fal'ik) *adj.* referring to the midbrain.

mesencephalon (mez"en-sef'ah-lon) *n.* the mid-portion of the brain. The midbrain.

mesenchyme (mes'eng-kīm) *n.* embryonic cells or connective tissue that may block the middle ear of infants as long as three or four weeks after birth.

mesial (me'ze-al) *adj.* medial—situated in the middle.

mesotympanum (ma"zo-tim-pah'num) *n.* the middle ear.

message control unit. an automatic means for typing out an identification message on a Telecommunications Device for the Deaf.

messages, competing. differing signals or messages presented at the same time. Often used as a test of a hearing aid fitting to demonstrate the advantage of binaural listening.

met-, meta- (met'ah). prefix meaning later, beyond, or behind.

metaplasia (met"ah-pla'ze-ah) *n.* abnormal conversion of one kind of cellular tissue into another.

metastasize (me-tas'tah-sīz) *v.* to spread from the original site of the disease, as might occur with a malignant tumor.

meter *n.* 1. device that measures and indicates amounts. 2. standard unit of linear measurement in the metric system. It equals 39.37 inches.

meter, decibel. instrument calibrated in decibels designed to measure voltage differences when the line impedance (in ohms) is known.

meter, impedance. electro-acoustic device designed to measure: 1. acoustic impedance at the drumhead—the ability of the eardrum and ossicular chain to transmit sound pressure waves. 2. the stapedius muscle reflex. 3. the compliance of the tympanic membrane.

meter, otoadmittance. electro-acoustic device similar to the impedance meter and designed to perform the same functions.

meter, sound level. electronic device made up of a microphone, an amplifying network, and a meter to indicate the r.m.s. (root-mean-square) value of the sound pressure in a complex sound wave. In addition to a flat C scale, it usually includes two other scales—A and B—which attenuate the low frequencies in various degrees. Sometimes referred to as a pressure meter, or sound pressure meter. In

15. Determine proper amount of masking by the "plateau method" (ALS Vol. 1 - #4). (a) present weak masking to non-test ear (b) determine threshold in test ear (c) increase masking 5 db steps until test tone remains in test ear.

16. Place bone receiver carefully in most sensitive position on mastoid bone. If mid-line positioning is preferred (ALS Vol. 4-#2) a special holder is available from Maico. Use PLATEAU masking method but apply following corrections for transcranial loss.

17. 500 cps and below - deduct 10 db from reading - (read 20, write 10) 1000 and 2000 -deduct 5 db from reading - (read 20, write 15) 3000 and 4000 no correction necessary (read 20, write 20)

18. The SAL technique may be employed to validate questionable bone levels (MA-8, MA-10, MA-24 only).

SPEECH TESTS

19. The next logical step in "office audiometry" is the performance of the three speech tests suggested on the audiogram card. SRT (Speech Reception Threshold), MCL (Most Comfortable Loudness), and TD (Threshold of Discomfort). Speech pads are available from your Maico dealer for this purpose.

20. A speech discrimination score may be desired next. This is done by speaking the PB-50 Word Lists (Speech Pad) into microphone and delivering to patient at MCL.

Other test procedures such as SISI, Malingering tests, etc., should be carefully practiced before presentation to patient. The manual accompanying your audiometer will explain these in detail.

AUDIOMETRIC HINTS - Arne Darbo

1. Test in a quiet place – use Maico AURALDOMES.

2. Seat patient comfortably – behind audiometer.

3. Instruct patient how to indicate "when sound is first heard".

AIR CONDUCTION PURE TONE TESTS

4. Place receivers, carefully, directly over ears.

5. Test better ear first so you will know if masking is necessary.

6. The "WINCHESTER TRICK" acquaints you quickly with the problem.

7. Start pure tone test at 1000 cps -use ascending technique; 125 may be eliminated.

8. Mask better ear when difference exceeds 40 db – allow 5 db credit for masking effect.

9. Ordinarily an amount of masking comfortable to the good ear is sufficient, however, there are instances when more must be used.

BONE CONDUCTION PURE TONE TEST

10. Determine if bone conduction test is indicated by inspection of air test.

11. If air level is 20 db or better in the low frequencies (ISO) do not attempt bone test under "office" conditions as unoccluded ear will reflect room masking.

12. Always mask contralateral ear during bone test.

13. Allow 5 db credit to test ear ONLY if your audiometer is not calibrated "HAIC INTRIM" for bone. No credit if HAIC INTRIM calibrated.

14. Test bone 500-600 cps - do not use 250 or lower because of feeling curve (ALS Vol. 4 - #3).

some instruments there is also a D weighting scale to measure the annoyance level of "fly-over" noise.

meter, VU (volume units). device used to monitor voice or music intensity levels. *syn*: volume-level indicator.

method, ascending. determining an audiometric threshold by increasing the intensity of the stimulus until it is identified. The opposite of the descending method.

method, bimodal. combination of manual and oral education of the deaf child. *syn*: simultaneous method.

method, descending. determining an audiometric threshold by decreasing the intensity of a previously identified stimulus until it is no longer audible. The opposite of the ascending method.

method, equation. procedure for determining thresholds by which the subject varies the intensity of a stimulus to match or barely differ from a reference stimulus. *syn*: method of adjustment, method of equivalent stimuli.

method, Feré. electrodes are attached to the skin to measure the change in resistance to a minute external electric current that results from a sound stimulus—as in GSR or EDR audiometry.

method, frequency. procedure for measuring the thresholds by which the one being measured responds after each discrete stimulus presentation. *syn*: method of constant stimuli.

method of adjustment. procedure for measuring the absolute or differential threshold. The one being measured controls the intensity of the stimulus and sets it according to instructions from the examiner. Just barely heard, for example. *syn*: method of average error.

method of constant stimuli. procedure for measuring the threshold by which the one being measured responds verbally after each discrete stimulus presentation.

method of limits. procedure for measuring the threshold by which the one being measured is given a tone at an intensity high enough to be definitely identified. The intensity of the tone is then lowered until no longer heard and raised again until the threshold is determined by bracketing it. *syn*: method of serial exploration.

method, Rainville. procedure for determining the conductive loss by comparing the masking effect on air-conducted tones produced by bone-conducted noise at the mastoid between normal listeners and the patient under test.

method, Rochester. method of teaching the deaf in which oral methods are supplemented by fingerspelling.

method, simultaneous. communication by means of the manual alphabet, signs and speech.

method, stimulation. system of speech correction in which major emphasis is placed on teaching the correct speech sounds by having the patient listen to them.

method, Tarchanoff (Tarchanow). electrodes are attached to the skin to measure the changes in electrical potential of the sweat glands that result from a sound stimulus as in EDR audiometry (compare Feré method). The T effect is sometimes referred to as the galvanic skin response.

method, Verbotonal. system of teaching the deaf devised by P. Guberina of Yugoslavia.

methyl ethyl ketone. MEK. solvent sometimes used to polish soft plastic earmolds.

Metropolitan achievement test. reading test that has been revised for use with the deaf.

Metz recruitment test. (Otto Metz, Swedish audiologist). acoustic impedance measurement that may indicate recruitment in a patient with a hearing impairment if a stapedius reflex is elicited by a stimulus smaller than 60 to 70 dB above threshold.

Meyerson group speech test. (Lee Meyerson, PhD). a number of children are screened simultaneously by having them point to the appropriate picture in response to the word.

mho (mo) *n.* the practical unit of electrical conductance; the reciprocal of the ohm.

Michel's syndrome. described in 1863, it includes among its symptoms, failure of the inner ear to develop.

micro- often symbolized by the lower case Greek letter Mu "μ". A prefix meaning tiny or minute. In connection with numbers it indicates one millionth.

microbar, μbar. dyne per square centimeter. The basic unit of measurement of sound pressure. It represents the amount of energy required to move a mass of one gram a distance of one centimeter in one second. In pressure it equals one millionth of normal atmospheric pressure at sea level.

micrognathia (mi"kro-na'the-ah) *n.* the condition of having abnormally small jaws.

micron. one-thousandth of a millimeter, the millionth part of a meter, one twenty-five thousandth of an inch.

micronewton. one-millionth of a newton.

micropascal, μpascal (pas-kal') (Blaise Pascal, 17th century French scientist). new international term intended to replace the microbar as the zero reference level for sound pressure.

microphone *n.* device, transducer, which converts sound pressure waves into electrical energy. *adj*: **microphonic.**

microphone, carbon. device for converting sound pressure waves into electrical energy that utilized the unique properties of carbon.

microphone, condenser. device for converting sound pressure waves into electrical energy by utilizing a vibrating diaphragm as one plate of a condenser.

microphone, crystal. device for converting sound pressure waves into electrical energy by utilizing the unique properties of a piezoelectric crystal.

microphone, diabow. diagonally bowed ceramic substrate microphone.

microphone, directional. microphone designed for ear-level aids with two openings so there will be greater sensitivity to sounds coming from the front (or direction toward which the head is turned). Sounds from the rear are attenuated in various ways.

microphone, dynamic. device for converting sound pressure waves into electrical energy as a thin diaphragm is moved, causing an alternating current to flow through a connecting wire coil suspended in a magnetic field.

microphone, electret. condenser microphone that has been miniaturized to the point it can be used in hearing aids.

microphone, probe-tube. tiny microphone attached to a flexible plastic tube. A variant of the sound-probe microphone.

microphone, sound-probe. tiny microphone on a thin rod or cylinder designed to study sound waves in small confined spaces with a minimum of disturbance to the wave form.

microphonia, microphony *n.* abnormally soft voice.

microphonic, cochlear. electrical voltage produced by the hair cells of the cochlea. The electrical response follows the wave form of the acoustic stimulus in a manner similar to the action of a microphone.

microphonic potential. electrical voltage produced by the hair cells of the cochlea. *syn*: cochlear microphonic.

microphonics, microphonic effects. unwanted sound generated in a loudspeaker or in an electrical circuit by mechanical movements of normally non-moving parts.

microphonoscope *n.* stethoscope with a diaphragm designed to intensify body sounds.

microscope, electron. microscope that can magnify up to 100,000 times by using electron beams with wave lengths thousands of times shorter than visible light in place of light.

microscope, phase-contrast. microscope equipped with a special condensor to make details of objects visible through a change in phase; e.g., of color or brightness.

microscope, scanning. type of electron microscope involving a moving electron beam.

microsurgery *n.* surgery made possible by the use of a microscope; e.g., stapedectomy.

microtia (mi-kro'she-ah) *n.* abnormally small pinna.

microtrauma (mi"kro-traw'mah) *n.* bodily damage resulting from the cumulative effect of minute injuries. Noise-induced hearing loss has been referred to as acoustic microtrauma.

microvolt *n.* one-millionth of a volt.

microwave *n.* an extremely short electromagnetic wave.

middle ear. auris media, or tympanic cavity. The portion of the hearing mechanism between the outer and inner ears. Consists of the eardrum, the ossicles, the opening of the eustachian tube, the oval window, and the round window.

middle ear cavity, middle ear cleft. cavity in the temporal bone about ½ inch (1.25 cm) from front to back and roof to floor. Wall to wall distance varies from less than ⅛ inch (2 mm) to about ⅜ inch (6 mm) obliquely about ⅓ inch (8 or 9 mm). Capacity less than 2 cm³ (2 cc). Contains the middle ear mechanism.

middle ear effusion. an accumulation of thin, watery fluid in the middle ear. Sometimes called serous otitis media; less often called catarrhal otitis media.

middle ear impedance. resistance of the drumhead, the oval window, and the ossicular chain to acoustic stimuli.

mike *n.* 1. altered and shortened term for microphone. 2. used in communications as a code word for the letter m (when capitalized).

milli- prefix for one-thousandth.

milliampere *n.* one-thousandth of an ampere—abbrev: ma.

millisecond *n.* one-thousandth of a second. msec.

millisone *n.* one-thousandth of a sone, a unit of loudness.

millivolt *n.* one-thousandth of a volt.

mimic speech. involuntary repetition of words or phrases just spoken by someone else. *syn*: echo speech, echolalia, echologia, echophasia, and echophrasia.

mind deafness. 1. cortical deafness. 2. auditory aphasia. 3. functional or nonorganic deafness.

mini-CROS. hearing aid system with the microphone on one side and the amplifier on the other, with a short plastic tube (or none) from the receiver spout to the ear.

minimal change. term synonymous with difference limen, just noticeable difference, or minimum perceptible difference.

minimum audible field. MAF. the threshold of hearing measured under controlled sound field conditions.

minimum audible pressure. MAP. threshold of acuity expressed in SPL or re .0002 dynes/cm².

minimum auditory capabilities battery. MAC. a group of 14 tests designed to determine individual auditory rehabilitative potential prepared under the supervision of Elmer Owens, PhD.

minimum masking level. MML. as used in tinnitus studies, the lowest level of intensity of the selected band or bands of noise that will effectively mask out the tinnitus.

minimum perceptible difference. MPD.

Minnesota Multiphasic Personality Inventory. MMPI. personality test sometimes used in cases of functional deafness.

mitosis (mi-to'sis) *n.* process of cell reproduction. *adj*: **mitotic.**

mixed hearing loss. hearing impairment resulting from malfunction of both the conductive and sensorineural pathways.

MLB. monaural loudness balance.

MLV. monitored live voice.

MMC. "Monday morning clubber."

MML. minimum masking level.

MMPI. Minnesota Multiphasic Personality Inventory.

mnemonics (ne-mon-iks) *n.* a method of improving the memory. The art of association in recall.

mobilization of stapes. surgical procedure designed to loosen the footplate of the stapes in the oval window, now largely superseded by stapedectomy.

modality (mo-dal'ĭ-te) *n.* that characteristic of a sensation by which it is distinguished from all other sensations.

modality, sense. grouping of sensory receptors serving a common purpose, e.g., hearing, vision.

mode *n.* 1. the manner by which a sensation reaches the brain, e.g., audition, vision. 2. the number that occurs most often in a frequency distribution.

mode of oscillation. the fundamental frequency with its natural harmonics—multiples of the fundamental.

modification (mod"ĭ-fĭ-ka'shun) *n.* a change in the designed response, e.g., by the use of filters or dampers.

modified Rainville (test). M-R. the masking noise is introduced through the forehead, rather than at the mastoid (as in the Rainville test).

modified rhyme test. MRT. multiple-choice speech test in which the listener is asked to circle the word spoken. The vowel nucleus in each set is the same but the consonants differ.

modified Stenger test. speech is used instead of pure tones for the Stenger test of malingering.

modified tone-decay test. MTDT. a pure tone is presented 5 dB above the threshold level. If and when the tone disappears the intensity is increased 5 dB. The number of

times this increase must be repeated (the shifts in one minute, for example) is noted as an index of the degree of tone decay at that frequency.

modiolus (mo-di'o-lus) *n.* bony axial pillar that supports the structures within the cochlea. The columella cochleae.

modiolus base. base of the modiolus, the part that rests on the bony structure between the oval and round windows.

modiolus, spiral canal of. tiny spiral canal within the modiolus that allows for the transmission of nerves and blood vessels.

modular *adj.* assembled from standardized units, e.g., some kinds of audiometers.

modular hearing aid. usually refers to a hearing aid built into a case designed to fit into the ear with a standard ear-tip, stock earmold, or earmold prepared for the purpose by the dispenser.

modulate *v.* to modify the frequency or amplitude.

modulation *n.* a controlled change in amplitude or frequency.

modulation, amplitude. variation of the amplitude of a radio carrier wave in relation to the strength of the audio or other signal.

modulation, frequency. variation of the frequency of a radio carrier wave in accordance with an audio or other signal.

module *n.* standardized electronic sub-assembly made up for use with other sub-assemblies to constitute an audiometer, for example.

modulus *pl.* **moduli** *n.* number used to express a relative physical effect.

mold *n.* earmold.

mold, CROS. earmold with minimal frame designed to hold a plastic tube in place in the external ear canal. At the same time the ear canal is left as open as possible.

monaural *adj.* pertaining to one ear.

monaural diplacusis. one tone appears to have two pitches in the same ear. Sometimes known as diplacusis uniauralis. The tone may just appear to be a noise.

monaural hearing. hearing with one ear.

monaural hearing aid. hearing aid designed to present amplified sound to only one ear.

monaural loudness balance test. a test for recruitment by comparing judgments of loudness between the frequencies in the same ear. A pure tone of a better (lower, preferably normal or nearly normal) frequency is presented at successively increasing levels above its threshold. A pure tone of a higher frequency is adjusted each time until the tones are judged to be equally loud. The values are plotted at the increasing levels of intensity to see if the differences decrease with the changes. *syn*: monaural bi-frequency equal loudness level test.

Monday morning clubber. MMC. one who seems to appear in the hearing aid dispenser's office with complaints every Monday morning.

Mondini's syndrome. symptoms include incomplete development or malformation of the inner ear.

mongolian *adj.* pertaining to the congenital form of mental deficiency known as mongolism—Down's syndrome.

mongolism, mongolianism *n.* a type of congenital mental deficiency with physical anomalies.

monitor *n.* a device to measure and indicate or control the intensity of speech sounds, (e.g., sound level meter or VU meter).

monitor *v.* to control the intensity of speech sounds for testing purposes.

monitored live voice. MLV. presentation of speech test materials by a vocal speaker who controls (monitors) the level of his voice through observation of a VU Meter.

monitoring audiometry. periodic retests of hearing to detect possible hearing loss from noise exposure, ototoxic drugs, and other causes.

mono- prefix meaning one.

monochord test. early device for testing hearing. It consisted of a taut wire activated by a hammer or a violin bow.

monomeric *adj.* concerning the hereditary or genetic control of a single part of the body, e.g., the ear.

monopack. hearing aid that combines the microphone, amplifier, and battery in a single case (as opposed to the early types in which these parts were separate).

monophasia *n.* type of aphasia in which speech is limited to a single word or phrase.

monophonic *adj.* pertaining to a recording or reproduction involving a single transmission path.

monosyllabic (mon″o-sĭ-lab′ik) *adj.* having only one syllable.

monosyllable (mon″o-sil′ă-bul) *n.* a word with only one syllable.

monotic (mon-o′tik) *adj.* one-eared.

monotone (mon′o-tōn) *n.* literally one tone. Speech in unchanging pitch.

monotonous (mo-not′ah-nus) *adj.* spoken in unchanging pitch.

monotony (mo-not′o-ne) *n.* unvaried pitch or sound.

monozygotic (mon″o-zi-got′ik) *adj.* developing from a single fertilized ovum, as an identical twin.

Moro's reflex or **response** (Ernst Moro, German physician, 1874-1951). a physical startle reaction to a stimulus in which the newborn tends to withdraw to the position in which it was carried in the womb.

Moro reflex test. the presentation of a sound stimulus to observe the reaction of a newborn.

morpheme (mor′fēm) *n.* the smallest meaningful unit of speech. It may be a word, as pan; or part of a word, as the "s" is pans. It is also sometimes used to refer to the basic signs used in sign language.

morpheme, free. one that is a complete word, e.g., pan, cat, ban.

morphology (mor-fol′o-je) *n.* the study of word formation. In biology, the study of the form and structure of animals and plants.

Mortimer audiometer (Hector Mortimer, Canada). early type of automatic or patient-controlled audiometer, which utilized a typewriter for recording responses to tone stimuli.

most comfortable loudness. MCL. range of intensity of sound (usually vocal) that an individual finds most pleasing.

most comfortable range. MCR. span of intensities of sound that an individual finds most acceptable.

motoneuron (mo″to-nu′ron) *n.* nerve cell that activates a muscular reaction. *syn:* motor neuron.

motor alexia. condition in which one can understand what he reads silently, but cannot read aloud.

motor aphasia. form of aphasia in which a person can understand, but cannot express himself in words, or read aloud.

motorboating. the "putt putt" sound that sometimes occurs in a hearing aid as the battery weakens.

moving coil or **dynamic earphone.** earphone with a diaphragm (of an especially thin sheet of metal) activated by an alternating signal current flowing through a connecting wire coil suspended in a magnetic field. The diaphragm thus activated changes (transduces) the electrical current to sound pressure waves for introduction directly into the ear canal.

moving coil loudspeaker. loudspeaker with a diaphragm activated by a moving coil in a fixed magnetic field.

moving coil microphone. microphone with a diaphragm that responds to sound pressure waves in activating a moving coil in a fixed magnetic field.

moving-iron receiver. magnetic receiver.

MPD. minimum perceptible difference. *syn:* DL. difference limen.

MPO. maximum power output. (Same as MDP).

MR. mentally retarded.

M-R. modified Rainville (test).

MRT. modified rhyme test.

msec. millisecond.

MTDT. modified tone decay test.

MTP. maximum tolerable pressure.

mucoid (mu'koid) *n.* resembling mucous.

mucoid (mucous) otitis media (mu'koid o-ti'tus me'de-ah). disease in which the middle ear is filled with thick, gummy fluid. In advanced stages adhesions develop around the eardrum, the windows, and the ossicles. *syn:* "glue ear", or chronic adhesive otitis media.

mucopereosteum (mu"ko-per"e-os'te-um) *n.* fibrous tissue covering bone that secretes mucous.

mucopurulent (mu"ko-pu'roo-lent) *adj.* mixture of mucous and pus.

mucosa (mu-ko'sah) *n.* the mucous membrane.

mucous (mu'kus) *adj.* pertaining to mucus.

mucous membrane. thin layer of tissue, containing fluid-secreting cells, which lines passages or cavities connecting with the air.

mucous otitis. commonly called glue ear and also known as adhesive otitis media. Chronic disease in which the middle ear is filled with thick gummy fluid. Since there is seldom any inflammation involved, many physicians refer to "otic transudates."

mucus *n.* sticky or gummy fluid produced by the mucous membrane and glands.

muffler, ear. device, such as a cotton-filled glass tumbler, formerly used to minimize transient masking noise during hearing tests.

Mueller tube. type of ear trumpet used by physicians to determine possible effect of surgery.

Mueller-Walle (Julius Mueller-Walle). German developer of an analytic method of teaching speechreading in which sounds in isolation are taught first. The patient then progresses to words, phrases, sentences, and finally paragraphs.

multi- (mul'ti). prefix meaning many—at least more than two.

multi-CROS. A CROS-BICROS hearing aid combination with a switch to make either arrangement easily available.

multiple-cueing. refers to the fact that speech understanding is unaffected for the normal ear when some of the frequencies are filtered out under controlled conditions.

multiple echo. reflections of an original sound wave stimulus that occur in separately distinguishable intervals. Echoes that occur more rapidly are called flutter echoes.

multiple sclerosis. brain or spinal cord damage resulting from excessive growth of fibrous tissues or patches of hardened tissue. It is characterized by paralysis, tremors, and jerky muscular action.

multisensory approach. teaching of communicative skills through the use of eyes (visual), ears (auditory), touch (tactile), and feel (kinesthetic).

MUM. maximum usable masking.

mumps *n.* infectious fever or inflammation of the parotid gland. When deafness occurs it is usually unilaterally sensorineural. Sometimes one ear is totally deaf and the other is perfectly normal. It may involve one or both parotid glands and one or both submaxillary saliva glands. Mumps virus sometimes causes damage called endolymphatic labyrinthitis. *syn:* epidemic parotitis or parotiditis.

murmur *n.* a usually soft, but sometimes rasping, or blowing continuous sound as heard on auscultation.

murmurs, aural. tinnitus. Noises originating within the ear.

muscle, stapedius. tiny muscle connected to the neck of the stirrup from the wall of the middle ear.

musculoplasty *n.* surgical reconstruction of the external auditory canal.

music deafness, musical deafness. inability to produce or understand music or musical sounds.

musical paracusis. a shift in the pitch of tones generally associated with threshold shifts in a limited frequency range.

mutant *adj.* concerning or produced by mutation.

mutation *n.* a basic change in genes that may be transmitted to offspring.

mute *adj.* unable to speak. Dumb. *n:* **muteness, mutism.**

mute *n.* a person who cannot speak.

mute *v.* to reduce the intensity of sound.

muteness *n.* condition of being unable to speak.

mutism *n.* condition of being unable to speak.

mutism, deaf. lack of speech resulting from inability to hear.

mycomyringitis (mi"ko-mir"in-ji'tis). inflammation of the eardrum resulting from the growth of a fungus. *syn:* myringomycosis.

mycosis (mi-ko'sis) *n.* any disease caused by a fungus. *adj:* **mycotic.**

mycotic otitis. inflammation of the ear caused by fungus.

mycotic otitis, external. inflammation of the outer ear canal caused by fungus or microorganisms. *syn:* myringomycosis.

myelin, myeline *n.* fatty insulating substance that covers most nerve fibers. *adj:* **myelinic.**

myelinated neuron. nerve cell covered by a myelin sheath.

myelin sheath. insulating nerve cover that speeds up the nerve impulse. *syn:* medullary sheath.

myelination (mi″ĕ-lĭ-na′shun), **myelinization** (mi″e-lĭ-nĭ-za′shun) *n.* the development of a fatty insulating substance (medullary or myelin sheath) around a nerve fiber.
myelitis (mi″ĕ-li′tis) *n.* inflammation of either the spinal cord or the bone marrow.
myeloencephalitis (mi″ĕ-lo-en-sef″ah-li′tis) *n.* inflammation involving the brain and spinal cord at the same time. *syn:* encephalomyelitis.
myelogram (mi′ĕ-lo-gram) *n.* a radiologic dye study—especially of the spinal cord.
myo- (mi′o). prefix meaning muscle.
myoclonus, palatal. spasms of the soft palate. A possible cause of objective tinnitus.
myofunctional (mi″o-funk′shun-al) *adj.* concerning muscular activity.
myogram (mi′o-gram) *n.* tracing made by a myograph.
myograph (mi′o-graf) *n.* instrument that makes tracings of muscular contraction. *adj:* **myographic.**
myringectomy (mir″in-jek′to-me) *n.* surgical removal of a part or all of the eardrum. *syn:* myringodectomy.
myringitis (mir″in-ji′tis) *n.* inflammation of the eardrum.
myringitis, bullous. viral infection of the eardrum that may cause it to split open. *syn:* myringodermatitis.
myringodectomy (mĭ-ring″go-dek′to-me) *n.* surgical removal of a part or all of the eardrum. *syn:* myringectomy.
myringodermatitis (mĭ-ring″go-der″mahti′tis) *n.* inflammation of the outer surface of the eardrum. *syn:* bullous myringitis.
myringomycosis (mĭ-ring″go-mi-ko′sis) *n.* condition resulting from the growth of a fungus in the external ear canal.
myringoplasty (mĭ-ring′go-plas″te) *n.* surgical correction (rebuilding) of defective eardrum.
myringostapediopexy (mĭ-ring″go-stah-pe′de-o-pek″se) *n.* fixation of the head of the stapes to the tense portion of the eardrum. *syn:* stapediomyringopexy.
myringoscope (mĭ-ring′go-skōp) *n.* instrument for viewing the eardrum. An otoscope.
myringotome (mĭ-ring′go-tōm) *n.* knife designed for opening the eardrum.
myringotomy (mir″in-got′o-me) *n.* surgical opening of the eardrum. *syn:* tympanotomy.
myxedema (mik″sĕ-de′mah) *n.* disorder caused by thyroid deficiency. Symptoms include subcutaneous edema, drying of skin, loss of hair, and muscular weakness. A possible cause of tinnitus.

N

N. international hearing aid symbol for normal tone-control position.
n. number (included in a report) or norm.
NAD. National Association of the Deaf. nothing abnormal detected (as used in Britain).
NAEL. National Association of Earmold Laboratories.
NAHSA. National Association of Hearing and Speech Agencies.
nano- (na′no). prefix indicating dwarfed. 2. prefix indicating one-billionth (10^{-9}). Sometimes called milli-micro-.
nanogram (na′no-gram) *n.* one-billionth of a gram.
nanoliter (na″no-le′ter) *n.* one-billionth of a liter.
nanosecond (na″no-sek′ond) *n.* one-billionth of a second.
nanovolt (na′no-volt) *n.* one-billionth of a volt.
narco- (nar′ko). prefix referring to sleep.
narcosynthesis (nar″ko-sin′thĕ-sis) *n.* type of therapy utilizing hypnosis or narcotics to induce sleep. *syn:* narcotherapy.
nares (na′rēz) *n.* (*pl.*) nostrils.
naris (na′ris) *n.* (*sing.*) nostril.
narrow band masking. use of filtered bands of white noise for masking purposes. Special circuits designed to present a mixture of tones centering around each test frequency may also be used.
narrow band noise. sound made up of a narrow range of frequencies of equal intensity.
narrow range audiometer. one designed to test the response to one, two, or three pure tone frequencies at limited sound pressure levels for hearing screening purposes.
NAS. National Academy of Sciences.
nasal (na′zal) *n.* consonant sound made by using the resonant chambers of the nasopharynx: m, n, ng.
nasal *adj.* pertaining to the nose.
NASC. National Alliance of Senior Citizens.
naso- (na′zo). prefix meaning the nose.
nasopharyngeal (na″zo-fah-rin′je-al) *adj.* concerning the area adjoining the nose and throat.
nasopharynx (na″zo-far′inks) *n.* upper part of the throat continuous with the nasal passage.
natal (na′tal) *adj.* concerning birth.

natal hypoxia (hi-pok'se-ah) *n.* hypoxia that occurs during the birth process.

National Academy of Sciences. NAS.

National Alliance of Senior Citizens. NASC.

National Association of the Deaf. NAD.

National Association of Earmold Laboratories. NAEL.

National Association of Hearing and Speech Agencies. NAHSA.

National Bureau of Standards. NBS.

National Captioning Institute. NCI.

National Hearing Aid Society. NHAS.

National Institute for the Deaf (Great Britain). NID.

National Institutes of Health. NIH.

National Institue of Mental Health. NIMH.

National Institute for Neurological Diseases and Blindness. NINDB.

National Rehabilitation Association. NRA.

National Research Council. NRC.

National Science Foundation. NSF.

National Technical Institute for the Deaf. NTID.

natural communication. method of teaching deaf and hearing-impaired children to hear and speak by providing consistent, continuous, and appropriate binaural amplification. Auditory training is carried on in a natural manner, through the child's own hearing aids, using an orderly arrangement of teaching/learning experiences.

natural or normal frequency. number of cycles per second at which it is easiest for a mass to vibrate—whether gas, liquid, or solid. *syn*: resonant frequency.

natural pitch. fundamental frequency that appears most often in a class of musical instruments or voices: about 100 Hz for men's voices and about 200 Hz for women's and children's voices. *syn*: optimal pitch.

NBM. narrow band noise.

NBS. National Bureau of Standards.

NCI. National Captioning Institute.

NDT. noise detection threshold.

near ear. ear on the same side of the head as the signal source.

Nebraska test. test of hearing or understanding of verbal directions that also indicates levels of intelligence. *syn*: Hiskey-Nebraska Test of Learning Aptitude.

necr-, necro- (nek'ro). combining form relating to death or a corpse.

necrosis (ně-kro'sis) *pl.* **necroses** *n.* death or mortification of cells or tissue. *adj*: **necrotic.**

necrosis of the incus. death or mortification of the incus.

necrosis of the ossicular chain. death or mortification of the ossicular chain.

necrotize (ně'kro-tīz) *v.* to become mortified.

necrotizing otitis media. destruction of the eardrum as a result of infection.

negative electrode. 1. cathode or element that releases electrons when heated in a vacuum tube. 2. cathode of a hearing aid cell that releases negative ions.

negative feedback. results when an out-of-phase (or inverted) signal of an amplifier is fed back to a previous stage to reduce amplification or harmonic distortion. *syn*: out-of-phase, degenerative, or inverse feedback.

NEL. noise exposure level—term replaced by PEL: permissible exposure limit.

neo- combining form meaning new.

neologism (ne-ol'o-jizm) *n.* 1. a new meaning given to an old word or phrase or the creation of a new word, common in new fields such as audiology. 2. meaningless words coined or used by the mentally unbalanced.

neomycin (ne'o-mi"sin) *n.* an antibiotic—one that may impair hearing through damage to the hair cells.

neomycin sulfate. a form of the antibiotic neomycin.

neonatal (ne"o-na'tal) *adj.* concerning the newborn. *n.* **neonate.**

neonatal hemolytic disease. HDN. hyperbilirubinemia.

neonatal jaundice. icterus neonatorum or hemolytic disease of the newborn (HDN). It results from abnormal amount of bile pigment (bilirubin) in the blood. A cause of sensorineural deafness.

neonate, neonatus *n.* newborn baby.

neonatology (ne"o-na-tol'o-je) *n.* study of the diseases of the newborn.

neo-oralism *n.* name given to a method of teaching speech and language in Russian schools.

neophobia *n.* fear of new things or change.

neoplasia *n.* new (neo) growth of abnormal tissue, as in a tumor.

neoplasm *n.* new growth, a tumor. *adj*: **neoplastic.**

neostomy (ne-os'to-me) *n.* creation of a new or artificial opening by surgery.

neper (ne'per) *n.* unit of logarithmic ratio devised by John Neper (Napier), Scottish mathematician (1550-1617). It is used in some European countries. One neper equals 8.686 dB.

nephritis (ně-fri'tis) *pl.* **nephritides** *n.* inflammation of the kidneys, more commonly known as Bright's disease. In some cases, especially in the hereditary form, it is associated with a sensorineural hearing impairment.

nephritis, hereditary. a type of familial kidney disease which may be accompanied by sensorineural hearing loss.

nerve, acoustic (auditory). the eighth (VIIIth) nerve, or eighth cranial nerve; the cable of nerve fibers that carries impulses between the inner ear and the brain. It consists of two branches—vestibular (balance) and cochlear (hearing).

nerve, afferent. one that carries impulses toward the central nervous system or brain. *syn*: centripetal nerve.

nerve, auditory. the acoustic nerve.

nerve, balance. vestibular nerve that joins with the cochlear nerve to become the auditory or acoustic nerve (VIIIth cranial nerve).

nerve, cochlear. branch of the eighth cranial (acoustic) nerve that arises in the cochlea and conveys sound stimuli to the brain. The nerve of hearing.

nerve, cranial. cerebral nerve.

nerve deafness. obsolete term for sensorineural hearing loss.

nerve, efferent. one that carries impulses away from the brain or central nervous system. *syn*: centrifugal nerve.

nerve, eighth. the VIIIth cranial nerve combines fibers of the cochlear and vestibular nerves. *syn*: acoustic or auditory nerve.

nerve, facial. the VIIth cranial nerve. It accompanies the VIIIth nerve through the internal auditory canal. Some of its branches control muscles of the external and middle ear; e.g., the chorda tympani.

nerve fiber. the long process of a nerve cell; the axon.

nerve, fifth. the Vth cranial nerve serves part of the head, jaws, and eyes. A branch connects with the tensor tympani. *syn*: trigeminal nerve.

nerve force. ability of nerve fibers to transmit stimuli.

nerve impulse. the successive changes in the protoplasm of a nerve cell that result from stimulation and transmit a sensation.

nerve, Jacobson's. the tympanic nerve—an afferent nerve that serves the eardrum and the middle ear.

nerve loss. old term for sensorineural hearing impairment.

nerve, mixed. nerve cable that contains both afferent and efferent nerve fibers.

nerve, motor. efferent nerve cell that activates a muscular reaction. *syn*: motor neuron.

nerve pulse. burst of electrical energy that moves along the nerve fiber in response to a stimulus.

nerves, cerebral (ser′ĕ-bral, sĕ-re′bral). also known as cranial nerves, 12 major pairs arise in the brain. The two pair that go through the internal auditory canal are of special audiologic interest. They are the VIIth, known as the facial nerve; and the VIIIth, variously known as the auditory, acoustic, or vestibulo-cochlear nerves—the nerves of hearing and balance.

nerve, sensory. afferent nerve that carries a stimulus toward the central nervous system or brain.

nerves, radial. neurons that separate from the cochlear nerve and move out from the center of the cochlea to connect with some of the hair cells.

nerve, seventh. the VIIth cranial or facial nerve.

nerve, space. branch of the vestibular nerve that connects with the semicircular canals for orientation in space.

nerves, spiral. neurons that separate from the cochlear nerve and move along the perimeter of the cochlea and branch inward to serve some of the hair cells.

nerve, stapedial (stah-pe′de-al). branch of the facial nerve (VIIth cranial) that connects with the stapedius, the muscle controlling the stapes.

nerve, trigeminal (tri-jem′ĭ-nal). the Vth cranial nerve that serves part of the head, jaws, and eyes. A branch connects with the tensor tympani.

nerve, tympanic (tim-pan′ik). an afferent nerve that serves the eardrum and the middle ear. *syn*: Jacobson's nerve.

nerve, vestibular (ves-tib′u-lar). branch of the VIIIth cranial nerve that serves the utricle and the semicircular canals.

nerve, vestibulocochlear. acoustic or auditory nerve.

nerve, Voit's (voit). branch of the auditory nerve that serves the saccule.

neural epithlium. surface layer of cells that contain nerve endings of special sense, e.g., the hair cells of the inner ear.

neurepithelium (nūr″ep-ĭ-the′le-um) *n.* neural epithelium—the hair cells of the inner ear.

neurinoma, acoustic (nu″rĭ-no′mah). tumor of the VIIIth cranial nerve. *syn*: acoustic neuroma.

neurocirculatory (nu″ro-cir′cu-lah-to″re) *adj.* pertaining to both the nervous system and the blood circulatory system.

neurocyte (nu′ro-sīt) *n.* a neuron or nerve cell.

neurocytoma (nu″ro-si-to′mah) *n.* tumor involving nerve tissue.

neuroepithelial (nu″ro-ep-ĭ-the′le-al) *adj.* pertaining to neuroepithelium.

neuroepithelioma (nu″ro-ep″ĭ-the″le-o′mah) *n.* tumor arising in neuroepithelium.

neuroepithelium *n.* variant of neurepithelium, e.g., the hair cells of the inner ear.

neurofibril *n.* tiny fiber within a nerve cell that may be a conducting element *adj*: **neurofibrillary.**

neurofibroma (nu″ro-fi-bro′mah) *n.* tumor involving nerves—usually nerve endings—which may affect the acoustic nerves.

neurofibromatosis (nu″ro-fi″bro-mah-to′sis) *n.* disease characterized by numerous tumors involving nerve endings or the connective tissue of nerves. *syn*: von Recklinghausen's disease.

neurogenic (nu″ro-jen′ik) *adj.* arising in the nervous system.

neurogenous (nu-roj′ĕ-nus) *adj.* relating to the nervous system.

neuroglia (nu-rog′le-ah) *n.* cells that support nerve tissue in the brain and spinal cord. *adj*: **neuroglial, neurogliar.**

neuroglioma (nu″ro-gli-o′mah) *n.* an uncontrolled new growth of tissue (neoplasm or tumor) within the brain tissue (parenchyma). *syn*: gliomatosis, glioma.

neurohumor *n.* a chemical released at a nerve-ending which helps in the transmission of a nerve impulse. *adj*. **neurohumoral.**

neurologic, neurological *adj.* concerning the study of nervous diseases.

neurology (nu-rol′o-je) *n.* the study of the nervous system and its diseases.

neurolymph *n.* the cerebrospinal fluid.

neurolysin *n.* poison that affects nerves.

neuroma (nu-ro′mah) *pl.* **neuromas, neuromata** *n.* a tumor involving a nerve or the nervous system.

neuroma, acoustic. tumor of the VIIIth cranial nerve.

neuromast (nu′ro-mast) *n.* nerve receptor with cilia or hair-like projections enclosed in a flexible mass of gelatinous material, e.g., into the cupola of the ampullary crest.

neuromotor (nu″ro-mo′tor) *adj.* pertaining to a motor or efferent nerve.

neuromuscular (nu″ro-mus′ku-lar) *adj.* pertaining to nerves and muscles together.

neuron (nu′ron) *n.* a nerve cell. *adj*: **neuronal.**

neuron, myelinated (mi′ĕ-lĭ-nāt″ed). nerve cell covered by a myelin sheath.

neuron, second-order. nerve cell lying beyond at least one synapse from the specialized nerve ending or receptor.

neuronitis, vestibular. inflammation of the vestibular nerve cells of the ear. A possible cause of tinnitus. Dizziness may accompany this disorder. There is seldom a hearing loss.

neuropathology (nu″ro-pah-thol′o-je) *n.* study of diseases of the nervous system.

neuropathy (nu-rop′ah-the) *n.* disease involving the nervous system.

neurophonia *n.* rare disorder of the speech muscles that causes involuntary cries and other spasmodic sounds.

neurophysiological *adj.* concerning the study of the physical structure of the nervous system.

neurophysiology *n.* study of the physical composition of nerves and the nervous system.

neuropsychiatry (nu″ro-si-ki′ah-tre) *n.* NP. science devoted to the treatment of nervous and mental disease—either functional or organic. *adj*: **neuropsychiatric.**

neurosensory (nu″ro-sen′so-re) *adj.* involving the nervous pathways and/or the brain. *syn*: sensorineural (used more often).

neurotherapeutics (nu″ro-ther″ah-pu′tiks) **neurotherapy** (nu″ro-ther′ah-pe) *n.* treatment of diseases of the nerves.

neurotic (nu-rot′ik) *adj.* emotional instability connected with an affliction of the nervous system.

neurotic profit. unconscious use of an impairment to excuse lack of achievement or to gain attention.

neurotoxic (nu″ro-tok′sik) *adj.* poisonous to the nerves. *n*: **neurotoxicity.**

neurotoxin (nu″ro-tok′sin) *n.* a poison that affects nerves.

neurovascular (nu″ro-vas′ku-lar) *adj.* concerning both the nerves and blood system.

nevus (ne′vus) *n.* a mole or vascular tumor that may occur in the ear.

newton *n.* (Sir Isaac Newton, English mathematician, 1642-1727). a unit of physical force. It would cause a mass of one kilogram to accelerate at the rate of one meter per second. One newton equals 10^5 dynes.

NHA. National Hearing Association.

NHAS. National Hearing Aid Society. Formerly SHAA, Society of Hearing Aid Audiologists.

niacin (ni′ah-sin) *n.* nicotinic acid—an acid of the vitamin-B complex. Used in some cases of deafness, tinnitus, and Meniere's syndrome.

niacinamide (ni″ah-sin′am-īd) *n.* a nicotinic acid similar to niacin but causes less flushing. *syn*: nicotinamide.

nicotinamide (ni″ko-tin′ah-mīd) *n.* one of the vitamin-B complexes used in the same manner as nicotinic acid. *syn*: niacinamide.

nicotinic acid (nik″o-tin′ik). an acid of the vitamin-B complex. A vasodilator used in some cases of deafness, tinnitus, and in Meniere's syndrome.

NID. National Institute for the Deaf (Great Britain).

nidus (ni′dus) *n.* 1. a nest or cluster of cells. 2. focal point of infection. 3. point of origin or nucleus of a nerve.

Nielsen group test (Svend F. Nielsen, U.S.). The hearing sensitivity of a number of children is determined at the same time by scoring their indicated responses as intensities decrease during the random presentation of a series of long and short tones.

NIH. National Institute of Health.

NIHL. noise-induced hearing loss.

NIL. noise interference level.

NIMH. National Institute of Mental Health.

NINDB. National Institute for Neurological Diseases and Blindness.

Nitchie, Edward B. developer of the synthetic method of teaching speechreading in which the patient begins by learning to recognize the meaning of whole paragraphs. Compare Mueller-Walle.

noci- (no'se). combining form meaning painful.

nociceptive (no"se-sep'tiv) *adj.* painful or responding to a painful stimulus. (As used in some types of evoked response audiometry).

nociceptor *n.* a sense organ that reponds to painful stimuli.

node *n.* 1. a point in a standing wave that has no amplitude. 2. a point in a vibrating system that is free of vibration. 3. a knot of one type of tissue enclosed in tissue of another type, e.g., lymph node. 4. a firm tumor.

node, partial. a portion of a standing wave system that has minimum amplitude but is not zero.

node of Ranvier. one of the spots along a nerve cell where the myelin sheath is broken and the nerve is exposed. The nerve impulse jumps from node to node—thus speeding it up.

nodule (nod'ūl) *n.* A small node or lump.

no-echo chamber. an anechoic room—one without echoes or reverberations.

noise *n.* unwanted sound. Random irregularity of wave-form.

noise *v.* to make a sound or to talk loudly.

noise, ambient. surrounding sounds of the environment or sounds in an amplifying system which are not part of the wanted signal. *syn:* background noise.

noise analyzer. an instrument designed to determine the frequency components of a particular noise; e.g., the sound levels in bands one-third, one-half, or one octave, in widths may be measured.

noise audiogram. an audiogram based on the use of narrow bands of white noise.

noise, background. the surrounding sounds of the environment. Ambient noise.

noise box, Barany. device operated by a key-wound spring to produce complex noise for masking purposes.

noise, broad-band. sound containing a wide range of frequencies.

noise, clothing. noise produced in a body-worn hearing aid by clothes rubbing across the microphone.

noise, complex. as used in masking for bone conduction tests, complex noise consists of a fundamental frequency of 120 Hz and numerous harmonics. It is sometimes called sawtooth masking.

noise detection threshold. NDT.

noise, extraneous. the sounds of the environment. *syn:* ambient noise.

noise floor. 1. the level of ambient noise below which accurate sound measurements should not be expected. 2. the basic circuit noise of a hearing aid or audiometer. *syn:* circuit noise.

noise, Gaussian (gow'shun). white noise—a sound that contains equal amounts of energy in all frequencies.

noise, impact. see noise, impulse.

noise, impulse. transient noise with a sharp rise and fall time around a peak of high intensity; e.g., gunfire and explosions. *syn:* impact noise.

noise-induced hearing loss. NIHL. hearing loss that develops gradually from continuous exposure to noise above acceptable levels.

noise interference level. NIL. sound pressure level at which noise interferes with the understanding of speech. *syn:* speech interference level. SIL.

noise level. the sound pressure level of a noise as indicated by a sound level meter. If measured on a weighted scale the weighting should be indicated.

noise level, perceived. a comparison of the sound pressure level of the 910-1090 Hz band and another sound as measured in units known as PNdBs. See noy.

noise, narrow-band. sound made up of a narrow range of frequencies of equal intensity.

noise, pink. random noise similar to white noise but whose spectrum level decreases with increase in frequency (3 dB per octave) to provide constant energy per octave of bandwidth.

noise pollution. ambient or background noise of sufficient intensity to damage hearing or cause stress.

noise, random. a complex sound wave whose instantaneous amplitudes vary in time according to a normal distribution curve.

noise reduction rating. NRR.

noise, saw-tooth. a sound made up of a fundamental frequency of about 60 or 120 Hz with all its harmonics to 10,000 Hz in random phase. *syn:* complex noise.

noise, speech. a wide band of noise utilizing the frequencies between 500 and 2000 Hz—sometimes used for masking during speech audiometry.

noise, white. sound that contains equal amounts of energy in all frequencies. *syn:* Gaussian noise.

noise, wide-band. sound containing a wide range of frequencies. *syn:* broad-band noise.

noises, ear. noises originating within the ear itself. *syn:* tinnitus; susurrus aurium (ear whispers); or tinnitus cerebri.

noisy (noi′ze) *adj.* consisting of unwanted sound.

nomograph, audiometric (nah′mo-graf). graphic representation of the audiometric results to be expected from a surgical procedure.

non- (non). prefix meaning no, not, or none.

nonauditory effects of noise. the stress, fatigue, breakdown of work efficiency and health, which are among the harmful effects of continuous exposure to noise that is above acceptable levels.

nonconductor *n.* a material that is a poor conductor of sound, heat, or electricity.

nonconsensual *adj.* concerning a reflex that has no direct relationship to the stimulus.

nonlanguage scale test. test that depends upon standardized pantomime and gestures to transmit instructions.

nonlinear distortion (non-lin′e-ar). inexact reproduction of a sound wave pattern that results when the output of an electroacoustical system is not proportional to the input. *syn:* amplitude distortion.

nonoccluding earmold (non″ŏ-klōōd′ing). a tubing-type earmold that leaves the ear canal open to the outside air.

nonorganic deafness (non-or-gan′ik). deafness or hearing loss that has little or no physical damage as a basis. It may be: 1. a purposeful effort to show a worse-than-actual hearing loss, as in malingering—feigned or simulated deafness. 2. a subconscious effort to show a worse-than-actual hearing loss, as in psychogenic or hysterical deafness. Either type may also be referred to as functional hearing loss.

nonperiodic (non-pe″re-od′ik) *adj.* occurring at irregular intervals. *syn:* aperiodic.

nonpurulent (non-pu′roo-lent) *adj.* containing no pus.

nonsense syllable. monosyllable that has no meaning. Used in difficult speech discrimination tests.

nonsuppurative (non-sup′u-ra″tiv) *adj.* not pus-forming.

nonsyllabic (non-sĭ-lab′ik) *adj.* concerning a speech sound that does not constitute a syllable or the important part of a syllable.

nonverbal (nonverb′al) *adj.* unable to talk.

nonvibratory tinnitus. subjective tinnitus—head noises that can be heard only by the patient.

norepinephrine (nor″ep-ĭ-nef′rin) *n.* a chemical transmitter of a nerve impulse.

no response. NR. lack of reaction to a stimulus.

norm (norm) *n.* standard established for a homogeneous group—the average or mean of any qualification or quantification of the group.

Northampton charts. charts of consonants and vowels that have secondary spellings to indicate the pronunciation.

noso- (nos′o). prefix referring to disease.

nosography (no-sog′rah-fe) *n.* symptomatic description of diseases.

nosological (nos″o-loj′e-kal) *adj.* concerning the classification of diseases.

nosology (no-sol′o-je) *n.* the study and classification of diseases.

notch, Carhart. a dip in the bone conduction audiogram of 5 dB at 500, and 4000 Hz, 10 dB at 1000 dB, and 15 dB at 2000 Hz. It results from the inability of the fluids to move freely in the cochlea when the footplate of the stapes is firmly fixed in the oval window.

notch, Rivinus'. a niche in the upper part of the annular ring that contains the flaccid part of the eardrum.

noy *n.* unit of subjective measurement of perceived noisiness. One noy is the subjective sensation of loudness given by listeners to the band of frequencies from 910 to 1090 Hz at a sound pressure level of 40 dB. Suggested by Karl D. Kryter.

NP. neuropsychiatry, or neuropsychiatric.

NR. no response.

NRA. National Rehabilitation Association.

NRC. National Research Council.

NRR. noise reduction rating.

NSF. National Science Foundation.

NTID. National Technical Institute for the Deaf.

nuclear hearing loss. hearing loss resulting from a lesion within the dorsal and ventral cochlear nuclei. It is said to be a result of RH incompatibility.

nucleus (nu′kle-us) *n.* 1. the central bit of different protoplasm that serves as the control center of a cell. 2. a mass of nerve cells in any part of the brain or spinal cord.

nucleus, cochlear. the collective terminations of the cochlear nerve fibers in the brain stem and from which the central auditory pathways arise.

Nuel's space (Jean P. Nuel, Belgian otologist, 1847-1920). a cleft or intermediate tunnel between the inner and outer tunnels of the organ of Corti. These spaces provide a passageway for nerve fibers and the endolymph which bathes and nourishes the inner cells.

null *v.* to cancel the magnetic spillover of an electrical system; e.g., the cancelling—or nulling—loop that may be used to confine the signal of an induction loop system to the room of initial installation.

null hypothesis. a tentative assumption made for the sake of discussion that a statement is not true in order to test its validity. A reverse hypothesis.

nyctaphonia (nik″tah-fo′ne-ah) *n.* nonorganic or functional loss of voice during the night.

nyctophonia (nik″to-fo′ne-ah) *n.* nonorganic or functional loss of voice only during the day.

nystagmogram (nis-tag′mo-gram) *n.* a chart of the involuntary movements of the eyeball in caloric tests of nystagmus.

nystagmograph *n.* an instrument for recording the involuntary movements of the eyeball in tests of nystagmus.

nystagmus (nis-tag′mus) *n.* involuntary movements of the eyeball. They may be constant, as the result of disease, or induced, as in caloric tests of nystagmus.

nystagmus, audiokinetic. involuntary movements of the eyeball that may result from sudden loud sounds or the touching of the canthus.

nystagmus, aural. nystagmus resulting from labyrinthine disturbances. It is characterized by involuntary eyeball movements— first rather slowly in one direction, then by quick jerking movements in the opposite direction.

nystagmus test. Water or gas is used alternately above and below body temperature to irrigate the external ear canal. The resulting involuntary eye movements are studied in relation to vestibular or labyrinthine function.

O

O. international hearing aid symbol for off. (Out of operation, as opposed to I: In operation.)

OBA. octave band analyzer.

objective (ob-jek′tiv) *adj.* responses unaffected by voluntary control. The opposite of subjective.

objective tests of hearing. a measurement of hearing sensitivity that does not depend on a voluntary response from the testee.

objective tinnitus. head noises arising from muscular spasms or blood-flow disturbances within the external or middle ear. Rare in occurrence, they may be audible to the examiner. *syn:* clicking tinnitus, Leudet's tinnitus; vibrating tinnitus.

obmutescence (ob″mu-tes′ens) *n.* loss of ability to speak. *syn:* aphonia.

obstruction, earwax. the problem caused by wax obstructing the ear is technically known as ceruminosis.

obstructive deafness. conductive deafness.

obturator foramen (ob′tu-ra″tor fo-ra′men). The closure for an opening; e.g., the stapes as a closure for the oval window.

occipital (ok-sip′ĭ-tal) *adj.* pertaining to the back of the head. *n:* **occipital.**

occlude *v.* to close tightly, obstruct or join together. *adj:* **occludent, occlusive.**

occlusion *n.* the condition of being closed or of fitting together.

occlusion of the eustachian tube. closure of the eustachian tube. *syn:* acute eustachian salpingitis.

occlusion test. a comparison of the response to a bone vibrator stimulus when the external ear canal is left open and then closed. Also known as the Bing test, the comparison of absolute and relative bone conduction thresholds is essentially an occlusion test.

occult (ŏ-kult′) *adj.* 1. not obvious 2. symptoms only recognized by special examination or study of familial or personal history.

occupational deafness. more commonly known as noise-induced hearing loss— from industrial noise.

Occupational Safety and Health Act. OSHA.

octave *n.* the interval between two frequencies, one of which is twice as large as the other.

octave band. a spread of frequencies whose upper limit is twice the lower.

octave band analyzer. an instrument that has a number of electronic filters to provide for the measurement of noise in selected frequency spreads (octave bands).

octave band filter. electronic instrument designed to allow preselected frequencies to be heard or measured at octave intervals.

ocular audition. old term for speechreading (John Bulwer, 1644).

oculogyric reflex. (ok″u-lo-ji′rik). a movement of the eyeball, e.g., one that might result from an auditory stimulus.

OD. outside diameter.

odynacousis, odynacusis (o″din-ah-ku′sis). an unusual sensitivity of hearing so that noises cause pain.

oedema (edema) (ĕ-de′mah) *n.* abnormal accumulation of fluid in body tissues or cavities. *syn:* hydrops, as in endolymphatic hydrops—Meniere's.

OEM. opposite ear masked.

oersted (er′sted) (Hans Christian Oersted— Danish physicist, 1777-1851). a unit of measurement of intensity of a magnetic field.

ogive (o′jiv) *n.* statistically, a curve of numerical frequencies that rises slowly, then steeply, then slowly to 100 per cent. *adj:* **ogival.**

OHC. outer hair cell.

ohm *n.* unit of measurement of electrical resistance.

ohm, acoustic. unit of measurement of resistance to the flow of sound pressure waves through a medium. The unit is equal to a pressure amplitude of one dyne per square centimeter per second of flux amplitude.

ohm, mechanical. the unit of mechanical impedance. It is equal to the force of one dyne divided by a velocity of one centimeter per second.

ohmmeter (ōm′me-ter) *n.* instrument for measuring electric resistance in ohms.

Ohm's law (George Simon Ohm, German physicist, 1787-1854). 1. the human ear perceives the components of a complex wave stimulus separately, not as a single sound. 2. the intensity of an electric current (in amperes) is equal to the electromotive force (emf-in volts) divided by the resistance.

olivacochlear (o″li-vah-kok′le-ar) *adj.* pertaining to the bundle of nerve fibers between cochlea and olivary nucleus.

olivacochlear bundle. an olive-shaped group of nerve cells that carry impulses from the brain to the cochlea.

olivary complex. a junction of nerve fibers on their pathway to the brain. See superior olivary complex.

olophonia (ol″lo-fo′ne-ah) *n.* unnatural speech due to malformation of the vocal organs.

omnidirectional *adj.* refers to a microphone that picks up sound from all directions.

onomatomania (on″o-mat″o-ma′ne-ah) *n.* uncontrollable impulse to repeat certain words or sounds.

onomatophobia (on″o-mat″o-fo′be-ah) *n.* abnormal fear of hearing certain words or names because of imaginary evils attached.

onomatopoeia (on″o-mat″o-po-e′-ah) *n.* the echoic principle in language; that is, the formation of a word (buzz) or a name (bobwhite quail) to imitate a sound. *adj:* **onomatopoeic, onomatopoetic.**

onomatopoiesis (on″o-mat″o-poi-e′sis) *n.* the formation of words that have no meaning—in imitation of sounds.

onychodystrophy (on″ĭ-ko-dis′tro-fe) *n.* congenital defect or weakening of fingernails often associated with congenital deafness.

opeidoscope (o-pi′do-skōp) *n.* a device using a mirror to reflect rays of light altered by voice vibrations on a screen.

open BICROS. BICROS arrangement that utilizes open earmolds or tubing alone to the aidable ear.

open syllable. syllable that ends in a vowel or diphthong.

opisthotic (o″pis-thot′ik) *adj.* located behind or within the inner ear.

opposite phase. two tones of the same frequency and intensity are said to be in opposite phase or out of phase when their cycles of compression and rarefaction are opposite each other (or separated by ½ cycle). These tones then cancel each other out so there is zero amplitude.

optimal pitch. the fundamental frequency that appears most often in a class of musical instruments or voices: about 100 Hz for men's voices and 250 Hz for women's and children's voices. *syn:* natural pitch.

optokinetic (op″to-kĭ-net′ik) *adj.* concerning eye movements in response to a stimulus. Nystagmus.

orad *adv.* near the mouth.

oral *adj.* 1. spoken or using speech as in the oral method of teaching the deaf. 2. involving the mouth.

oral cavity. the mouth—especially when considered as a resonator for speech.

oral method. teaching the deaf to communicate in as nearly normal a manner as possible using amplification, speech, and speechreading.

oralism *n.* training the deaf to communicate by word of mouth—including speechreading.

orancusis, orankusis (or″an-ku′sis) *n.* total lack of ability to hear.

orbicular (or-bik′u-lar) *adj.* circular or spherical.

orbicularis oculi reflex. the auropalpebral reflex—a twitch of the eyelid or corner of the eye resulting from a stimulus such as a loud sound.

ordinate (or′dĭ-nāt) *n.* the vertical coordinate of a graph; e.g., intensities on an audiogram.

organ *n.* a part of the body performing a special function; e.g., the ear is the organ of hearing.

organ, acoustic. uncommon name for the organ of Corti.

organ (end). the specialized termination of a system of nerve fibers that serves as a receptor; e.g., the organ of Corti is considered the end-organ of hearing.

organ of balance. the semicircular canals of the internal ear. Situated at right angles to each other in three planes, movement of the fluid (endolymph) within the canals activates the hair cells that initiate nerve impulses. These nerve impulses are conducted along the vestibular nerve to the cortex to be interpreted by the brain for orientation in space, and thus help to maintain equilibrium.

organ of Corti. a structure resting on the basilar membrane within the cochlear duct (scala media). It contains the essential sensory elements of hearing, the hair cells, and their supporting cells. The function of the hair cells is to convert sound pressure

97

waves into nerve impulses, which are transmitted by way of the VIIIth cranial nerve to the brain. It is the end-organ of hearing. *syn*: organum spirale.

organ spirale. the organ of Corti. *syn*: acoustic papilla.

organic (or-gan'ik) *adj.* concerning an organ of the body.

organic defect. an impairment resulting from a structural alteration or weakness. There may be a functional overlay that compounds the problem psychologically.

organoleptic (or″gah-no-lep'tik) *adj.* affecting one of the special sense organs.

organon auditus. Latin: auditory system. *syn*: the organ of hearing.

organon spirale. Latin: spiral organ in the cochlea. *syn*: organ of Corti.

organum (or'gah-num) *n.* an organ—as in organum spirale (organ of Corti). *syn*: organon.

orifice (or'ĭ-fis) *n.* an opening to any body cavity.

origin (or'ĭ-jin) *n.* the point of attachment of a muscle to the relatively fixed portion of the anatomy.

oro- (o'ro). prefix meaning mouth.

orolingual (o″ro-ling'gwal) *adj.* pertaining to the mouth and tongue.

oronasal (o″ro-na'zal) *adj.* pertaining to the mouth and nose.

oropharynx (o″ro-far'inks) *n.* portion of the pharynx below the soft palate and above the larynx.

orosensory (o″ro-sen'so-re) *adj.* concerning the sense associated with oral stimulation—hearing and speechreading.

orotund (o'ro-tund) *adj.* speech distinguished by fullness, clarity, and strength.

orthoepic (or″tho-ep'ik) *adj.* concerning the study of pronunciation.

orthoepist (or″tho-ep'ist) *n.* a specialist in pronunciation.

orthoepy (or″tho-ep'e) *n.* the study of word pronunciation.

orthogenics (or″tho-gen'iks) *n.* the study of the treatment of mental or physical defects that retard normal development. *adj*: **orthogenic, orthogenetic.**

orthotelephonic gain (or″tho-tel-ĕ-fon'ik). the additional sound pressure reaching the eardrum when a hearing aid is used—compared to the sound pressure reaching the eardrum without a hearing aid. *syn*: real ear, etymotic, or insertion gain.

oscillate (os″ĭ-lāt) *v.* to vibrate or move back and forth between two points.

oscillation (os″ĭ-la'shun) *n.* vibration—moving back and forth between two points.

oscillation, mode of. the fundamental frequency with its natural harmonics—multiples of the fundamental.

oscillator (os'ĭ-la″tor) *n.* an electronic device to produce tones of a desired frequency.

oscillator, pure tone. a device designed to produce a tone of one frequency without harmonics.

oscillogram *n.* a graphic recording of sound waves or vibrations made by an oscillograph. Less often a picture of sound waves as they appear on an oscilloscope.

oscillograph *n.* a device that records vibrating wave forms—especially those made by sound waves.

oscilloscope *n.* a vacuum tube similar to a television tube, designed to make sound waves visible.

OSHA. Occupational Safety and Health Administration.

-osis (o'sis). suffix indicating an abnormal condition or disease.

osseous *adj.* bony.

osseous labyrinth. the bony labyrinth—the cavity in the petrous portion of the temporal bone that contains the inner ear.

osseous spiral lamina. the bony plate that extends outward from the modiolus. It is part of the structure that divides the cochlea into sections. It extends for 2¾ turns and is about 32 mm long. *syn*: ossicula auditus.

ossicle (os'sĭ-k'l) *n.* a small bone, especially one of the bones in the middle ear.

ossicles, auditory. the small bones of the middle ear that convey sound impulses from the eardrum to the oval window. They are known as the hammer (malleus), anvil (incus), and stirrup (stapes).

ossicle vibrator. an instrument devised to free the stapes in the oval window in the stapes mobilization operation.

ossicular chain. the ossicles, the three small bones in the middle ear that convey sound waves from the drumhead to the oval window of the inner ear—the malleus (hammer), the incus (anvil), and stapes (stirrup).

ossiculoplasty (os″ĭ-ku-lo-plas'te) *n.* surgical repair of the ossicular chain.

ossiculotomy (os″ĭ-ku-lot'o-me) *n.* surgical removal of one or more of the ossicles of the ear.

ossiculum (o-sik'u-lum) *n.* Latin: tiny bone.

ossification *n.* conversion of tissue into bony substance. *adj*: **ossificatory.**

ossify (os'ĭ-fi) *v.* to become bone or bone-like.

osteal *adj.* bonelike.

osteitis (os″te-i'tis) *n.* bone inflammation.

osteitis deformans. thickening of skull bones. *syn*: Paget's disease.

osteoblast (os'te-o-blast″) *n.* an embryonic bone cell. *adj*: **osteoblastic.**

osteogenesis imperfecta (os″te-o-gen'ĕ-sis). abnormal bone development such as may affect the ossicular chain; may be congenital.

osteoma (os″te-o′mah) *n.* a benign bonelike tumor that forms a lump under the skin of the ear canal or on the eardrum.

osteomalacia (os″te-o-mah-la′she-ah) *n.* a disease that causes softening of the bones.

osteomyelitis (os″te-o-mi″ĕ-li′tis) *n.* an inflammatory disease of bone marrow.

osteopetrosis *n.* brittle bones that result in spontaneous fractures. This condition may result in disarticulation of the ossicular chain from a comparatively light blow.

osteoporosis. otosclerosis.

osteosarcoma (os″te-o-sar-ko′mah) *n.* a malignant bony growth. A tinnitus suspect.

ostium (os′te-um) *n.* a small opening, as in the eustachian tube.

ostium pharyngeum (far-in-je′um). the pharyngeal opening of the eustachian tube.

ostium tympanicum (tim-pan′ĭ-cum). the opening of the eustachian tube in the middle ear.

ot, oto- combining form referring to the ear.

otacoustic (o″tah-kōōs′tik) *adj.* pertaining to or helping the hearing.

otacousticon *n.* old term for ear trumpet.

otalgia *n.* earache.

otantritis. (o″tan-tri′tis) *n.* inflammation of the opening in the temporal bone behind the ear.

otaphone *n.* a hearing aid, especially nonmechanical.

otaudion *n.* an early electric audiometer (Schwartz 1920).

otectomy, ossiculectomy. surgical removal of ossicles.

othelcosis (ot″hel-ko′sis) *n.* running ear.

othematoma (ōt″he-mah-to′mah) *n.* bloody tumor of the ear sometimes found in the insane. *syn*: asylum ear, hematoma auris.

othemorragia *n.* bleeding from the ear.

othemorrhea (ōt″hem-o-re′ah) *n.* bleeding from the ear.

othygroma (ōt″hi-gro′mah) *n.* a fluid-filled swelling of the ear.

otiatrics (o″te-at′riks) *n.* treatment of disorders of the ear.

otic (o′tik) *adj.* having to do with the ear.

-otic. suffix pertaining to the ear.

otic barotrauma. injury to the ear caused by excessive changes in atmospheric pressure as may occur in flying or deep sea diving. The damage may be to the walls of the ear canal or eardrum. Such injury may occur when there is a substantial difference between the pressure in the external auditory canal (atmospheric pressure) and the pressure in the middle ear. *syn*: aero-otitis.

otic capsule. the membranous sac that contains the inner ear.

oticodinia (o″tĭ-ko-din′e-ah) *n.* dizziness resulting from an ear disorder.

otic transudates. fluids that pass through membranes or capillary walls. They fill the middle ear when the eustachian tube is blocked, preventing drainage into the pharynx.

otic vesicle. embryonic cell structure that becomes the inner ear.

otitic herpes. a rash in and around the ear that may result in deafness from the spread of the virus infection that caused the rash.

otitis (o-ti′tis) *n.* a broad term for inflammation of the ear.

otitis, aviation. dysfunction of the middle ear caused by the changes of atmospheric pressure while flying. *syn*: barotrauma.

otitis externa. inflammation of the walls of the external auditory canal.

otitis exudate. the fluid, pus, or serum that oozes into the middle ear during the course of otitis media.

otitis, furuncular. an abscess in the external auditory canal.

otitis interna. inflammation of the inner ear. Endolymphatic labyrinthitis.

otitis labyrinthica. disease affecting the labyrinth.

otitis, mastoidal or **mastoideal.** inflammation of the mastoid.

otitis media. inflammation involving the middle ear.

otitis media, catarrhal. a disorder in which the middle ear is filled with thin and watery fluid. More commonly known as serous otitis or middle ear effusion.

otitis media, serous. accumulation of thin, watery fluid within the middle ear cavity; *syn*: middle ear effusion or catarrhal otitis media.

otitis media, suppurative (sup′u-ra″tiv). continually running ears as a result of infections.

otitis, mucous. chronic disease in which the middle ear is filled with thick gummy fluid. Since there is seldom any inflammation involved, many physicians refer to otic transudates. *syn*: glue ear, adhesive otitis media.

otitis, mycotic. inflammation of the ear caused by fungus.

otitis, parasitical. ear inflammation caused by a parasite.

otitis, sclerotic. hardening of inner ear tissues and structures as a result of inflammation.

otitis, serous. an accumulation of fluid in the middle ear that is thinner and more watery than in mucous otitis.

otitis, viral. inflammation attributed to a virus infection.

otoadmittance meter. an electro-acoustic device similar to an impedance meter and designed to perform the same functions.

otoantritis *n.* inflammation involving the mastoid antrum.

otoblennorrhea (o″to-blen″o-re′ah) *n.* inflammation of the external ear canal with mucous discharge. *syn*: otorrhea.

otocatarrh *n.* discharge from the ear resulting from inflammation of the mucous membrane.

otocerebritis (o″to-ser″ĕ-bri′tis) *n.* inflammation of the brain connected with ear disorders. *syn:* otoencephalitis.

Oto-Check. trade name for a limited-frequency audiometer designed to specifications proposed by Drs. Aram Glorig and Howard P. House.

otocleisis (o″to-kli′sis) *n.* 1. closure of the external ear canal (by wax or a growth). 2. closure of the eustachian tube.

otocist *n.* otocyst.

otoconia (o″to-ko′ne-ah) *sing.* otoconium *n.* minute crystalline particles of aragonite (a type of calcium carbonate—CaCO₃). Also known as ear crystals, ear dust, or otoliths (ear stones). By pressure upon the hair cells of the semicircular canals, these particles help activate the sense of balance. *adj:* otoconial.

otocyst (o′to-sist) *n.* the otic or auditory vesicle—the embryonic cell body from which the ear develops. *adj:* otocystic.

otodynia. earache.

otoencephalitis (o″to-en-sef″ah-li′tis) *n.* brain inflammation resulting from ear disorders. *syn:* otocerebritis.

otogenic (o″to-jen′ik) otogenous (o-toj′ĕ-nus) *adj.* originating within the ear.

otography (o-tog′rah-fe). description of physical features of the ear.

otohemineurasthenia (o″to-hem″e-nu″ras-the′ne-ah) *n.* a disorder in which hearing is limited to one ear, without evidence of any material damage to the auditory apparatus.

otolaryngologist (o″to-lar″in-gol′o-jist) *n.* medical doctor specializing in diseases of the ear, throat, and nose.

otolaryngology *n.* medical specialty devoted to the ear, and throat. It usually includes the nose as a short term for otorhinolaryngology.

otolith, otolite *n.* ear stone or crystal.

otolith apparatus. portion of inner ear (semicircular canal) that responds to gravity.

otologist (o-tol′o-jist) *n.* medical doctor specializing in problems of the ear. *syn:* aurist—seldom used.

otology *n.* divison of medicine specializing in the study and treatment of diseases of the ear. *adj:* otological.

otomandibular dysostosis (o″to-man-dib′u-lar dis″os-to′sis). otomandibular syndrome.

otomandibular syndrome. incomplete development of the lower jaw, accompanied by malfunctions of the ear. *syn:* otomandibular dysostosis.

otomassage *n.* an early treatment for ear problems. It was felt that hearing could be improved by exercising the ear muscles

and ossicular chain by means of pulsed sound waves, jets of air, or mechanical vibration of the eardrum.

otometrist *n.* one who practices otometry.

otometry (o-tom′ah-tre) *n.* (John A. Victoreen, LLD., U.S. physicist.) the science that deals with the sensation of loudness created by sound pressures. It is concerned with residual hearing and the determination of most comfortable loudness sound pressures and their ranges.

otomucormycosis *n.* an infection of the ear caused by fungi of the family mucoraceae.

-otomy. suffix indicating surgical procedure.

otomyasthenia (o″to-mi″as-the′ne-ah) *n.* impaired hearing resulting from weakened condition of tensor tympanic and stapedius muscles.

otomyces (o″to-mi′sēz) *n.* a fungus growth in the external ear canal. Otomyces hageni—a green variety, and otomyces purpureus—a dark red variety.

otomycosis (o″to-mi-ko′sis) *n.* (oto = ear; mycosis = disease caused by fungus). condition resulting from the growth of a fungus or bacteria in the external ear canal.

otoncus (o-tong′kus) *n.* an ear tumor.

otonecrectomy, otonecronectomy (o″to-nĕ-krek′to-me) *n.* surgical removal of necrosed (dead) tissue from the ear—especially the middle ear.

otoneuralgia *n.* earache originating in the nerves but not caused by inflammation.

otoneurasthenia *n.* 1. nervous irritability and weakness appearing as a functional overlay to ear disease. 2. hearing deficiency associated with a functional nervous disease—dependent upon no evident disorder.

otoneurology *n.* the study of the nervous system, and its disorders as related to hearing.

otoneurotic *adj.* term used to describe a person with a hearing loss who is more distressed by the loss than audiometric test results would suggest. The word was coined by David M. Lipscomb, Ph.D.

otopalatal (o″to-pal′ah-tal) *adj.* concerning the ears and palate—usually as a part of a syndrome.

otopalatodigital *adj.* concerning the ears, palate, and fingers, especially as part of a syndrome.

otopathology *n.* study of diseases affecting the ear.

otopathy (o-top′ah-the) *n.* any disease involving the ear.

otopharyngeal (o″to-fah-rin′je-al) *adj.* involving both the ear and the pharynx.

otopharyngeal tube. canal that connects the middle ear with the pharynx—the eustachian tube.

otophone (o′to-fōn) *n.* a type of ear trumpet.

otopiesis (o"to-pi'ĕ-sis) *n.* 1. depression of the eardrum caused by external atmospheric pressure which is not equalized through the eustachian tube. 2. hearing disorder resulting from pressure on the labyrinth.

otoplasty *n.* surgery intended to correct defects of the external ear.

otopolypus (o"to-pol'ĭ-pus) *n.* a polyp or growth in the external ear canal often arising from the middle ear.

otoparosis. otosclerosis.

otopyorrhea (o"to-pi"o-re'ah) *n.* discharge of pus from the ear. More commonly known as suppurative otitis media.

otopyosis *n.* discharge of pus as a result of ear disease.

otorhinolaryngologist (o"to-ri"no-lar"in-gol'o-jist) *n.* medical doctor specializing in diseases of the ear, nose, and throat.

otorhinolaryngology *n.* study of the diseases of the ear (oto), nose (rhino), and throat (laryngo).

otorhinology *n.* study of the diseases of the ear and nose.

otorrhagia (o"to-ra'je-ah) *n.* bleeding from the external ear canal.

otorrhea (o"to-re'ah) *n.* inflammation of the external ear canal with mucous discharge. *syn:* blenorrhea, otorrhoea.

otosalpinx *pl.* **otosalpinges.** the eustachian tube (tuba auditiva) connecting the middle ear cavity with the pharynx.

otosclerectomy, otoscleronectomy *n.* surgical removal of ear ossicles.

otosclerosis (o"to-skle-ro'sis) *n.* bony disease involving the middle ear, with the progressive loss of hearing; characterized by the growth of spongy bone around the stapes and oval window. *adj:* **otosclerotic.**

otosclerosis, cochlear. growth of spongy bone on the cochlear side of the oval window. Stapes fixation may or may not be involved. *syn:* labyrinthine otosclerosis.

otosclerosis, labyrinthine. growth of bony tissue within the inner ear. *syn:* cochlear otosclerosis.

otoscope (o'to-skōp) *n.* an instrument for making a visual examination of the external ear canal and eardrum. *syn:* auriscope, myringoscope.

otoscope, pneumatic. an otoscope with a bulb attachment to provide air pressure to cause movement of the eardrum. *syn:* Siegle's otoscope.

otoscopy (o-tos'ko-pe) *n.* inspection of the external ear canal and eardrum by means of the otoscope. *adj:* **otoscopic.**

otosis (o-to'sis) *pl.* **otoses.** 1. mishearing or misunderstanding of spoken sounds. 2. mispronunciation of words resulting from faulty hearing.

otospongiosis *n.* otosclerosis. (Term considered by some authorities to be more accurate).

otosteal (o-tos'te-al) *adj.* pertaining to the ossicles of the ear.

otosteon (o-tos'te-on) *n.* 1. any of the ossicles of the middle ear. 2. an ear stone (otolith) sometimes larger than a grain of ear dust (otoconia).

ototomy (o-tot'o-me) *n.* 1. surgical cutting or dissection of the ear. 2. surgical opening of the eardrum; myringotomy.

ototoxic (o"to-tok'sik) *adj.* poisonous to the ear. Some ototoxic drugs that may adversely affect hearing are kanamycin, streptomycin, dihydrostreptomycin, aspirin, and quinine. A more complete list of ototoxic drugs will be found in Appendix No. XIII, Page 187.

ototoxicity (o"to-toks-is'ĭ-te) *n.* the quality of being ototoxic.

OUT. Organization for Use of the Telephone, Inc.

outer ear. external ear—the portion of the hearing mechanism made up of the external ear flap (auricle or pinna) and the external auditory canal terminating at the eardrum (tympanic membrane).

outer hair cells. the hair cells in the organ of Corti that rest on the outer edge of the basilar membrane; i.e., the edge away from the modiolus. There are about 20,000.

outer rod of Corti. outer leg of cartilaginous structure resting on the basilar membrane that supports several rows of hair cells and the cells of Hensen.

out of phase. see opposite phase.

out-of-phase feedback. the result when an out-of-phase (or inverted) signal of an amplifier is fed back to a previous stage to reduce amplification or harmonic distortion. *syn:* degenerative, inverse, or negative feedback.

output *n.* power or energy released by an instrument after the input signal has been amplified or altered by electronic circuitry.

output, acoustic. the sound pressure resulting from the increase in intensity of an input signal as measured at the speaker, earphone, or receiver of an electronic amplifying system.

output, HAIC. the average of the three saturation output pressures of the hearing aid at 500, 1000, and 2000 Hz.

output, maximum power. in hearing aids this term is usually used to express the average of the saturation output pressures at 500, 1000, and 2000 Hz. It is more often referred to as the output of the hearing aid. *syn:* maximum deliverable pressure, maximum acoustic output.

output, peak. the highest point in the curve of saturation output of an amplifying system. *syn:* peak sound pressure.

output, saturation. the greatest sound intensity an amplifying system can produce. It usually varies with frequency. *syn*: maximum acoustic output, maximum deliverable pressure.

oval fossa. depression in which the oval window rests.

oval window. resting place for the footplate of the stapes, the oval window allows the mechanical action of the ossicles to be translated into fluid waves in the perilymph of the cochlea beginning in the scala vestibuli. *syn*: fenestra ovalis, fenestra vestibuli.

over-damping. mechanically decreasing the amplitude of vibrations or waves to the point that the wave form is altered or distorted.

overlay, functional. an inability to operate normally that arises from a mental (psychical) exaggeration of the results of a physical disability.

overload. distortion of a sound signal when the intensity of the signal exceeds the capacity of the amplifier.

overload, aural. distortion of a sound signal by the ear itself when the intensity of the sound exceeds the limit of the individual's hearing mechanism.

over-masking. the use of a level of intensity of masking noise that is so high it produces an inaccurately increased threshold of sensitivity in the opposite ear.

overrecruitment *n.* the sensation of loudness of a tone in the poor ear exceeds the sensation of loudness in the good ear at higher intensity levels. *syn*: hyper-recruitment.

overt (o-vert') *adj.* 1. open or apparent. 2. symptoms of hearing impairment that are easily recognized.

overtone. a multiple of the fundamental tone produced (simultaneously) by a musical instrument. *syn*: harmonic or upper partial.

overt response. reaction that can be easily observed.

OVR. Office of Vocational Rehabilitation.

oxy- prefix meaning sharp, keen, shrill, quick.

oxyacoia, oxyakoia (ok'se-ah-koi'ah) *n.* unusual sensitivity to noise resulting from paralysis of the stapedius muscle that may accompany facial paralysis.

oxyacusis (ok-se-ah-ku'sis) *n.* unusually sensitive to sound.

oxyecoia *n.* oxyacoia.

oxylalia (ok-se-la'le-ah) *n.* abnormally rapid speech.

oxyphonia (ok"se-fo'ne-ah) *n.* abnormal shrillness of voice.

P

PA. power amplifier. public address (system).

pachy- (pak'e). prefix meaning thick.

pachyotia (pak"e-o'she-ah) *n.* abnormal thickness of the external ears.

paed-, paedo-, ped-, pedo- prefix referring to infants and children.

paedoaudiologist (pe"do-aw"de-ol'o-jist) *n.* an audiologist engaged primarily in working with infants and children. *syn*: pediatric audiologist.

paedoaudiology (pe"do-aw"de-ol'o-je) *n.* specialty devoted to the hearing problems of infants and children. *syn*: pediatric audiology.

page printer. a type of teletypewriter in which the message is printed on paper.

Paget's disease (paj'ets) (Sir James Paget, English physician, 1814-1899). thickening and inflammation of the skull bones. *syn*: osteitis deformans.

pain, threshold. the level of intensity at which sound becomes painful—about 140 dB SPL for the average ear.

PAL. Psycho-Acoustic Laboratory (Harvard University).

palatal myoclonus. muscular spasm of the soft palate. It may be heard through an ear to ear tube as a click within the patient's ear and may be a symptom of a brain stem lesion. A type of objective tinnitus.

palate (pal'at) *n.* the roof of the mouth. The hard palate is in front and the soft palate in back.

palate, cleft. congenital lack of closure of the roof of the mouth. On occasion it may extend to a harelip.

palate, soft. the muscular, rearward portion of the roof of the mouth. It helps to separate the nose, mouth, and throat.

palatoplasty (pal'ah-to-plas"te) *n.* surgical repair of cleft palate. *syn*: uraniscoplasty, uranoplasty.

palatum fissum. cleft palate.

palilalia (pal"i-la'le-ah) *n.* involuntary repetition of spoken words or phrases. *syn*: palinphrasia, paliphrasia.

palinphrasia, paliphrasia (pal"in-fra'ze-ah) *n.* palilalia.

pallesthesia (pal"es-the'ze-ah) *n.* the sensation of movement without accompanying sound when a vibrating tuning fork or bone vibrator touches the body.

pallium (pal'e-um) *n.* the mantle of the brain: the cerebral cortex and its underlying white substance. *adj*: **pallial.**

palpebral, reflex (pal'pĕ-bral). eyeblink.

palsy, Bell's (Sir Charles Bell, Scottish physician, 1774-1842). facial paralysis caused by a lesion of the VIIth cranial nerve. Hearing impairment may accompany the facial distortion. *syn*: facial palsy.

pan- prefix meaning all or whole.

pancochlear (pan-kok'le-ar) *adj.* involving all of the cochlea.

pancochlear hearing loss. hearing loss typified by an elevated threshold of sensitivity at all frequencies.

panendoscope (pan-en'do-skōp) *n.* instrument designed to allow visual study of interior surfaces. *adj*: **panendoscopic.**

papilla (pah-pil'ah) *n.* a nipple or nipple-like projection.

papilla, acoustic. the organ of Corti.

papilla, basilar. the organ of Corti—the specific receptor organ of hearing.

para- (par'ah). prefix meaning 1. almost or nearly—a variant of the normal. 2. close to or near. 3. involving two like parts.

paracentesis (par"ah-sen-te'sis) *n.* surgical opening of a membrane to allow drainage or equalization of pressure.

paracentesis tympani. surgical opening of the eardrum to provide drainage. *syn*: myringotomy, tympanotomy.

paracousis (par-ah-ku'sis) *n.* variation of paracusis—abnormal hearing.

paracusia (par-ah-ku'se-ah) *n.* an abnormality in the sense of hearing.

paracusia or **paracusis acris.** abnormally acute hearing. *syn*: hyperacusia.

paracusia duplicata. one tone is heard as two; diplacusis.

paracusia imaginaria. head noises; tinnitus.

paracusia localis (loci). lack of ability to determine direction of sound. Usually occurs when two ears hear unequally.

paracusia obtusa. Blunt hearing—hard of hearing.

paracusis (par-ah-ku'sis) *n.* abnormal hearing.

paracusis, false. sensation of improvement in hearing when others speak loudly because of noisy surroundings.

paracusis loci, localis. impairment of ability to localize sound.

paracusis, musical. a shift in the pitch of tones generally associated with threshold shifts of hearing in a limited frequency range.

paracusis Willisiana, paracusia Willisii, Willis' paracusis. apparent ability to hear (understand) better in noisy surroundings.

paradigm (par'ah-dīm) *pl.* **paradigms, paradigmata.** a model, design, example, or pattern. *adj*: **paradigmatic.**

paradoxical deafness. the paradoxical ability of many who have a conductive hearing loss to hear better in noisy places: Paracousia Willisiana or Willis' paracusis.

para-equilibrium. dizziness due to a disorder of the vestibular apparatus of the ear.

paralanguage. Body language (gestures, postures, etc.), or tone and stress variations that communicate meaning.

paralysis, acoustic. sensorineural deafness.

parameter (pah-ram'ĕ-ter) *n.* 1. a basic element or principal characteristic. 2. a quantity defining a statistical population. *adj*: **parametric.**

parasalpingitis (par"ah-sal"pin-ji'tis) *n.* inflammation involving tissues near the eustachian tube.

parasitical otitis. ear inflammation caused by a parasite.

parasynthesis (par"ah-sin'the-sis) *n.* the formation of a new word from an old one, e.g., prefixing a particle and adding a derivative ending to a familiar word; deemphasize. Communicology is another example—as a combination of an old word with a new suffix. *adj*: **parasynthetic.**

paries (pa're-ez) *n.* a wall of a hollow in the body, paries caroticus cavi tympani—the wall of the middle ear that contains the opening of the eustachian tube.

parietal (pah-ri'ĕ-tal) *adj.* concerning the wall of a cavity or organ.

parotic (pah-rot'ĭk) *adj.* beside or near the ear.

parotid (pah-rot'id) *adj.* near the ear—usually refers to the parotid gland.

parotid duct. tube that conveys saliva from the parotid gland to the mouth. *syn*: Stensen's duct.

parotid gland. large salivary gland near the ear.

parotiditis (pah-rot"ĭ-di'tis) *n.* parotitis or inflammation of the parotid gland. Also called mumps, it may involve other glands of the body.

parotitis, epidemic. mumps.

paroxysmal dysacusis. (par"ok-siz'mal dis-ah-ku'sis). hearing impairment resulting from a sudden change in blood circulation to the ear.

pars flaccida (flak'sĭ-dah). the small thin, triangular portion of the eardrum located in the upper part of the membrane. It is not as tense as the rest of the eardrum and is called the flaccid part. *syn*: Rivinus' ligament and Shrapnell's membrane.

pars tensa. the larger portion of the eardrum. It is tense in contrast with the small triangular flaccid part.

partial *n.* a sound pressure wave that is a portion of a complex sound. It may be either higher or lower in frequency than the fundamental, and does not necessarily have an arithmetical relationship to it.

partial deafness. old term for hearing loss.
partial node. a portion of a standing wave system that has minimum amplitude but is not zero.
partial recruitment. the sensation where loudness of a tone in the poorer ear approaches, but does not equal, the sensation of loudness in the better ear at high intensity levels. *syn*: incomplete recruitment.
partial reinforcement. not all responses in a conditioning pattern are reinforced.
partial stapedectomy. one leg of the stapes, with part of the footplate attached, is used instead of total replacement of the stapes by plastic or wire prosthesis.
partially deaf units. PDU. British term for classes of hard-of-hearing students partially integrated with regular schools.
particle velocity. the speed of movement of an individual particle of the medium through which a sound wave is passing, compared to the movement of the medium as a whole. The unit of measurement is the centimeter per second (cps).
PAS. para-aminosalicylic acid, a drug used to inhibit the growth of the bacteria responsible for tuberculosis.
pass band. an electrical filter that allows a fixed or preselected band of frequencies to pass—to be transmitted. Acoustic signals or frequencies above or below the band-pass filter are rejected, not transmitted or amplified.
passive filter. an electric filter made up only of passive elements such as resistors or capacitors.
patent (pa'tent) *adj.* open and unobstructed. A patent eustachian tube opens to allow air to move freely between the middle ear and throat.
pathogen (path'o-jen) *n.* the agent or microorganism that is the direct cause of disease.
pathogenesis (path"o-jen'ĕ-sis) *n.* the development and progress of a disease. *adj*: **pathogenetic, pathogenic.**
pathognomonic (path"og-no-mon'ik) *adj.* pertaining to a symptom or distinguishing indication of a particular disease.
pathologist (pah-thol'o-jist) *n.* a specialist in the study of the changes in tissue caused by disease.
pathology (pah-thol'o-je) *n.* the study of the cause, progress, and effects of disease. *adj*: **pathologic, pathological.**
pathometer (pah-thom'ĕ-ter) *n.* device used to measure changes in the body's electrical conductivity.
pattern, sound (pat'ern). a pictorial display of the spectrum of a sound as revealed by a spectrograph.
patterns, interference. the intricate pressure wave systems resulting from the introduction of sounds of the same frequency from two or more sources.

patulous (pat'u-lus) *adj.* open or patent, especially as referring to the eustachian tube.
PB. phonetically balanced.
PB word list. a list of one-syllable words used in speech discrimination tests. The words were selected and arranged so that the speech sounds are represented in the same frequency in which they appear in conversational speech. The list is thus phonetically balanced.
PBF. phonetically balanced familiar word lists.
PBK. phonetically balanced kindergarten word lists.
PB max. the discrimination score determined through use of a speech audiometer under the most favorable levels of amplification.
PC. international hearing aid symbol for peak clipping.
PD. potential difference.
PDU. partially deaf units—British term for hard-of-hearing classes.
PE. probable error. physical education. polyethylene.
PE tube. a polyethylene tube placed surgically in the eardrum to drain and ventilate the middle ear.
peak clipping. a method of limiting the output (e.g., through a hearing aid) which prevents transmission of intensities that exceed a predetermined maximum level.
peak clipping, hard. type of peak clipping that occurs in a hearing aid as the maximum acoustic capacity of the system is reached.
peak clipping, soft. a phrase sometimes used to refer to any method of circuit limitation of the output of a hearing aid below the maximum acoustic capacity of its transducers.
peak gain. the highest point on the frequency response curve of the amplifier.
peak output. the highest point in the curve of saturation output of an amplifier. *syn*: peak sound pressure.
peak sound pressure. the maximum pressure point of any sound or pure tone wave. *syn*: peak output.
pediacoumeter (pe-de-ak'u-me-ter) *n.* instrument designed by Olaf Haug, Ph.D. It utilized a peep-show technique in testing the hearing of children 20 to 48 months of age.
pediatric audiologist (pe"de-at'rik aw"de-ol'o-jist). an audiologist engaged primarily in working with infants and children. *syn*: paedoaudiologist.
pediatric audiology. specialty devoted to the hearing problems of infants and children. *syn*: paedoaudiology.
pediatrician (pe"de-ah-trish'un) *n.* a physician specializing in diseases of infants and children.

pediatrics (pe″de-at′riks) *n.* the branch of medicine concerned with the care and treatment of children and their diseases.
PEL. permissible exposure limit. (This term should replace NEL—noise exposure level—in general usage).
PEM. predictable earmold modification.
Pendred's syndrome. a congenital glandular deficiency characterized by goiter. The accompanying deafness is sensorineural.
penetrance (pen′ĕ-trans) *n.* the relative number of people who display the characteristic effect of a mutant gene.
penicillin *n.* one of a group of antibiotics formed from molds.
penicillium *n.* a genus of molds used to produce penicillin and that occasionally cause infections of the external ear.
pennate *adj.* ribbed like a feather. The stapedius and tensor tympani are pennate muscles.
perceived noise decibels. PNdB. a unit of measurement of the sound pressure level of a band of noise from 910 to 1090 Hz when compared with another sound.

perceived noise level. PNL. a comparison of the sound pressure level of the 910 to 1090 Hz band and another sound as measured in units known as PNdBs. See noy.
percentage of hearing handicap. the AAO Committee on Hearing and Equilibrium revised its formula for calculating the percentage of hearing handicap in 1979 to produce Table 4. (The complete report is in Appendix II, Page 168).
percent impairment of hearing. (percent of hearing loss). an estimate of ability to understand speech based on the pure tone audiogram. The formula used for calculation according to rule of law varies from state to state.
perceptibility, threshold of. seldom used term for the level of intensity at which sounds begin to be perceived as words. It is between the threshold of detectability and the threshold of intelligibility.
perception (per-sep′shun) *n.* awareness of a stimulus.
perceptive (perception) deafness. sensorineural hearing loss—one not involving the

Table 4. Monaural Hearing Impairment*

DSHL†	%	DSHL†	%
100	0.0	240	52.5
105	1.9	245	54.4
110	3.8	250	56.2
115	5.6	255	58.1
120	7.5	260	60.0
125	9.4	265	61.9
130	11.2	270	63.8
135	13.1	275	65.6
140	15.0	280	67.5
145	16.9	285	69.3
150	18.8	290	71.2
155	20.6	295	73.1
160	22.5	300	75.0
165	24.4	305	76.9
170	26.2	310	78.8
175	28.1	315	80.6
180	30.0	320	82.5
185	31.9	325	84.4
190	33.8	330	86.2
195	35.6	335	88.1
200	37.5	340	90.0
205	39.4	345	90.9
210	41.2	350	93.8
215	43.1	355	95.6
220	45.0	360	97.5
225	46.9	365	99.4
230	48.9	370	100.0
235	50.6	(or greater)	

*1. From the audiogram or numerical record of the audiometric test, find the decibel sum of the hearing threshold levels (DSHL) of 500, 1000, 2000, and 3000 Hz. Example:

500	20
1000	25
2000	35
3000	40

Total 120 DSHL
2. Under the DSHL heading 120 DSHL (column 1, line 5) equals 7.5%.
3. Computation of percent of hearing handicap. If the monaural percent figure is the same for both ears, that figure expresses the percent hearing handicap. If the percent monaural hearing impairments are not the same, apply the formula:

$$\frac{(5 \times \%[\text{better ear}]) + (1 \times \%[\text{poorer ear}])}{6} =$$

% hearing handicap

Audiometers are calibrated to ANSI 1969 standard reference levels.
†Decibel sum of hearing threshold levels at 500, 1000, 2000, and 3000 Hz.

Previous methods of calculation were as follows: AAOO method of calculation (1959): monaurally, compute the average air conduction threshold at 500, 1000, and 2000 Hz; subtract 26 dB (ANSI) and multiply the remainder by 1½%. Binaurally, multiply the percentage of impairment of better ear by 5 and add the percentage for poorer ear—then divide the result by 6.
AMA method (1947): Calculation was made from weighted values assigned as follows: 500 Hz, 15%; 1000 Hz, 30%; 2000 Hz, 40%; 4000 Hz, 15%.

conductive mechanism. Formerly known as nerve deafness.

perceptive loss. hearing impairment now referred to as a sensorineural loss.

percutaneous (per″ku-ta′ne-us) *n.* through unbroken skin. *syn:* transcutaneous.

perflation (per-fla′shun) *n.* the process of blowing air through a cavity, canal, or tube to expand its walls or to force out pus or other material.

perforate (per′for-āt) *v.* to puncture or create a hole in a surface. *n:* **perforator.**

perforated eardrum. an eardrum that has been ruptured by accident or disease. The reduction in hearing sensitivity usually amounts to about 5 or 10 dB.

perforation (per″fo-ra′shun) *n.* 1. a hole. 2. the process of making a hole. *adj:* **perforate.**

perforation, Bezold's. perforation of the inner surface of the mastoid caused by breakthrough of pus from Bezold's abscess.

peri- (per′e). prefix meaning around or about.

periconchal (per″ĭ-kong′kal) *adj.* near the concha of the ear.

periconchal sulcus. groove under the helix of the pinna.

perifascicular sheath (per″e-fah-sik′u-lar). connective tissue surrounding a bundle of nerve fibers. *syn:* perineurium.

perilabyrinthine (per″ĭ-lab-ĭ-rin′thīn) *n.* concerning the tissues surrounding the labyrinth of the ear.

perilabyrinthitis (per″ĭ-lab″ĭ-rin-thi′tis) *n.* inflammation of tissues around the labyrinth.

perilymph (per′ĭ-limf) *n.* portion of cerebrospinal fluid contained within the scala vestibuli and the scala tympani of the cochlea and between the membranous and bony portion of the semicircular canals.

perilymphatic duct. the tiny canal that allows the perilymph to be replenished from the cerebrospinal fluid that surrounds the brain.

perinatal (per″ĭ-na′tal) *adj.* pertaining to the time of birth, or near the time of birth.

perineuritis (per″ĭ-nu-ri′tis) *n.* inflammation of the sheath surrounding nerve fibers.

perineurium (per″ĭ-nu′re-um) *n.* the connective tissue sheath surrounding a bundle of nerve fibers. *syn:* perifascicular sheath. *adj:* **perineurial.**

period (pe′re-od) *n.* time interval involved in the regular repetition of a cycle of sound or some other event or function.

period, refractory. time between firings of nerve pulses. During this time the ions of the nerve return to their prefiring or resting position.

periodic (pe″re-od′ik) *adj.* occurring at regular intervals; e.g., constant repetitions of the same basic waveform.

periodic sounds. sounds that repeat themselves regularly as a function of time; e.g., musical sounds.

periodic wave. a waveform that repeats regularly in a time period.

periodicity (pe″re-o-dis′ĭ-te) *n.* the attribute of regular recurrence of various characteristics of a wave form.

periodicity pitch. the sensation of hearing a pitch that has no direct relationship with the sound waves presented, which results from the summation of the regular recurrence of the peaks of acoustic pressure.

periodicity of sound. the regular recurrence of wave forms in mathematical relationship to the fundamental (harmonics) that makes sound musical.

periorbital muscles (per″e-or′bĭ-tal). the muscles that surround the eye and react in the auropalpebral reflex.

periosteum (per″e-os′te-um) *n.* the fibrous tissue that covers a bone except at articulation points. It contains the nerves and blood vessels supplying the bone.

periostitis (per″e-os-ti′tis) *n.* inflammation involving the tissue surrounding a bone.

periotic (per″e-o′tik) *adj.* around the ear, more specifically, the bony structure surrounding the inner ear.

periotic bone. the petrous and mastoid (petromastoid) portions of the temporal bone.

peripheral (pĕ-rif′er-al) *adj.* toward the outer part—away from the center.

peripheral deafness. impaired hearing resulting from a lesion affecting the sensorineural or conductive mechanism. Indicates deafness that is not central in origin.

periphery (pĕ-rif′er-e) *n.* the outer part or on the external surface.

permanent threshold shift. PTS. an irreversible loss of sensitivity. The term usually relates to noise-induced hearing loss.

permissible exposure limits. PEL. (Formerly noise exposure levels—NEL). Set by OSHA 1910.95c Federal Register. See Table 5, page 107.

perseveration (per-sev″er-a′shun) *n.* the continuing sensation of hearing a sound after the stimulus has ceased. Also known as "after" hearing, it is similar to the after image in vision.

perstimulatory fatigue (per″stim′u-lah-tor-e). the apparent diminishing of the loudness of a stimulus when presented continuously at an intensity level which is above threshold. A type of tone decay.

petro- prefix meaning stone—as indicating the hardest (petrous) part of the temporal bone.

petromastoid (pet″ro-mas′toid) *adj.* concerning both the petrous and mastoidal portions of the temporal bone.

petrosa (pĕ-tro′sah) *n.* the hard (petrous) part of the temporal bone.

Table 5. Permissible Exposure Limits

A-weighted Sound Level L(decibel)	Reference duration time, T(hour)
85	16.0
86	13.9
87	12.1
88	10.6
89	9.2
90	8.0
91	7.0
92	6.2
93	5.3
94	4.6
95	4.0
96	3.5
97	3.0
98	2.6
99	2.3
100	2.0
101	1.7
102	1.5
103	1.4
104	1.3
105	1.0
106	.87
107	.76
108	.66
109	.57
110	.50
111	.44
112	.38
113	.33
114	.29
115	.25

petrosal *adj.* stonelike or very hard. *syn*: petrous.

petrositis (pet″ro-si′tis) *n.* inflammation involving the petrous portion of the temporal bone.

petrosphenoid (pet″ro-sfe′noid) *adj.* concerning the petrous portion of the temporal bone and sphenoid bone.

petrosquamous (pet″ro-skwa′mus) *adj.* concerning the petrous and squamous portions of the temporal bone.

petrotympanic fissure. a groove between the tympanic and squamous portions of the temporal bone. It provides space for the chorda tympani nerve.

petrous (pet′rus) *adj.* stonelike or very hard.

-pexy (pek′se). suffix indicating a fixation—usually surgical.

PGA. psychogalvanic audiometry (commonly called PGSR).

PGR. psychogalvanic reflex or response.

PGSR. psychogalvanic skin reflex or response.

phalangeal cells (fah-lan′je-al). cells that support the inner hair cells of the organ of Corti.

phalangeal cells, outer. cells that support the outer hair cells in the organ of Corti. *syn*: Deiter's cells.

phalanx (fa′lanks) *n.* one of the sets of plates made up of phalangeal cells (inner and outer) that form the supporting structure of the hair cells in the organ of Corti.

pharyngeal (fa-rin′je-al) *adj.* concerning the pharynx or throat.

pharyngeal recess. depression in the wall of the pharynx above and behind the eustachian tube. *syn*: Rosenmuller's fossa.

pharyngeal tonsil. adenoid. Lymphoid tissue growing around the nasopharyngeal opening of the eustachian tube.

pharyngitis (far″in-ji′tis) *n.* inflammation of the mucous membrane of the pharynx.

pharyngotympanic tube. auditory or eustachian tube.

pharynx (far′inks) *pl.* **pharynges, pharynxes.** the part of the digestive tube between the mouth and the nasal cavities above and the esophagus below. *adj*: **pharyngeal.**

phase *n.* a distinctive point or fraction of a recurring cycle of sound; e.g., the peak in a pure tone sine wave. "In phase" indicates that two sound pressure waves reach corresponding points (or phases) at the same time. "Out of phase" or "opposite phase" indicates that the waves tend to cancel each other at certain points. *adj*: **phasic.**

phase-contrast microscope. a microscope equipped with a special condensor to make details of objects visible through a change in phase; e.g., of color or brightness.

phase difference. the relative locations of two pressure waves at a point in time.

phase meter. device used to measure phase relationships between alternating oscillations of the same frequency.

phase relations. the connection measured in time periods between fractions (usually crests) of a sound wave.

phase theory of binaural localization. differences in time of arrival of wave peaks to each ear makes possible localization of sound—most effectively at frequencies below 1000 Hz.

-phasia. suffix indicating a disorder affecting speech.

phenotype (fe′no-tīp) *n.* a grouping based on one or more genetic traits; e.g., blood types or physical appearance. *adj*: **phenotypic, phenotypical.**

phenylalanine (fen″il-al′ah-nīn) *n.* one of the amino acids. Congenital deficiency is characteristic of phenylketonuria.

phenylketonuria (fen″il-ke″to-nu′re-ah) *n.* PKU. a metabolic disorder characterized by an inability to assimilate certain types of protein foods and resulting in retarded or undeveloped mentality. *syn:* phenylpyruvis oligophrenia.

-phobia *n.* suffix indicating unreasoning dread or fear; e.g., phonophobia, an exaggerated fear of sound or speaking above a whisper.

phon-, phone-, phono- (fo'no). combining form indicating voice, speech, or sound.

phon (fōn) *n.* the unit for measuring the loudness level of a sound in comparison with a 1000 Hz tone. The loudness level in phons is numerically equal to the SPL of the 1000 Hz tone, while the SPL at other frequencies will vary for the same number of phons.

phonacoscope (fo-nak'o-scōp) *n.* a device for increasing the intensity of voice sounds or percussion notes with the physician's ear or stethoscope placed on the opposite side of the chest.

phonacoscopy *n.* examination of the chest with the phonacoscope.

phonate *v.* to voice sounds.

phonation *n.* vibration of vocal cords in the larynx. The production of voiced sounds. *adj:* phonal, phonic, phonatory.

phonautograph (fōn-aw'to-graf) *n.* a device for registering voice and other sound vibrations.

phone *n.* a single voiced sound.

phoneme (fo'nēm) *n.* 1. one of the smallest units of speech (or class of phones) that distinguishes one word from another; e.g., p, b, and f in pan, ban, and fan. 2. hearing of imaginary voices.

phoneme, nonsense. a small unit of speech that lends no intelligibility to a syllable.

phonemic analysis. study of speech sounds.

phonemic composition. the manner in which speech sounds are put together to form words.

phonemic regression. deterioration in discrimination ability without lessening of sensitivity that sometimes accompanies the aging process.

phonemics *n.* the study of phonemes in relation to the formation of words.

phonendoscope (fōn-en'do-skōp) *n.* a stethoscope designed to mechanically amplify sounds—one designed to mechanically intensify (not just isolate) body sounds.

phonetic *adj.* pertaining to speech, the voice, or the symbols representing speech sounds.

phonetically balanced. containing all the phonetic elements of general American English speech balanced in relationship to occurrence in normal speech. Usually referring to monosyllabic word lists prepared to meet such criteria.

phonetically balanced familiar word lists. PBF. developed at Clarke School for the Deaf by C. V. Hudgins for young children and people with limited vocabularies.

phonetically balanced kindergarten word lists. PBK. developed by Harriet Haskins for use with very young children.

phonetic alphabet. 1. a system of individual symbols for distinctive speech sounds. 2. a method of identifying letters of the alphabet by the use of code words; e.g., "able" for a.

phonetic alphabet, international. IPA. a system of symbols for speech sounds adopted by the International Phonetic Association. Each speech sound is represented by a distinctive symbol.

phonetic elements. phonemes.

phonetician *n.* a student of phonetics or the elements of speech and voice.

phonetic power. relative energy of a phoneme (speech sound).

phonetics *n.* the study of the smallest speech units that make up words. Sometimes known as phonics, which, however, is more directly involved with reading.

phonetics, acoustic. the study of the composition of the sound pressure waves produced as speech sounds are voiced. *syn:* physical phonetics.

phonetics, physical. acoustic phonetics.

phonetype *n.* a teletype-telephone network combination for communication by the deaf. It utilizes an acoustic converter to enable a regular telephone to carry teletypewriter signals.

phoniatrics (fo"ne-at'riks) **phoniatry** (fo-ni'ah-tre) *n.* the study of speech and voice disorders.

phonic (fon'ik) *adj.* pertaining to speech and the voice.

phonics *n.* the study of speech sounds as an aid to reading and word pronunciations.

phonism (fo'nizm) *n.* the subjective sensation of hearing sound or voices when another sense is stimulated. A form of synesthesia.

phono- (fo'no). prefix meaning sound, speech, voice, or tone.

phono-audiologist (fono-audiologist). in Latin America, a specialist in the problems of hearing and deafness who does not have a degree in medicine—as the title audiologist implies in Europe and Latin America.

phonocardiograph *n.* an instrument for graphically recording the sounds of the heart.

phonocardiography (fo"no-kar"de-og'rah-fe) *n.* graphic recording of heart sounds made possible by use of a microphone and galvanometer.

phonodeik (fo'no-dēēk) *n.* an instrument that records air waves in the form of a graph.

phonogram *n.* 1. a graphic curve showing the duration and intensity of a sound. 2. symbol representing a speech sound or combination of speech sounds. 3. a combination of letters representing the same sound in various words (as ove in dove, love, shove, etc.)

phonograph *n.* a device designed to transform the mechanical vibration of a needle following a groove into electric and acoustic signals. *adj*: **phonographic.**

phonography *n.* 1. the use of phonics in establishing spelling and pronunciation. 2. a shorthand method based on sound.

phonology *n.* 1. the study of speech sounds as related to language. 2. the study of the development of a language in terms of its changes in speech sounds. *syn*: phonetics. *adj*: **phonologic, phonological.**

phonomassage *n.* an attempt to stimulate the eardrum and restore ossicular movement (therefore hearing) by means of alternating noise or mechanical pressure and suction applied to the external ear canal.

phonometer (fo-nom′ĕ-ter) *n.* a device for measuring intensity or frequency of vocal sounds.

phonopathy (fo-nop′ah-the) *n.* any disease of the vocal organs that affects speech.

phonophobia *n.* 1. an abnormally acute sense of pain caused by sounds far above the individual threshold of hearing. 2. abnormal feeling of discomfort caused by loud sounds. *syn*: hyperacusia dolorosa. 3. morbid dread of speaking aloud.

phonopsia *n.* the subjective sensation of color or when some people hear certain sounds.

phonoreception *n.* the recognition of vibrating motion as hearing.

phonoreceptor *n.* the mechanism of the ear.

phonovision *n.* picturephone.

photism *n.* the subjective sensation of color or light produced under certain conditions as the result of the stimulation of another sense: hearing, smell, touch, or taste.

photoelectric cell. an electrical device that reacts to light.

photophone *n.* an instrument invented by A. G. Bell to transmit sound by light-beam vibrations.

phrase, carrier. a phrase preceding the test word in speech audiometry; e.g., "You will say-." It is used both to instruct the patient and monitor the speaker's voice.

PHS. Public Health Service.

phylogenic *adj.* pertaining to evolution or racial history.

physiatrics (fiz″e-at′riks) *n.* the practice of physical medicine. Physiotherapy.

physics *n.* the branch of science concerned with the interaction of the mass and energy of matter without loss of chemical identity.

physiogenic *adj.* arising from physiologic causes—changes in the normal living processes, as opposed to psychogenic, arising from mental or emotional problems.

physiological audiometry. test of hearing that depends upon the measurement of changes in electrical response from either the skin (electrodermal) or the brain (electroencephalic).

physiologist *n.* a scientist specializing in the study of living matter.

physiology *n.* the branch of science dealing with living matter. *adj*: **physiologic, physiological.**

PICA. Porch Index of Communicative Ability.

pick up. 1. a device for changing mechanical vibrations into electrical signals, as in a phonograph. 2. a device for changing sound waves into electrical signals—a microphone.

picturephone *n.* an attachment to a telephone (sometimes called "phonovision") that allows communication by speechreading or sign language.

picture, sound. a spectrogram or photograph of the pressure waves of a particular sound.

Pierre Robin syndrome (ro-ba′). a complex of symptoms including incomplete jaw development, cleft palate, tongue anomalies, and eye defects.

piezo- (pi-e′zo). prefix indicating pressure.

piezoelectric *adj.* concerning the production of electricity by pressure—usually on a crystal.

piezoelectric or crystal microphone. a device for converting sound pressure waves into electrical energy by utilizing the unique electrical voltage-generating property of a piezoelectric crystal.

piezoelectricity *n.* the electricity resulting from pressure on a crystal.

pillar cell. a cell that supports the walls of the inner tunnel of Corti.

pillar, Corti's. the inner and outer rod cells that line the tunnel of Corti.

pink noise. random sound similar to white noise, but whose spectrum level decreases with increase in frequency (3 dB per octave) to provide constant energy per octave of bandwidth.

pinna *n.* the portion of the ear that is visible on the side of the head. *adj*: **pinnal;** *syn*: auricle.

pip *n.* a brief high-frequency tone.

pit, auditory. a depression on either side of the head of the embryo where the ear will develop.

pitch *n.* 1. the auditory sensation in response to frequency. 2. the differences in basic vocal chord vibratory patterns that characterize different voices. 3. the changes in vibration frequency that contribute to the total communicative speech pattern.

pitch, absolute. the ability to identify unerringly the fundamental frequency of a tone that is heard.

pitch, click. a sharp sound that lasts long enough to give an auditory sensation of tonality.

pitch discrimination. the ability of the ear to distinguish slight differences in frequency.

pitch level. pitch level varies with intensity and is numerically equal to the frequency of a 40-phon pure tone whose pitch is judged equal to that of the sound in question. The unit of this subjective measurement of differences in pitch is the mel.

pitch, natural. the fundamental frequency that appears most often in a class of musical instruments or voices—about 100 Hz for men's voices and about 250 Hz for women's and children's voices. *syn*: optimal pitch.

pitch, optimal. natural pitch.

pitch, periodicity. the sensation of hearing a pitch having no direct relationship with the sound waves presented, which results from the summation of the regular recurrence of the peaks of acoustic pressure.

pitch pipe. small tube or combination of cylinders designed to produce one or more tones when blown. It is used to establish pitch in singing or tuning a musical instrument.

pitch scale. an arbitrary scale relating frequency to pitch. On the scientific scale, 256 Hz equals middle C. On the musical scale, middle C equals 261.6 Hz.

pitch, subjective scale for. the unit of measurement is the mel.

pitch, volley theory of perception. the theory that pitch is determined by the brain's interpretation of sequences (volleys) of electrical impulses carried by different groups of neurons within a nerve.

PK. psychokinesis.

PKU. phenylketonuria.

place *v.* to control the voice to produce the desired pitch.

place theory of hearing. belief that pitch discrimination is dependent upon the response to the stimulation of localized areas along the basilar membrane within the cochlea. The theory is often considered to extend to places within the brain.

placode (plak′ōd) *n.* a platelike thickening of embryonic cells that develops into an organ or structure.

placode, auditory. collection of embryonic cells that develop into the internal ear.

planigraphy (plah-nig′rah-fe) *n.* a method of x-ray photography that provides focus on a particular layer of tissue. *syn*: tomography, polytomography.

-plasia (pla′ze-ah). suffix meaning development or formation.

-plasty. suffix indicating surgical repair or replacement of a body part; e.g., tympanoplasty.

plate, auditory. bony roof of the external ear canal.

play audiometry. technique for measuring the hearing of young children by rewarding a correct response to an auditory stimulus by allowing the child to see a picture, activate a mechanical toy, or do something equally interesting.

play therapy. method of treatment that allows a child to play with preselected toys or equipment.

pleio-, pleo- (ple′o). prefix meaning more.

pleiomorphic (ple″o-mor′fik) *adj.* appearing in more than one form—as the various configurations of otosclerosis.

plethysmograph (ple-thĭz′mo-graf) *n.* instrument for measuring changes in the volume of a body part or organ due to changes in the blood supply.

plexus *n.* a network of interlacing nerves, veins, or lymphatic vessels; e.g., the network of nerve fibers surrounding the hair cells. *adj*: **plexal.**

plexus tympanicus (tympanic plexus, Jacobson's plexus). network of nerves that serve the eardrum, eustachian tube, middle ear, and mastoid.

plosive *n.* speech sound made by suddenly releasing air pressure in the voice tract as p, b, d, t, g, and k. *syn*: stop consonants.

plugs, ear. devices intended to be inserted in the external ear canal to protect the ear from loud noises or water.

PMI. pressure measuring instrument. Sometimes called a master hearing aid.

PNdB. perceived noise decibels.

pneumatic otoscope. an otoscope with a bulb attachment to provide air pressure to cause movement of the eardrum. *syn*: Siegle's otoscope.

pneumatization (nu″mah-ti-za′shun) *n.* degree to which the cells of the mastoid process are filled with air.

pneumococcal, pneumococcic arthritis (nu″mo-kok′al, nu″mo-kok′sik). an arthritis sometimes following lobar pneumonia, affecting one or more joints and the middle ear.

PNL. perceived noise level.

pockets, pouches of Troltsch. narrow slits in the wall of the tympanum forward (anterior) and behind (posterior) the handle of the malleus. More commonly referred to as the anterior and posterior recesses of the tympanic membrane.

Pohlman prosthesis (A. G. Pohlman, U.S. physician). a diaphragm of plastic in which a bristle was imbedded. The patient inserted the device into the outer ear canal until the bristle made contact with the stapes.

point, auditory. the lowest point of the notch between the tragus and the rim of the concha.

point, auricular. center of external entrance to the auditory canal. *syn*: auriculare.

Point-eight rule, Fletcher's. a seldom used formula to determine a percentage for hearing loss: the average of the hearing levels at 500, 1000, and 2000 Hz is multiplied by 0.8.

point source. a source that radiates sound uniformly in all directions in free-field conditions. *syn*: simple sound source.

polarity *n.* the state of having two opposite poles, as in a magnet.

pole *n.* one of the terminals of a battery.

pole, negative. the terminal of a battery that releases negative ions. *syn*: cathode.

pole, positive. the terminal of a battery that collects ions released by the negative terminal (cathode). *syn*: anode.

Politzer bag (Adam Politzer, Austrian otologist, 1835-1920). a pear-shaped rubber bulb used for forcing air through the eustachian tube into the middle ear.

politzerization *n.* forced expansion of the eustachian tube and inflation of the middle ear by means of a Politzer bag at the instant the patient swallows. *syn*: Politzer's method.

Politzer's cone of light. an area on the drumhead shaped like a triangle, which appears brighter than the rest of the membrane. *syn*: Politzer's luminous cone.

Politzer's luminous cone. Politzer's cone of light.

poly- (pol'e). prefix meaning several.

polycythemia (pol"e-si-the'me-ah) *n.* too many red blood cells. Sometimes held responsible for sudden deafness.

polyethylene (pol"e-eth'ĭ-lēn) *n.* PE. a type of plastic (polymer) sometimes used in surgical procedures; e.g., as a prosthesis in the stapedectomy operations.

polyethylene strut. a prosthetic device used to replace the stapes in the stapedectomy operation.

polyethylene tube. a plastic tube placed surgically through the eardrum to drain and ventilate the middle ear.

polyotia *n.* a condition in which there is an extra pinna on one or both sides of the head.

polyp, raspberry. a chronically inflamed and reddish mass of tissue that may hang within the external auditory canal.

polysyllable *n.* word containing more than three syllables.

polysyllabic *adj.* containing more than three syllables.

polytomography (pol"e-to-mog'rah-fe) *n.* a method of x-ray photography that provides focus on a particular layer of tissue. *syn*: tomography or planigraphy.

polytomogram (pol"e-to'mo-gram) *n.* an x-ray picture of a particular layer of tissue.

pons (ponz) *n.* a protruding bundle of nerve fibers on the lower rear surface of the brain. It contains (among others) nuclei of the VIIIth cranial nerve. Also referred to as the pons varolii, named for Costanza Varolio, Italian anatomist, 1544-1575.

pore (pōr) *n.* a tiny opening in the skin or other anatomic surface.

pore, auditory. the opening of the external ear canal in the pinna. *syn*: porus acusticus externa.

porus (po'rus) *n.* pore. A small opening in a tissue may also be known as a meatus or a foramen.

porus acusticus externus. the opening of the external ear canal in the pinna. *syn*: auditory pore.

porus acusticus internus. the opening of the internal ear canal into the cranial cavity.

positive electrode. 1. the anode or element that collects the free electrons released by the negative electrode (cathode) in a vacuum tube. 2. the anode of a hearing aid cell.

positive feedback. the result of a portion of the output voltage being returned and added to the input voltage. *syn*: in-phase or regenerative feedback.

positive Schwartze sign. reddish color of the promontory as seen through the intact tympanic membrane. An indication of possible cochlear otosclerosis.

post- prefix meaning behind, after, later, or as a result of.

postauricle *adj.* behind the ear.

postauricle hearing aid. hearing aid worn behind the ear and coupled to the ear by tubing attached to an earmold. *syn*: BTE (behind the ear) hearing aid.

postauricular tympanoplasty. repair of the eardrum by an approach from behind the pinna.

posterior (pos-tēr'e-or) *adj.* behind, toward the back or rear.

posterior vertical canal. one of the semicircular canals—part of the human balance mechanism.

postlingual deafness. loss of hearing occurring after the acquisition of speech and language.

postnatal (pōst-na'tal) *adj.* after birth.

postrhinoscopic (post-ri"no-skop'ik) *adj.* in back of the nose.

poststimulatory threshold shift. the phenomenon by which a sound continues to be masked (not heard) for a brief period after the masking noise is discontinued. *syn*: forward or residual masking.

postulate (pos'tu-lāt) *n.* a supposition assumed to be true without proof.

potential difference. PD.

potential, electrical. the amount of electrical pressure (electromotive force measured in volts) potentially available in an electrically charged body.

potential, endolymphatic (en"do-lim-fat'ik). energy in the form of steady voltage between the endolymph inside the cochlear partition and the perilymph outside.

potential, evoked. EP. electrical potential generated by brain activity in response to a stimulus; e.g., sound.

potential, intracellular. the negative internal polarizations of cells in relation to adjacent tissue fluids. Within the cochlea, intracellular potentials are from −20 to −80 millivolts in relation to the perilymph.

potential, microphonic. the electrical voltage produced by the hair cells of the cochlea. *syn*: cochlear microphonic.

potentiometer (po-ten"she-om'ĕ-ter) *n.* an instrument designed to measure electromotive force.

power (pow'er) *n.* the amount of energy used or generated in a given unit of time; usually expressed in watts.

power, acoustic. the square root of the pressure generated by a tone or combination of tones.

power CROS. a hearing aid amplifying system that provides a microphone at one ear with a wire leading to an amplifier and receiver at the other ear. It is designed to allow the use of greater power through ear-level aids.

power law. an equation formulated to relate loudness to intensity. Loudness is proportional to the 0.3 power of the intensity (energy flux density).

power level. in decibels, is 10 times the logarithm to the base 10, of the ratio of a given power to a reference power. The reference power must be indicated.

power of sound waves. proportional to the square of the pressure; also proportional to the square of the velocity.

power output meter. an instrument designed to measure power. The input impedance is varied by means of a selector switch. The scale may be calibrated both in milliwatts and decibels.

power pack. a device for supplying or converting energy for use in a hearing aid or audiometer.

power, phonetic. relative energy of a speech sound (phoneme).

power unit. the unit for measuring power is the watt.

pps. pulses per second.

pragmatic (prag-mat'ik) *adj.* concerning knowledge gained from practical experience as opposed to theoretical speculation.

pragmatics *n.* study of the practical application of the rules of syntax as affected by common or local usage.

prate (prāt) *v.* to speak nonsense or to babble.

prattle (prat'al) *n.* meaningless speech.

prattle *v.* to voice meaningless sounds. *n*: **prattler.**

pre- prefix meaning before, in front of, or in advance of.

preauricular (pre"aw-rik'u-lar) *adj.* near or in front of the pinna (auricle).

preauricular appendages or tags. either protuberances or pits that occur in front of the pinna. They may be indicative of other disorders or abnormalities.

preauricular tags. preauricular appendages.

precedence effect (prĕ'sĭ-dence). when the same sound reaches the ear from two sources at different distances, the precedence effect results from the sound being heard as coming from the nearer source rather than from both.

precedent masking. a louder noise is introduced within 100 milliseconds after a short pure tone test is presented. The louder noise masks out (makes inaudible) the pure tone even though the louder sound is presented after the test tone. *syn*: backward masking.

precipitating factor. element that causes or accelerates a condition.

precipitous (pre-sip'ĭ-tus) *adj.* sharply falling—loss increases about 15 to 20 dB in the higher frequencies.

precondition *n.* a state of circumstance that must precede an action.

precondition *v.* to prepare or induce a state of mind that will allow something to happen as a result of another action.

predisposing factor. genetic or environmental element that inclines a person toward a condition.

preferred frequencies. series of frequency bands recommended by the American National Standards Institute for acoustical measurements. The cut-off frequencies are 45, 90, 180, 355, 710, 1400, 2800, and 5600 Hz. Corresponding midfrequencies are 63, 125, 250, 500, 1000, 2000, and 4000 Hz.

prefix (pre'fiks) *n.* a portion of a word—constant in its meaning (as hemo, blood)—attached to the beginning of other words to influence their meaning.

prelingual (pre-ling'gwal) *adj.* preceding the establishment of speech. *syn*: preverbal.

prelingual deafness. hearing impairment occurring before the development of speech and language. May be either adventitious or congenital.

premature (pre-mah-tūr') *adj.* before maturity. A pregnancy that does not run full term may result in a high-risk birth; that is, there may be a predisposition to birth defects.

premise (pre'mis) *n.* a supposition used as the basis for debate or inference.

premise *v.* to set forth a supposition as a basis for discussion.

prenatal (pre-na'tal) *adj.* before birth.

preplacement audiogram. in industrial audiometry, an audiogram resulting from a hearing test that preceded employment in a particular job.

presby- (pres'be). prefix referring to the aging process.

presbycusis, presbyacousis, presbyacusis (pres"be-ku'sis) *n.* the loss of hearing sensitivity associated with the aging process.

presence *n.* the sensation of realism created by the midrange (frequencies) that the listener is in the presence of the performer. (Usage with hearing aids introduced by E. Robert Libby.)

presenter switch. switch that presents a tone from an audiometer. *syn:* interrupter switch.

pressure (presh'ur) *n.* a measure of force divided by the area to which the force is applied. In audiology it is measured in dynes per square centimeter.

pressure, acoustic radiation. tiny increase in atmospheric pressure on a surface resulting from sound waves.

pressure hearing aid. hearing aid using a so-called nondirectional microphone. It is said to be sensitive only to the sound pressure at the location of the microphone opening.

pressure measuring instrument. PMI. generic term intended to include all the master hearing aids made by various hearing aid manufacturers.

pressure meter. electronic device made up of a microphone, an amplifying network, and a meter to indicate the r.m.s. (root-mean-square) value of the sound pressure in a complex sound wave. In addition to a flat C scale, it usually includes two other scales, A and B, which attenuate the low frequencies in various degrees. *syn:* sound level meter, sound pressure meter.

pressure, peak sound. maximum pressure point of any sound or pressure wave. *syn:* peak output.

pressure phase. two tones of the same frequency and intensity are said to be in pressure phase when their cycles of compression and rarefaction are identical. The resulting tone will be twice the amplitude of either one. *syn:* in phase.

pressure, sound. changes in the molecular pattern of a medium caused by the energy or force of sound. Measurement is in dynes per square centimeter.

pressure spectrum level. American standard acoustical terminology: the pressure spectrum level of a sound at a specified frequency is the effective sound pressure level for the sound energy contained within a band 1 cycle per second wide, centered at a specified frequency. Ordinarily this has significance only for sound having a continuous distribution of energy within the frequency range under consideration. The reference pressure should be explicitly stated.

pressure, static. constant and unchanging pressure.

pressure waves. successions of compressions and rarefactions of the air caused by a vibrating body.

preverbal (pre-ver'bal) *adj.* before speech has been established. *syn:* prelingual.

PRF. pulse recurrence frequency, pulse repetition frequency.

primary auditory cortex. the part of the cortex of the brain that receives nerve impulses from the ear.

primary centers in the brain. the areas or portions of the brain where sensory associations are stored.

printed circuit. a circuit printed, etched, or built up with a conductive material to include the necessary wiring, condensers, and resistors for an electronic device such as a hearing aid.

prints, voice. a picture of the spectrum of a voice as revealed by a spectrograph.

probable error. PE. percentage of expected deviation from predicted result caused by uncontrollable factors.

probe (prōb) *n.* 1. a device designed to test the ability of various portions of the ossicular chain to transmit sound pressures. 2. pointed metal rod for making electrical contact with a circuit element being checked.

probe, acoustic. device utilizing a long thin rod to compare the sensation of loudness when various parts of the conductive mechanism are touched.

probe, sound. tiny microphone on a thin rod or cylinder designed to study sound waves in small confined spaces with a minimum of disturbance to the wave form.

probe-tube microphone. tiny microphone attached to a flexible plastic tube. A variant of the sound-probe microphone.

procaine *n.* a drug used as a local anesthetic or, intravenously, to increase blood flow.

process *n.* a protuberance, projection, or outgrowth—as of bone; e.g., the mastoid process behind the ear.

process, auditory. the edge of the tympanic plate to which the cartilage of the external ear canal is attached.

process, cochlear. a thin plate of bone that separates the eustachian tube from the canal, through which the tensor tympani muscle passes to the malleus.

process, lenticular. a knob at the tip of the long process of the incus (anvil) into which the head of the stapes fits.

process, long. a comparatively long projection of bone; that is, long compared to other projections of the same bone; e.g., the long process of the malleus.

process, long, of the incus. the arm of the incus (anvil) that articulates (moves) the stapes.

process, mastoid. the rounded bony structure behind the outer ear usually honeycombed by air cells.

process, postglenoid. portion of the temporal bone that almost separates the jawbone from the external ear canal.

process, short. opposite of long process.

prodrome (pro'drŏm) *n.* early symptom of disease. *adj:* **prodromal, prodromic, prodromous.**

profound deafness. extreme hearing impairment bordering on total deafness. A degree of loss so severe that hearing aid amplification must be supplemented by speechreading at all times to be effective. Numerically, it is generally considered to be an average of over 90 dB at 500, 1000, and 2000 Hz audiometrically (ANSI).

prognosis (prog-no'sis) *n.* forecast or prediction of the course of a disease or disability.

progressive matrices test. a test of intelligence sometimes used with deaf and hard-of-hearing adults.

prolapsed *adj.* closed—as by a breakdown of tissue around the external auditory canal.

prominence, spiral. a ridge in the cochlea on the inner surface of the spiral ligament that contains blood vessels.

promontory (prom'on-to"re) *n.* bony structure that protrudes into the middle ear cavity between the oval and round windows. It is formed by the first turn of the cochlea.

prootic (pro-ot'ik) *adj.* in front of the ear.

prophylactic (pro"fi-lak'tik) *adj.* pertaining to prophylaxis—the prevention of disease.

prophylactic *n.* a method (such as vaccination) or device used for the prevention of disease.

prophylaxis *n.* following rules, systems, or methods that will prevent disease.

proportional liability. a legal rule based on the principle that several employers may be held responsible for loss of hearing due to noise exposure.

proprioception (pro"pre-o-sep'shun) *n.* the awareness of position, balance, and movement that arises from within the ear. *adj:* **proprioceptive.**

proprioceptive impulses. nerve impulses leading toward the brain (afferent) that originate in sensory end-organs (proprioceptors) in the ear as well as in muscles, tendons, and joints.

proprioceptor *n.* a sensory end-organ that reacts to stimuli within the body itself—especially pressure or stretch.

prosody (pros'o-de) *n.* 1. the use of rhythmic material or versification in aural education. 2. refers to stress and intonation patterns of speech. *adj:* **prosodic.**

prosthesis (pros-the'sis) *n.* 1. hearing aid. 2. device to supplement or replace a damaged or missing part of the body. *adj:* **prosthetic.**

protectors, ear. devices to insert into the ear canal (as an earplug) or to cover the outer ear (as a muff) to lessen the effect of loud noises.

Prussak's space (Alexander Prussak, Russian physician, 1839-1897.) space between the eardrum and the neck of the malleus.

PSB. Professional Services Board (ASHA).

psellism (sel'izm) *n.* 1. stuttering. 2. mispronunciation of words, especially when due to cleft palate.

pseud-, pseudo- prefix indicating false.

pseudacousma (su"dah-kōōz'mah) *n.* 1. condition in which sounds appear to be altered in pitch and quality. 2. condition in which one imagines he hears sounds. *syn:* pseudacusis.

pseudoatresia (su"do-ah-tre'ze-ah) *n.* false closure. Said of the effect of misplacing the earphone of the audiometer in such a manner that the ear canal is closed.

pseudobinaural. separation of amplified sound from one hearing aid to both ears—a Y-cord fitting.

pseudochromesthesia (su"do-kro"mes-the'ze-ah) *n.* color hearing. The sense of color that accompanies certain sounds for some people.

pseudohypacusis, pseudohypoacusis *n.* nonorganic or psychogenic hearing loss.

Pseudomonas (su"do-mo'nas) *n.* a form of bacteria sometimes found in cases of continually draining ears.

pseudothreshold (su"do-thresh'old) *n.* false threshold.

pseudotumor (su"do-tu'mor) *n.* a swelling resembling a tumor. Sometimes a cholesteatoma is referred to as a pseudotumor.

psi. per square inch.

psopholalia (so"fo-la'le-ah) *n.* vocalizing (babbling) with no attempt to make conventional speech sounds or to communicate with others. A normal stage in the development of speech. Lack of or early cessation of babbling may be indicative of hearing impairment in the infant.

psych-, psycho- prefix indicating the mind.

psychauditory (si-kaw'dĭ-tor-e) *adj.* concerning the perception and interpretation of sound.

psychic deafness. a type of deafness in which sounds are heard but not understood. Aphasia.

psychoacoustics *n.* the combination of psychology and acoustics referring to the study of man's response to sound.

psychogalvanic audiometry. PGA. commonly called PGSR (psycho-galvanic skin response). A method of determining hearing thresholds by measuring changes in skin resistance, associated with a conditioned response to sound stimulus. *syn*: electrodermal audiometry.

psychogalvanic reflex, skin response. PGSR. a change in electrical skin resistance resulting from a sensory stimulus.

psychogalvanic skin response (or resistance) test. PGSR or GSR test. An auditory stimulus is given (as a warning signal) followed by a mild shock. The change in electrical resistance of the skin is recorded automatically by a stylus on a moving roll of paper. After adequate conditioning, the shock is withheld and a response to an auditory stimulus alone may thus be measured. *syn*: psychogalvanometric test.

psychogalvanometer (si″ko-gal″vah-nom′ĕ-ter) *n.* a device that records changes in electrical skin resistance resulting from mental or emotional stimuli.

psychogenic (si″ko-gen′ik) *adj.* arising from mental or emotional problems—as opposed to physiogenic, arising from physiologic causes—that is, changes in the normal living processes.

psychogenic deafness. all-inclusive term used to refer to a deficiency in which hearing loss is psychological rather than organic in nature.

psychokinesis (si″ko-kĭ-ne′sis) *n.* PK. the influence of the mind upon matter. The movement of objects by the mind only.

psycholinguistics *n.* the study of language or articulate expression as psychologically influenced by contemporary culture.

psychologic, psychological *adj.* relating to the mind.

psychologist *n.* a specialist in the study of the mind and its functioning.

psychometer (si-kom′ĕ-ter) *n.* 1. a device to measure mental work accomplished, time consumed, or intelligence involved in a task. 2. an older term for psychogalvanometer.

psychometrics, psychometry *n.* measurement of mental processes.

psychomotor (si″ko-mo′tor) *adj.* relating to the mental origin of voluntary movement.

psychophysics *n.* the science that deals with the relations between sense organs and physical stimuli. *adj*: **psychophysical.**

psychophysiologist *n.* a specialist in the study of the effects of mental activity on the body.

psychosensory *adj.* relating to the conscious perception of sensory stimuli.

psychosomatic (si″ko-so-mat′ik) *adj.* concerning the interrelationships between mind and body.

psychosomatic disorder. a dysfunction caused or intensified by mental or emotional factors.

psychovoltaic response. (si″ko-vol-ta′ik). PVR. a change in electrical skin potential resulting from a sensory stimulus.

PTA. pure tone average; pure tone audiogram. Parent-Teacher Association.

pts. permanent threshold shift.

pulse *n.* rhythmical presentation of short bursts of a pure tone.

pulse, alternating. a series of short bursts of pure tones that vary in amplitude in regular cycles.

pulse code of ear. system of electrical impulses relayed along the auditory nerve in response to a stimulus that the brain decodes and identifies.

pulse generator. instrument that produces short bursts of tone.

pulse, nerve. the burst of electrical energy that moves along the nerve fiber in response to a stimulus.

pulses per second, pps. the number of times a burst of tone may be presented in a second.

pulse recurrence frequency, pulse repetition frequency. PRF. the rate per second in which bursts of tone are presented.

pulse repetition rate. the number of times a burst of sound is repeated in a second.

pulse-tone group test. another name for, or a variation of, the binaural group test.

pulse-tone techniques with tone interrupter. the use of the tone interrupter to present pulsed tones through the audiometer.

pulsed-tone threshold audiometry test. the determination of thresholds of hearing sensitivity by means of short bursts of pure tones.

pupillary reflex (pu′pĭ-ler-e). eye blink in response to a sound stimulus.

pure tone. a tone or note that has only one frequency with no harmonics or overtones. *syn*: sinusoidal wave form, sine wave.

pure tone audiogram. PTA. a graph or record of the threshold of hearing sensitivity as revealed by responses to pure tone stimuli.

pure tone audiometer. the basic type of audiometer. An instrument that generates pure tones of various frequencies and ranges of intensity, which can be controlled to measure hearing acuity or sensitivity.

pure tone audiometry. audiometry based on the use of pure tones of various frequencies and intensities as auditory stimuli to measure hearing. Included are comparisons of responses to pulsed and continuous tones and comparisons of results with earphones and bone oscillators.

pure tone average. PTA. the average of the pure tone thresholds at 500, 1000, and 2000 Hz. The Committee on Hearing and Equilibrium of the AAO-HNS recommends that 3000 Hz be considered when calculating the pure tone average.

pure tone oscillator. a device designed to produce a tone of one frequency without harmonics.

pure tone threshold. level of intensity at which pure tone is just barely recognizable.

purulence, purulency (pu′roo-lens) *n.* a condition characterized by pus.

purulent *adj.* containing pus.

push-pull. two transistors (or tubes) are placed in the circuit of a hearing aid so one is pulling on an alternating input signal and the other is pushing the signal.

PVR. psychovoltaic response.

PVV. positive venting valve.

PWL. power level (or power watt level).

py-, pyo- combining form indicating pus, the presence of pus, or a condition associated with pus.

pyocyanase (pi″o-si′ah-nās) *n.* an antibiotic produced from bacteria.

pyolabyrinthitis (pi″o-lab″ĭ-rin-thi′tis). inflammation with draining of pus from the labyrinth of the ear.

pyosalpingitis (pi″o-sal″pin-ji′tis). inflammation of the eustachian tube with draining pus.

pyramid (pēr′ah-mid) *n.* small bony projection in the posterior wall of the middle ear cavity to which the stapedius muscle is anchored. *adj*: **pyramidal.**

pyramidal eminence. the pyramid.

pyr-, pyro- combining form meaning heat or fire.

pyrogenic (pi″ro-jen′ik) *adj.* causing or caused by fever.

Q

quality *n.* the psychological sensation of the quality of sound results from the difference in overtones generated with the fundamental through varying resonators.

quasi-Moro reflex (kwa′zi). quasi—approximating. A reflexive muscular reaction on

the part of the infant to a stimulus that is not a complete withdrawal to the fetal position.

quiescent (kwi-ĕ′sent) *adj.* inactive, latent, or dormant.

quinine (kwin′in, kwi′nīn) *n.* a drug formerly used for the prevention of malaria. Now a part of many cold remedies and abortifacients, it may cause deafness in susceptible individuals.

quotient, achievement. AQ. a number given to represent the relationship between chronological age (set as 100—or 100%) and the skills exhibited.

quotient, educational. EQ. a number given to represent the relationship between chronological age and grade standing in school.

quotient, intelligence. IQ. the number resulting from dividing the score of a test designed to determine the relative mental capacity of a person by his chronological age and multiplying by 100.

R

radial nerves. neurons that separate from the cochlear nerve and move out from the center of the cochlea to connect with some of the hair cells.

radiation, auditory. the bundle of nerve fibers extending from the auditory centers of the brain to the first synaptic junction points (medial geniculate bodies) in the pathway to the ears.

radiation feedback. a type of acoustic feedback (hearing aid squeal) that may occur when the earmold is not snug enough, a vent is too large, or the coupling tubing is too thin for the intensity level produced by the hearing aid.

radiation pressure, acoustic. the tiny increase in atmospheric pressure on a surface resulting from sound waves.

radical mastoidectomy. surgical removal of the middle ear structures in addition to the removal of diseased mastoid cells.

radical surgery. surgery intended to be an absolute cure and not just to relieve symptoms—as opposed to conservative treatment.

radio- (ra′de-o). prefix referring to 1. radium or radiant energy (as in x-rays). 2. radius.

radiogram (ra′de-o-gram″) *n.* seldom used term for x-ray picture. (More commonly used to refer to a message sent by radiotelegraphy).

radiograph (ra′de-o-graf″) *n.* uncommon term for x-ray picture. *syn:* roentgenogram.

radiographer (ra″de-og′rah-fer) *n.* x-ray technician.

radiologist (ra″de-ol′o-jist) *n.* physician specializing in the use of x-rays and radioactive substances for pictures or therapy.

radiology (ra″de-ol′o-je) *n.* medical specialty involving the use of radiant energy (x-rays and radioactive substances) for diagnostic and treatment purposes. *syn:* roentgenology.

radiolus (ra-de′o-lus) *n.* a sound used as a probe.

radiotherapy (ra″de-o-ther′ah-pe) *n.* treatment of diseased tissue by x-rays or radioactive material applied locally.

Rainville method. a procedure for determining the conductive loss by comparing the masking effect on air-conducted tones produced by bone-conducted noise at the mastoid between normal listeners and the patient under test.

Rainville test. A bone-conduction test devised by M. J. Rainville about 1955. It involves a comparison of the air and bone masking intensities required to mask an air-conducted pure tone threshold.

Rainville test (modified). M-R. the masking noise is applied through the forehead rather than through the mastoid.

raised threshold. an indication of lessened hearing sensitivity—the intensity of the sound must be raised to be heard.

Ramsey-Hunt syndrome. a complex of symptoms of a viral infection of the VIIth (facial) nerve. Among the symptoms are earaches followed by aural (otitic) herpes—a rash of tiny blisters in and around the ear. (Sometimes spelled Ramsay-Hunt).

ramulus (ram′u-lus) *n.* a tiny branch or final division of a ramus.

ramus (ra′mus) *pl.* **rami** *n.* a branch, as of a blood vessel, nerve, bone, or a groove in the brain. For example, the caroticotympanic ramus is a branch of the carotid artery that serves the tympanic cavity.

Randall's Island performance test. a nonverbal test of intelligence suitable for preschool deaf and hard of hearing children. It involves performance and manipulative tasks.

random *adj.* concerning distribution by chance.

random noise. a complex sound wave whose instantaneous amplitudes vary in time according to a normal distribution curve.

randomization *n.* the arrangement of a sampling of the elements or numbers involved in a test in such a manner as to appear to be a chance distribution, reduce the effect of meaningless variables, and produce more reliable statistical data.

range *n.* the area or extent included between the lowest and highest in any set of variables.

range of comfortable loudness. RCL. a range of sound pressure intensities that are subjectively comfortably loud for the individual.

range, frequency. any series of frequencies between specified limits either controlled (as in an audiometer) or natural (as in the response of the human ear).

Ranvier, node of (Louis A. Ranvier, French histologist, 1835-1922). one of the spots along a nerve cell where the myelin sheath is broken and the nerve is exposed. The nerve jumps from node to node to node—thus speeding it up.

rapid random loudness judgments. RRLJ. a test of nonorganic deafness devised by Robert F. Nagel. It involves quickly presenting pure tones randomly to each ear at various frequencies and intensities to confuse the suspected malingerer into responding to better levels than previously indicated.

rapport (rah-por′) *n.* a relationship of sympathy, understanding, and confidence.

rarefaction *n.* decrease of pressure. Second half of the cycle of a sound wave. *adj:* **rarefactional, rarefactive.**

Rasmussen, bundle of (G. L. Rasmussen). A group of efferent nerve fibers running between the superior olivary complex and the cochlea.

raspberry polyp. a chronically inflamed and reddish mass of tissue that may hang within the external auditory canal.

rate of decay. the speed with which a tone (or other sound pressure level) is fading at a given place and time. The rate may be expressed in decibels per second.

rationale (rash″un-al′) *n.* the basis or reason for an action or opinion.

rayl *n.* (Lord John W. S. Rayleigh, 1842-1919). a unit of measurement of acoustic resistance.

RCL. range of comfortable loudness.

RDP. relative delivered pressure.

reactance (re-ak′tans) *n.* the portion of the resistance to the flow of an alternating current through a circuit, which is due to capacitance or inductance or both. It is computed by formula and expressed in ohms.

reactance, acoustic. the portion of acoustic impedance that results from a combination of the stiffness and mass of the eardrum and middle ear mechanism.

reactance, inductive. a measure of the resistance to electrical flow in an induction coil.

reaction *n.* the response to an auditory stimulus.

reaction, Herxheimer (Karl Herxheimer, German physician, b. 1861). syphilitic deafness resulting from insufficient doses of a remedy.

reactive *adj.* concerning the quality of compliance of the middle ear mechanism in response to a sound stimulus.

reading, speech. to understand by close observation of the speaker's lips, facial expression, and gestures; sometimes referred to as visual hearing.

real-ear attenuation. a measurement of the amount by which ear protectors lessen sound pressure reaching the eardrum of a particular observer. It is expressed in decibels of difference between thresholds of audibility when the ears are open and when they are protected.

real ear gain. the additional sound pressure reaching the eardrum when a hearing aid is used—compared to the sound pressure reaching the eardrum without a hearing aid. *syn:* etymotic, orthotelephonic, or insertion gain.

receiver *n.* a device that converts (transduces) electrical impulses into sound waves (or signals). *syn:* earphone.

receiver, air conduction. a device that receives the amplified electronic signal of the hearing aid circuit and converts it into sound pressure waves (acoustical energy) that activate the eardrum and start the hearing process.

receiver, bone conduction. a vibrator or oscillator designed to transmit sound pressure waves through the skull.

receiver earmold. a full, solid, direct-coupled type of mold with metal snap-ring or other attachment to hold receiver directly onto the earmold.

receiver operating characteristic. ROC. the relationship among hits, misses, and false positives, of a listener to the detection of a threshold signal. The relationship may be graphically represented by a curve known as a ROC curve.

receptive aphasia. lack of ability to understand spoken or written language.

receptor *n.* 1. a sense organ: the ear. 2. any cell or grouping of cells that receive stimuli.

receptor, auditory. a hair cell in the inner ear.

receptor, distance. a sense organ that can respond to a stimulus originating at a distance from the body; e.g., the ear. *syn:* telereceptor.

receptor, sensory. any cell or group of cells (as the hair cells of the ear) that respond to an external stimulus. They give rise to an afferent nerve impulse (leading to the brain).

recess (re′ses) *n.* a cavity, hollow, or depression; e.g., the tympanic recess of the middle ear containing the head of the malleus and the body of the incus.

recess, cochlear. a small depression between the oval and round windows that forms the vestibular end of the cochlear duct.

recess, elliptical. small cavity in the upper part of the wall of the vestibule in which the utricle is lodged. The utricular fossa.

recess, epitympanic (ep″ĭ-tim-pan′ik). attic or upper portion of the middle ear, the epitympanum.

recess, pharyngeal. depression in the wall of the pharynx above and behind the eustachian tube. *syn:* fossa of Rosenmuller.

recess, spherical. depression in the wall of the vestibule of the inner ear in which the saccule is situated.

recesses, tympanic membrane. narrow pockets in the wall of the tympanum forward (anterior) and behind (posterior) the handle of the malleus. *syn:* pouches, pockets, or recesses of Troltsch.

recessive gene. a mutant gene whose failure to transmit a normal hereditary characteristic is masked by the dominant gene of a pair.

recorded speech test. list of words that has been reproduced on records or tapes for the purpose of determining speech reception thresholds or discrimination abilities.

recruitment (re-krōōt′ment) *n.* phenomenon that sometimes accompanies a sensory impairment in which a relatively slight increase in the intensity of a sound results in a disproportionate increase in the sensation of loudness. It is considered to be indicative of end-organ deafness—a lesion of the organ of Corti.

recruitment, complete. the sensation of loudness of a tone in the poor ear equals the sensation of loudness in the good ear at higher intensity levels.

recruitment factor. RF. degree by which an abnormally rapid increase in the sensation of loudness affects the ability of an individual to handle loud or amplified sound.

recruitment, hyper- the sensation of loudness of a tone in the poor ear exceeds the sensation of loudness in the good ear at higher intensity levels. *syn:* overrecruitment.

recruitment, incomplete. the sensation of loudness of a tone in the poor ear approaches, but does not equal, the sensation of loudness in the good ear at high intensity levels.

recruitment, loudness. abnormal growth of the sensation of loudness. See recruitment.

recruitment, over- hyperrecruitment.

recruitment, partial. incomplete recruitment.

recruitment test, Metz. an acoustic impedance measurement that may indicate recruitment in a patient with a hearing impairment if a stapedius reflex is elicited by a stimulus smaller than 60 to 70 dB above threshold.

rectangular voltage pulse. a pulse that has an instantaneous rise and decay and remains at maximum for a measurable time.

rectifier *n.* device that converts alternating current into direct current.

rectify *v.* to convert alternating current into direct or unidirectional current.

rectrometer *n.* an instrument designed to transmit sound by light-beam vibrations. A photophone.

reduced screening test. a screening test limited to 1, 2, or 3 frequencies at preset levels of intensity. *syn:* limited frequency screening.

redundant (re-dun′dant) *adj.* unnecessary repetition of a word or phrase.

redundancy (re-dun′dan-se) *n.* the repetition of sounds within words or phrases that sometimes makes them understandable even to an entity with impaired hearing.

Reed's test. a rhyming word-picture test of discrimination devised by Michael Reed.

reference audiogram. 1. a pre-employment or pre-placement audiogram. 2. any base audiogram.

reference intensity. RI. the intensity to which another intensity is compared in a loudness balance test.

reference volume. the strength or intensity of a speech signal that will cause a VU meter to register zero.

reflected wave. a sound pressure wave moving toward the source. The opposite of an incident wave. Measurement of sound pressure waves reflected from the eardrum within the external ear canal is the basic function of tympanometry.

reflection of sound. the return of sound pressure waves toward their source.

reflex (re′fleks) *n.* an involuntary movement that results from the stimulation of a sensory nerve.

reflex, acoustic. the reflex contraction of the intra-aural muscles (tensor tympani and stapedius) in response to sound. *syn:* intra-aural reflex; cochlear reflex; auditory reflex.

reflex, acoustopalpebral. rapid and distinct closing of the eyelids, or twitch at the corner (canthus) of the eye resulting from a sudden loud stimulus. *syn:* auropalpebral reflex.

reflex, audito-oculogyric (aw″dĭ-to-ok″u-lo-ji′rik). quick movement of the head and eyes in the direction of a sudden loud sound.

reflex, auditory. acoustic reflex.

reflex, auriculopalpebral (aw-rik″u-lo-pal′pĕ-bral). closure or blink of an eye resulting from stimulation by sudden sound, heat, or some irritant touching the external auditory canal. *syn:* Kisch's reflex, auropalpebral reflex.

reflex, auropalpebral (aw″ro-pal′pĕ-bral). rapid and distinct closing of the eyelids, or twitch at the corner (canthus) of the eye resulting from a sudden sound stimulus. It is said to be closely related to the stapedius muscle reflex in the middle ear.

reflex, cochlear. more commonly called the acoustic reflex, it is the reflex contraction of the intra-aural muscles (tensor tympani and stapedius) in response to a sound stimulus. *syn:* intra-aural reflex; acoustic reflex; auditory reflex.

reflex, cochleo-orbicular. a wink or a twitch at the corner (canthus) of the eye as a result of a sudden sound near the ear. *syn:* acousticopalpebral reflex, auropalpebral reflex, or cochleopalpebral reflex.

reflex, cochleopalpebral. acousticoorbicular reflex, auropalpebral reflex, or cochleo-orbicular reflex.

reflex, Gault's. seldom used term for the auropalpebral (APR) reflex.

reflex, intra-aural. the reflex contraction of the intra-aural muscles (tensor tympani and stapedius.) in response to sound. *syn:* acoustic reflex.

reflex, Kisch's. auriculopalpebral reflex—closure or blink of an eye resulting from stimulation by sudden sound, heat, or some irritant touching the external ear canal.

reflex, light. a triangular bright area on the eardrum. Also known as the cone of light, its base is on the lower edge of the tympanic membrane with the apex pointing toward the center. (Its position to the right or left of the umbo indicates accordingly which eardrum is being pictured).

reflex, Moro's or response, Moro's. the startle reaction of a newborn to a stimulus. It is evidenced by any or all of various sudden grimacing or stiffening movements. Sometimes described as a defensive return to the fetal position.

reflex, oculogyric (ok″u-lo-ji′rik). a movement of the eyeball, e.g., one that might result from an auditory stimulus.

reflex, orbicularis oculi. the auropalpebral reflex—a twitch of the eyelid or corner of the eye resulting from a stimulus such as a loud sound.

reflex, psychogalvanic skin. PGSR. change in electrical skin resistance resulting from a sensory stimulus.

reflex, pupillary (pu'pĭ-ler-e). eye blink in response to sound stimulus.

reflex, quasi-Moro (kwa'zi). quasi—approximating. A reflexive muscular reaction of an infant to a stimulus that is not a complete withdrawal to the fetal position.

reflex, stapedius. SR. a contraction of the stapedius muscle in response to a loud sound.

reflex, startle. the startle reaction to a stimulus; evidenced by any or all of various sudden grimacing or stiffening movements.

reflex test. a broad term that usually refers to the observation of physiological reactions to sudden sound stimuli—especially of babies and young children.

refraction *n.* the deflection of sound waves around obstacles.

refractory period. the time between firings of nerve pulses. During this time the ions of the nerve return to their prefiring or resting position.

Refsum's disease. a syndrome characterized by hearing loss, progressive night blindness, polyneuropathy, retinitis pigmentosa, and ataxia. Usually appears in later childhood and is slowly progressive. *syn:* heredopathia atactica polyneuritoformis.

regenerate *v.* to add to the amplification of a current by using part of the power of the output circuit in the input circuit.

regeneration *n.* the addition of a portion of the output voltage to the input voltage. Positive feedback.

regenerative feedback. the result, for example, when a portion of the output voltage is returned and added to the input voltage. *syn:* positive or in-phase feedback.

Reger effect. the inadvertent closing or partial closing of the external ear canal by misplacement of the earphones. Referred to as "pseudoatresia" by Scott Reger, PhD.

regional deafness. hearing loss restricted to certain frequency regions; e.g., high frequencies.

register, high risk. 1. broadly speaking, a roll or record of the names of newborns who may possibly have auditory handicaps as the result of birth hazards such as anoxia, hyperoxia, or parental blood incompatibilities. 2. a list of the diseases, syndromes, and defects that may cause auditory handicaps in the newborn.

regression *n.* 1. return to an earlier mental or behavioral level. 2. gradual loss of function or progressive decline in ability. 3. either a subsidence or return of symptoms.

rehabilitation (re"hah-bil"ĭ-ta'shun) *n.* 1. re-education for social adequacy of one who

has become deaf or hearing impaired. 2. to train for gainful employment one who is handicapped by a hearing deficit.

rehabilitation, aural. re-education in the use of the sense of hearing, with or without the help of amplification.

Reid's base line (Robert W. Reid, Scottish anatomist, 1851-1938). a line extending from the lower edge of the eye socket through the center of the opening of the ear canal to the center of the occipital bone.

reinforcement (re"in-fors'ment) *n.* adding a stimulus or reward for an appropriate response or a punishment for an inappropriate response in order to condition the subject to respond correctly.

reinforcement, partial. not all responses in a conditioning pattern are reinforced.

Reissner's membrane (rīs'nerz) (Ernst Reissner, German physician, 1824-1878). membrane within the cochlea that separates the scala vestibuli from the scala media. *syn:* vestibular membrane; membrana vestibularis.

relative bone conduction. a test to establish levels of threshold sensitivity in response to the stimulus from a bone oscillator while the ears are open (unoccluded). Compare absolute bone conduction.

renal (re'nal) *adj.* concerning the kidneys.

replicate (rep'lĭ-kāt) *v.* to repeat or duplicate.

replication (rep"lĭ-ka'shun) *n.* one of a series of identical experiments. *adj:* **replicate.**

report, Beasley. common name for a portion of US Public Health survey of 1935-36 conducted by Dr. Willis Beasley that established a normal hearing reference zero or normal auditory threshold. This became the ASA 1951 audiometric zero and was based on the threshold of hearing of about 1200 normal hearers.

research audiologist. one engaged primarily in research concerning the function of the auditory system.

resect (re-sekt') *v.* to cut out part of an organ or tissue.

resection (re-sek'shun) *n.* an operation involving the removal of part of an organ or tissue. *adj:* **resectable.**

residual (re-zid'u-al) *adj.* concerning the part remaining after some portion is lost.

residual hearing. the range of hearing between the threshold of sensitivity and the threshold of discomfort.

residual inhibition. RI. term coined by Jack A. Vernon, PhD, to describe a phenomenon that may or may not occur after removal of a sound used to mask tinnitus: A partial attenuation or complete absence of tinnitus for periods of time that may vary with the individual.

residual masking. phenomenon by which a sound continues to be masked (not heard) for a brief period after the masking noise is discontinued. *syn:* forward masking; post-stimulatory threshold shift.

resistance (re-zis′tans) *n.* opposition to the flow of current through a material. Ohm's law: Resistance equals the voltage divided by the current.

resistance, acoustic. acoustic impedance measured in acoustic ohms. It differs in phase from acoustic reactance by one-quarter cycle.

resistance, ear. the opposition to free movement of the various parts of the middle ear as measured by impedance bridge or meter—the acoustic impedance of the ear.

resistivity *n.* opposition to movement.

resistor *n.* device used to control the flow of electricity, as in the circuit of a hearing aid.

resonance (rez′o-nans) *n.* the basic or natural frequency of vibration that is unique to an acoustic system, or an air-filled cavity. This attribute causes a modification of the sound signal by prolongation or intensification when the frequency of the input is the same as the natural frequency of the system.

resonance peak. the period of high sound pressure produced when the input signal combines with the natural (resonant) frequency of a system.

resonance theory. Helmholtz in 1857 advanced the theory that the hair cells within the organ of Corti act as resonators—each with its own natural period of vibration and each responding only to one tone of one particular frequency.

resonance theory (selective). an early version of the resonance theory of pitch perception involved various cavities thought to be behind the eardrum (Gaspard Bauhin, 1605). Later in 1683, Joseph G. Du Verney theorized that the bony lamina resonated to different frequencies in accordance with its varying width.

resonance, vocal. the sounds of the voice as heard through a stethoscope held to the chest.

resonant frequency. the number of cycles per second at which it is easiest for a mass to vibrate—whether gas, liquid, or solid. Also referred to as natural or normal frequency.

resonate *v.* to vibrate at the rate of natural frequency.

resonating. 1. vibrating at the rate of natural frequency in response to an indirect excitation of the same frequency. 2. continuing to vibrate after a stimulus has been discontinued.

resonator *n.* any structure, material, or device that can be set into vibration by sound

pressure waves of its natural frequency originating in another vibrating body.

resorb (re-sorb′, re-zorb′) *v.* to reabsorb, to create a negative pressure; e.g., oxygen in the middle ear is absorbed by the surrounding tissues when the eustachian tube is blocked—thus causing negative pressure at the eardrum (lower than the outside atmospheric pressure).

resound (re-zownd′) *v.* to reverberate or re-echo.

respiration audiometry. audiometry based on a recording of changes in respiration in response to sound stimuli.

response *n.* 1. reaction to a stimulus. 2. the pattern of output of a transducer (e.g., of a hearing aid) when measured at various frequencies after the input has been amplified.

response, arousal. increase in activity level as a result of stimulation, e.g., neonatal response to narrow-band noise.

response, cardioid (re-spons′ kar′de-oid). the heart-shaped pattern of sensitivity displayed by a directional microphone.

response, conditioned. trained or taught (conditioned) by a reward, shock, or punishment to do something (respond) when a stimulus, such as a sound, is presented.

response, covert (ko′vert). reaction that is invisible to an outside observer.

response curve. pattern of output of a hearing aid, measured at various frequencies, expressed graphically.

response, false-negative. 1. lack of reaction to a sound stimulus when it has actually been heard. For example, this term is used if an infant has not responded during a hearing screening test when his hearing is within normal limits as revealed by other tests. 2. the appearance of a reaction to a sound stimulus when it has not actually been heard. This term, for example, may be used if an infant has responded during a hearing screening test when his hearing is not within normal limits as revealed by other tests.

response, flat. amplification approximately equal at all frequencies within a stated range.

response, frequency. an expression of the electrical or acoustic reaction of a device in terms of cycles per second and in relation to an input signal.

response latency (la′ten-se). the delay between the stimulus pulse or click and the response.

response, galvanic skin (gal-van′ik). GSR. a change in skin resistance (the Feré effect) that results from a stimulus to the nervous system. *syn:* psychogalvanic skin response.

response, maladaptive (mal-a-dap′tiv). avoidance conditioning response; i.e., one where the reward is the lack (or avoidance of) a disagreeable stimulus.

response, overt (o'vert). reaction that can be easily observed.

response range, frequency. the generally accepted Hearing Aid Industry Conference method of expressing the frequency response range of a hearing aid is determined as follows: The HAIC gain is calculated and noted on the 1000 Hz vertical axis. A horizontal line is then drawn 15 dB below that point to intersect the two extremes of the hearing aid curve as plotted on the graph of frequency response. The frequency response range of the hearing aid is then expressed as from the lowest frequency point of intersection to the highest frequency point of intersection.

reticular (rĕ-tik'u-lar) *adj.* concerning a network—as of fibers or cells.

reticular formation. a network of gray matter and fibers of white matter found in the brain and spinal cord.

reticular lamina (lam'ĭ-nah). the platelike tops of cells in the organ of Corti that make up its upper surface.

retinitis pigmentosa (ret″ĭ-ni'tis pig″mento'sah). a degenerative disease of the eye. Symptoms include pigmentary changes in the retina of the eye. Sometimes coincidental with congenital hearing impairment.

retraction (re-trak'shun) *n.* a drawing back.

retraction of eardrum. the forcing inward of the eardrum that results from the loss of pressure within the middle ear when the eustachian tube is blocked.

retractor (re-trak'tor) *n.* 1. a muscle that pulls in an organ or part. 2. a surgical instrument designed to hold open the edge of a wound or incision.

retro- (ret'ro). prefix meaning backward or behind.

retroauricular (ret″ro-aw-rik'u-lar) *adj.* behind the ear.

retrocochlear (ret″ro-kok'le-ar) *adj.* behind the cochlea.

retrocochlear hearing loss. hearing impairment resulting from a lesion behind (retro) the cochlea. High frequencies are lost first and growth of the sensation of loudness is abnormally slow (recruitment) allowing loud sounds to be tolerated. The ear with this type of loss usually loses its ability to understand speech or discriminate. The pure tone loss, however, may be mild or moderate. Surgical intervention in cases of retrocochlear lesions may be helpful.

retrocochlear lesion. damage behind the cochlea (including the auditory nerve and the brain).

retrogress (ret″ro-gres') *v.* to degenerate or go backward.

retrogression (ret″ro-gresh'un) *n.* a rever-

sion or going backward. *adj:* **retrogressive.**

retrolabyrinthine hearing loss (ret″ro-lab″ĭ-rin'thĕn). hearing impairment resulting from damage behind (retro) the labyrinth. More commonly referred to as retrocochlear.

Retzius fibers (ret'ze-us fi'berz) (Anders A. Retzius, Swedish physician, 1796-1860). fibers in the outer phalangeal or Deiter's cells.

reuniens duct (re-ūn'yens dukt). the duct (or canal) of Hensen. A short membranous tube that allows the interchange of endolymph between the cochlear duct and the sacculus.

reverberant (re-ver'ber-ant) *adj.* tending to re-echo.

reverberant room. a room in which sounds tend to echo. A "live" room.

reverberate (re-verb'er-āt) *v.* to echo or resound.

reverberation (re-ver″ber-a'shun) *n.* the continued movement of sound pressure waves as the result of repeated reflections after the initiating stimulus has stopped.

reverberation chamber. an enclosure so designed that sound waves will reflect from all surfaces.

reverberation time. the time it takes for sound pressure waves to decrease 60 dB in a room after the initial impulse is stopped.

reverse switch. a switch that allows the tone in an audiometer to be kept on continuously or to be presented by the examiner.

revised Beta test. a nonlanguage test of intelligence suitable for use with deaf and hard of hearing adults.

RF. recruitment factor.

Rh. 1. Rhesus (Macaca rhesus). Species of monkey used in studies that resulted in blood incompatibility knowledge. 2. symbol for rhodium.

Rh (Rhesus) factor. a protein contained in most blood types. If the blood of the mother does not contain this protein and that of the father's does, the incompatibility may result in damage to the newborn. This factor was first described in 1940 and associated with deafness in 1950.

Rh negative. having no Rh factor in the blood.

Rh positive. having the Rh factor in the blood.

rhinitis (ri-ni'tis) *n.* inflammation involving the mucous membrane of the nose.

rhino- (ri'no). combining form indicating the nose.

rhinolaryngology (ri″no-lar″in-gol'o-je) *n.* medical specialty dealing with the nose and throat.

rhinopharyngitis (ri″no-far″in-ji'tis) *n.* inflammation involving the nose and throat.

rhyme test (rim). a test of speech discrimination involving the use of words whose vowel sounds are the same but the initial and/or final consonants differ.

rhythm, alpha (rith'm). a basic brainwave pattern of about 10 cycles per second on an electroencephalogram.

RI. residual inhibition; reference intensity.

ribonucleic acid (ri"bo-nu'kle-ik). RNA. a complex chemical structure composed of sugar (pentose), phosphoric acid, and nitrogen. It forms the base of the protein molecules within body cells.

right ear. auris dextra (AD).

right ear dominancy. dextraural.

right side of the body. dextral.

ring n. a sound that reverberates or re-echoes.

ring v. to reverberate, resound, or re-echo.

ring, tympanic. an embryonic bony structure that develops into the tympanic plate of the temporal bone.

Rinne test (rin'nēh) (Heinrich Adolf Rinne, German physician, 1819-1868). primarily a tuning fork test. After being struck lightly the fork is held alternately with its base on the mastoid process, then with its acoustic axis in line with the ear canal, until it is no longer heard in one position or the other. When the sound is heard longer by air it is described as a positive Rinne—(symbol +R). When the sound is heard longer by bone it is known as a negative Rinne—(symbol −R). A negative Rinne is also indicated by pure tone audiometry when there is an air-bone gap, i.e., when the bone oscillator produces a better threshold than by air. A negative Rinne may be indicative of a conductive hearing loss or a conductive component in a mixed loss.

rise time. the interval of time required for a signal to increase from a minimum to a specified maximum of intensity.

Rivinus's ligament (August Q. Rivinus, German physician, 1652-1723). a small thin triangular portion of the eardrum. It is in the upper part of the tympanic membrane. Since it is not as tense as the rest of the eardrum it is called the "flaccid part", pars flaccida. syn: Shrapnell's membrane.

Rivinus's notch. a niche in the upper part of the annular ring that contains the flaccid part of the eardrum.

rms. root mean square.

RNA. ribonucleic acid.

roar n. a loud continuous noise.

roar v. to make a loud continuous noise.

ROC. receiver operating characteristic.

Rochester method. a method of teaching the deaf in which oralism is supplemented by fingerspelling.

rods of Corti. long cells (pillar cells) that rest on the basilar membrane. The cells are joined at the top but spread at the bottom to form the arches of the tunnel of Corti.

roentgen (rent'gen). (Wilhelm Konrad Roentgen, German physicist, 1845-1923) n. a measurement of x-ray dosage.

roentgen ray. x-ray.

roentgenogram (rent-gen'o-gram") n. x-ray picture. Infrequently referred to as a radiogram.

roentgenology (rent"gĕ-nol'o-je) n. study of the use of x-ray radiation for diagnosis and therapy; syn: radiology.

roentgenotherapy (rent"gen-o-ther'ah-pe). use of x-ray radiation for therapeutic purposes. syn: radiotherapy.

Rolando's area. the motor area in the precentral area of the cerebral cortex.

room, dead. a room with a maximum degree of sound absorption. An anechoic chamber is the ultimate example of a dead room. syn: free field room.

room, free field. an anechoic chamber—a room especially built so that the sound waves generated within are almost totally absorbed by the material used to cover walls, ceiling, and floor. There must also be a high degree of isolation from external sounds; syn: dead room.

room, live. a room in which sounds tend to echo. A reverberant room.

room, sound. usually refers to a chamber that is sound-isolated or has been sound-treated (with sound-absorbent material) to minimize the effect of ambient noise.

root-mean-square. rms. the square root of the mean of a number of squared quantities or the square root of the mean of the squares of instantaneous values within a quantity.

Rorschach test (ror'shahk) (Herman Rorschach, Swiss psychiatrist, 1884-1922). a measurement of personality and intelligence based upon interpretation of the subject's explanation of or comments concerning inkblot designs.

Rosenmuller's fossa (Johann Christian Rosenmuller, German physician, 1771-1820). depression in the wall of the pharynx above and behind the eustachian tube. syn: pharyngeal recess.

Rosenthal's canal (canalis spiralis cochleae) (Isidor Rosenthal, German physician, 1836-1915). the membranous spiral tube of the cochlea that contains the scala media, the scala tympani, and the scala vestibuli.

roseola (ro-ze'o-lah) n. a rose-colored rash, typical of rubella or German measles. adj: roseolar.

rostral (ros'tral). pertaining to the head; cephalic.

rotary test. test of equilibrium. The patient is seated in a Barany chair that can be turned rapidly in a circular motion and stopped suddenly.

rotation test. the rotary test.

round window. covered by a flexible membrane, this opening in the bony casing of the cochlea allows movement of the perilymph in the scala tympani to compensate for movement caused by the stapes at the oval window. *syn*: cochlear window; fenestra cochleae; fenestra rotunda.

round window niche. depression (below and behind the promontory) in the bony casing of the inner ear that contains the round window.

RRLJ. rapid random loudness judgement.

RSA. Rehabilitation Service Administration.

RTL. reference threshold level.

rubella (roo-bel'ah) *n.* German measles. A viral disease that, during the first three months of pregnancy, can adversely affect the developing embryo. Congenitally impaired hearing is a common result.

rubeola (roo-be'o-lah) *n.* measles. (rubeola is sometimes used synonymously with rubella). *adj*: **rubeolar.**

Rudmose audiometer. automatic recording audiometer designed by Wayne Rudmose, PhD.

Rudmose group test. the use of the Rudmose audiometer with multiple attenuators and recorders to automatically test the hearing of several subjects at the same time.

running ear. suppurative otitis media is the most common term, but it may also be referred to as othelcosis, otoblennorrhea, otocatarrh, otopyorrhea, or otopyosis.

running speech test. a method of determining the speech reception threshold (SRT) by the use of unemotional connected discourse progressively reduced in intensity until it can no longer be understood.

Rutherford, telephone theory of. a discounted belief that the basilar membrane vibrates as a whole like the diaphragm of a telephone. W. Rutherford in 1886 said that the entire organ of Corti would be stimulated by each sound wave that would then be translated into a nerve impulse of corresponding frequency and amplitude.

S

sabin (sa'bin) *n.* unit of measurement of sound absorption. It is equal to the absorption of 1 square foot of surface that is completely sound absorbent.

sac, endolymphatic (sak en"do-lim-fat'ik). a pouch embedded in the mastoid filled with endolymph.

saccular macula (sak'u-lar mak'u-lah). a raised spot on the wall of the saccule where a portion of the vestibular nerve terminates.

saccule, sacculus (sak'ūl, us) *n.* a small pouch. The smaller of the two sacs that occupy a portion of the membranous labyrinth of the vestibule of the inner ear. (The larger sac is the utricle.)

sacculocochlear (sak"u-lo-kok'le-ar) *adj.* concerning both the saccule of the vestibule and the cochlea.

saddle-shaped audiogram. denotes less hearing loss at the low and high frequencies than in the middle range.

SAE. surgical auditory evaluation.

SAF. synchronous auditory feedback.

Saint Zachary's disease. a disease characterized by inability to speak—mutism.

SAI. social adequacy index.

SAL. sensorineural acuity level; speech awareness level. *syn*: speech awareness threshold; speech detection threshold.

salicylate (sal"ĭ-sil"āt, sah-lis'ĭ-lāt) *n.* a salt of salicylic acid.

salicylic acid (sal"ĭ-sil'ik as'id). as a water-soluble powder, it is the base for aspirin.

salicylism (sal'ĭ-sil"izm) *n.* poisoning caused by salicylic acid or one of its derivatives or salicylates. One symptom is tinnitus (head noises). Others include nausea and vomiting.

salping- or salpingo- (sal'pin). prefix meaning trumpet, used in anatomy to denote a tube, e.g., the eustachian or fallopian tubes.

salpingemphraxis (sal"pin-jem-frak'sis) *n.* obstruction of the eustachian tube that may cause a hearing loss.

salpingian (sal-pin'je-an) *adj.* relating to the eustachian tube.

salpingitis (sal"pin-ji'tis) *n.* inflammation of the eustachian tube. (Less commonly, the fallopian canal).

salpingocatheterism (sal-ping"go-kath'ĕ-ter-izm) *n.* inflation of the eustachian tube by means of a tubular device (catheter).

salpingoscope (sal-ping'go-skop") *n.* a tubular device for inspecting the nasopharynx and eustachian tube.

salpingostenochoria (sal-ping″go-sten″o-ko′re-ah) *n.* closure or constriction of the eustachian tube.

salpinx (sal′pinks) *pl.* **salsalpinges** (sal-pin′jes) *n.* the eustachian tube.

SAM. School of Aerospace Medicine. School of Aviation Medicine.

sand, auditory minute particles of calcium carbonate in the labyrinth of the ear; *syn:* otolith; otoconium.

sarcoidosis (sar″koi-do′sis) *n.* a disease characterized by nodules or tumors (often malignant) that may affect the ear.

SAT. speech awareness threshold; *syn:* speech detection threshold; speech articulation threshold; speech or standard articulation test.

saturation output. the greatest sound intensity an amplifying system can produce; *syn:* maximum acoustic output; maximum deliverable pressure.

saturation sound pressure level. SSPL. newer term for maximum power output (MPO).

saw-tooth noise. a sound made up of a fundamental frequency of about 60 or 120 Hz together with all its harmonics to 10,000 Hz in random phase.

SBA. Small Business Administration.

scala (sca′la) *n.* one of the three main subdivisions of the cochlea.

scala media (me′de-ah). the cochlear duct, or the membranous cochlea. The middle triangular tube of the cochlea. It contains the organ of Corti and is filled with endolymphatic fluid; *syn:* ductus cochlearis.

scala tympani (tim′pa-ne). the lower tube of the cochlea. It extends from the round window to the tip (helicotrema) of the cochlea and contains perilymph.

scala vestibuli. the upper tube of the cochlea, extending from the oval window to the tip of the cochlea and containing perilymph.

scale, A (weighted). the A weighted scale of a sound level meter attenuates (reduces) the lower frequencies about 5 dB per octave from 1000 Hz down to 250 Hz. Below 250 Hz sounds are attenuated another 10 dB per octave. References to the A weighted scale are commonly noted as dBA.

scale, B. the B scale of a sound level meter is weighted (sounds are filtered) to cut the frequencies below 300 Hz—increasing from about 4 dB per octave.

scale, C. the broadest and flattest scale of a sound level meter. It measures sound pressure levels in decibels relative to .0002 dynes cm² and is essentially equally sensitive to all frequencies from 20 to 10,000 Hz. Flat from 100 to 2000 Hz, the C scale has gradual dips that make it 6 dB less sensitive at 21 Hz and at 11,000 Hz.

scale, D. a special weighting network included in some sound level meters to measure aircraft noise as it affects listeners in a particular area—the annoyance level of flyover noise. The weighting scale is based on mirroring the 40 noy contour to approximate the perceived noise level (PNdB) scale.

scale, pitch. an arbitrary scale relating frequency to pitch. On the scientific scale 256 Hz equals middle C. On the musical scale middle C equals 261.6 Hz.

scanning microscope. a type of electron microscope involving a moving electron beam.

scaphoid fossa. a depression or boatshaped furrow beneath the ridge of the helix in the upper posterior portion of the external ear.

scarlatina *n.* scarlet fever. An acute contagious disease that may cause a loss of hearing sensitivity.

scarlet fever. scarlatina.

Scarpa's fluid (Antonio Scarpa, Italian physician, 1747-1832). endolymph. Sometimes also called Scarpa's liquor.

Scarpa's ganglion. a collection of nerve cells within the internal auditory canal from the semicircular canals. *syn:* vestibular ganglion.

Scarpa's membrane. the thin layer of tissue that covers the round window. Sometimes called the secondary tympanic membrane. Membrana tympani secundaria of the fenestra rotunda.

Scheibe's syndrome. abnormalities of the cochlear duct and saccule and degeneration of the membranous portion of the inner ear—said to occur in about 70% of cases of hereditary deafness.

schema (ske′mah) *n.* a diagram showing the parts which make up an electronic or mechanical device. *adj:* schematic.

schwa, (shwah) *n.* the most common vowel sound in the language. It may be represented by any vowel letter in an unaccented position; e.g., a—alone; e—the system; i—easily; o—gallop; u—circus. A lower-case "e" upside down and backward is used as the phonetic symbol for the schwa (ə).

Schwabach test (shwah′bak) (Dagobert Schwabach, German physician, 1846-1920). a bone conduction test using tuning forks. It is a comparison of the patient's bone conduction with that of a normally hearing person. The results are categorized as normal, increased, or decreased, and may be indicated in seconds of difference.

schwannoma (shwon-no′mah) *n.* a small tumor involving a nerve sheath.

Schwartze sign, positive (Hermann Schwartze, German physician, 1837-1910). reddish color of the promontory as seen through the intact tympanic membrane. An indication of otosclerosis.

sclerosis (skle-ro′sis) *n.* hardening of body tissues or organs as a result of chronic inflammation. *adj*: **sclerotic.**

sclerotic otitis. hardening of inner ear tissues and structures as a result of inflammation.

SCONII. Subcommittee on Noise in Industry (of the Committee on Conservation of Hearing of the American Academy of Ophthalmology and Otolaryngology).

scoop, ear. spoon-shaped instrument used for removing ear wax or middle ear granulations.

scoop, mastoid. a narrow spoon-shaped instrument designed to remove diseased air cells from the mastoid process.

screen *v.* to test hearing in a limited manner to establish groups that may or may not require further examination.

screening audiometer. any audiometer utilizing limited frequencies and intensities to make quick checks for hearing loss. For example, the audiometrist may sweep through selected frequencies at a pre-set level of intensity to determine the listener's ability to hear. Failure to hear one, two, or more tones is usually followed by referrals for more complete testing.

screening audiometry. technique involving checking large groups of people rapidly against a preestablished limit of normalcy regarding hearing. *syn*: identification audiometry.

screening test. test of hearing sensitivity designed to pick out (or screen) individuals who may need more careful testing or medical attention.

screening test, limited frequency. hearing screening test limited to one, two, or three frequencies at preset levels of intensity; *syn*: reduced screening.

screening test, reduced. limited frequency screening test.

screening test, single frequency. screening test limited to 4000 Hz or any one other frequency.

scroll ear (skrol). an outer ear in which the rim appears to be rolled forward and inward.

scute, tympanic (skūt). the thin bony plate that separates the middle ear from the mastoid process. More commonly known as tegmen tympani.

SD or sd. standard deviation.

SDS. speech discrimination score.

SDT. speech detectability threshold.

sebaceous (sĕ-ba′shus) *adj.* concerning sebum—fatty tallow-like matter.

seborrhea (seb″o-re′ah) *n.* oversecretion of the sebaceous glands. *adj*: **seborrheal, seborrheic.**

sebum (se′bum) **n.** a fatty tallow-like matter secreted by the sebaceous glands.

second harmonic. the (first) overtone, twice the frequency of the fundamental or lowest tone.

secondary tympanic membrane. the thin tissue that covers the round window.

second-order neuron. a nerve cell lying beyond at least one synapse from the specialized nerve ending or receptor.

secretory (se-kre′to-re) *adj.* pertaining to or promoting secretion.

section (sek′shun) *v.* to cut—as to section the stapedius.

sedate (se-dāt′) *v.* to quiet with drugs.

sedation (se-da′shun) *n.* calming or quieting with drugs.

sedative (sed′ah-tiv) *adj.* tending to quiet.

sedative *n.* a drug used to calm or quiet.

SE. Signed English.

SEE. Seeing Essential English; Signing Exact English. (sometimes Seeing Essential English—since it was offered first—is noted SEE₁, and Signing Exact English—which came later—is noted as SEE₂.)

Seeing Essential English. SEE₁. a modification of AMESLAN (American Sign Language) devised by David Anthony & Associates to more accurately reflect English syntax and grammar.

selective amplification. the amplification of certain frequencies more than, or to the exclusion of, other frequencies.

selective resonance theory. an early version of the resonance theory of pitch perception involved various cavities thought to be behind the eardrum (Gaspard Bauhin, 1605). Later, in 1683, Joseph G. Du Verney theorized that the bony lamina resonated to different frequencies in accordance with its varying width.

selector, frequency. a device—usually a dial but sometimes a series of buttons—on an audiometer to provide a means of selecting the frequency of the test tone; *syn*: frequency control.

semicircular canals three tubes of the balancing portion of the inner ear—the fluid-filled ducts, each describing a little more than half of a complete circle within the labyrinth of the ear. Together with the utricle and the saccule, they make up the organ of balance. The three canals, positioned at 90 degree angles to each other, are known as the superior, the posterior, and the lateral (or horizontal) semicircular canals.

semicircular duct (ductus semicircularis). one of the three membranous tubes in the bony labyrinth of the inner ear that participate in the sense of balance.

semicircular tube. membranous inner lining of the semicircular canal.

semiconductor (sem″e-con-duk′ter) *n.* a solid crystaline material that can be used to provide for the controlled flow of electrons.

semi-insert. no longer used, this device occluded the ear canal and was held in place by a headband. It was intended to protect the ear from noise exposure.

semi-skeleton earmold. consists of canal, bridge, and helix. No concha rim.

senescence (se-nes′ens) *n.* the aging process.

senesce (se-nes′) *v.* to grow old.

senescent (se-nes′ent) *adj.* elderly; aging.

sensation (sen-sa′shun) *n.* the feeling or impression that results from the action of a stimulus on a sensory receptor.

sensation area, auditory. 1. the region (on a graph of frequency of pure tones versus intensity of pure tones) between the curve representing the threshold of audibility and the curve representing the threshold of tickle. 2. the portion of the temporal lobe of the cortex that responds to sound.

sensation, Fechner's law of. a sensation resulting from a stimulus seems to increase by a constant amount (arithmetically by addition) as the intensity of the stimulus is constantly increased (logarithmically by multiplication).

sensation level. SL. the level of a tone, in decibels, above the individual threshold of sensitivity.

sensation unit. an old term for the decibel as referred to the normal threshold of hearing.

sense (sens) *n.* the ability to respond to a stimulus, e.g., by means of the ear.

sense *v.* to become aware through one of the senses.

sense, labyrinthine. the sense of balance.

sense modality (mo-dal′ĭ-te). a grouping of sensory receptors serving a common purpose, such as hearing or vision.

sense-organ dysacusis (dis″ah-koo′sis). loss of understanding resulting from a lesion involving the inner ear.

sense, vestibular. another term for labyrinthine sense.

sensitivity (sen″sĭ-tiv′ĭ-te) *n.* ability to respond to a stimulus.

senstivity index. SI.

sensitivity tests. tests of ability to respond to auditory stimuli.

sensitivity threshold the faintest sound that can be heard at 50% of presentations. Formerly referred to as threshold of acuity.

sensitization (sen″sĭ-ti-za′shun) *n.* the phenomenon by which a moderately intense click prepares the ear for another sound—which may have preceded as well as followed the click. Studies show the click may prepare and protect the ear against explosive sounds.

sensitometer (sen″sĭ-tom′ĕ-ter) *n.* a device to measure hearing sensitivity. *adj:* **sensitometric.**

sensiton (sen′si-ton) *n.* a device to measure hearing sensitivity by means of a damped wave train.

sensorinaural (sen″so-re-naw′ral) *adj.* seldom used alternative to sensorineural in referring to hearing impairment.

sensorineural (sen″so-re-nu′ral) *adj.* involving the nervous pathways and/or the brain.

sensorineural acuity level. SAL. threshold of sensitivity for hearing when the external and middle ear conductive mechanism is excluded.

sensorineural acuity level (SAL) test. bone conduction test that involves introducing a masking noise through a bone oscillator placed on the forehead while pure tones are presented through the earphones of the audiometer. The results are compared with those obtained with normal ears.

sensorineural hearing loss. SNHL. hearing loss that results from damage to the sensory mechanism internally from the oval and round windows. It was formerly known as nerve or perceptive deafness.

sensory-neural. alternative spelling for sensorineural.

sensorium (sen-so′re-um) *n.* the total sensory mechanism or the portion of the brain concerned with the reception of sensory nerve impulses.

sensory *adj.* concerning sensations or the senses.

sensory amusia. inability to recognize melodies or tones.

sensory aphasia. inability to understand spoken language.

sensory cells. a term sometimes used for the hair cells.

sensory impairment. inability of a sense to function normally.

sensory nerve. an afferent nerve that carries a stimulus toward the central nervous system or brain.

sensory receptor. any cell or group of cells (as the hair cells of the ear) that respond to an external stimulus. They give rise to an afferent nerve impulse (leading to the brain).

sequela (se-kwe′lah) *pl.* **sequelae** *n.* following, or the result of disease.

serendipitous (se″ren-dip′i-tus) *adj.* discovered by accident or as a sidelight of research in other areas.

serendipity *n.* the gift of discovering worthwhile things or uses that are not a part of the original objective.

ser-, sero- prefix referring to serum or serous.

serosa (se-ro′sah) *n.* a membrane that produces serum or a thin watery fluid. *adj:* **serosal.**

127

serosanguineous *adj.* concerning both serum and blood.

serous *adj.* appearing to be, or concerning serum that is usually thin and watery.

serous otitis media. accumulation of thin watery fluid within the middle ear cavity—sometimes known as middle ear effusion or catarrhal otitis media.

serum *pl.* **serums, sera** *n.* the watery portion of circulating fluid within an animal; e.g., blood serum.

serum globulin (glob'u-lin) *n.* another name for gamma globulin. A part of the blood serum that contains antibodies (substances that weaken or destroy bacteria or viruses).

seventh nerve. the VIIth cranial or facial nerve.

severe deafness. a hearing loss between 70 dB and 90 dB when the hearing threshold level at 500, 1000, and 2000 Hz in the better ear is averaged.

SF. sound field. This term usually refers to hearing tests through loudspeakers.

SGR. skin galvanic response. More commonly known as galvanic skin response.

SHAA. Society of Hearing Aid Audiologists—now National Hearing Aid Society (NHAS).

shadow curve. a false audiogram indicating a threshold of hearing sensitivity in the poorer ear that parallels that of the normal ear. It may occur as the sound waves go around or through the head, from the ear under test to the better ear. Sometimes known as cross hearing.

shadow, sound. another term for head shadow effect.

sharply falling audiogram. loss increases about 15 to 20 dB per octave at higher frequencies; *syn:* sharply or marked falling curve.

Shea's operation. now commonly called stapedectomy, J. J. Shea, Jr., MD of Memphis, TN, in 1958 described his technique of replacing the stapes with a plastic strut and a vein graft.

sheath of Schwann (Theodor Schwann, German physician, 1810-1882). the layer of myelin that surrounds some nerve fibers. *syn:* medullary sheath.

shell earmold. consists of canal and a thin shell covering bowl of ear. May be with or without helix.

Sheridan's test. a screening test of infant hearing, based on meaningful sounds, designed by Dr. Mary Sheridan (Eng.)

SHHH. Self Help for Hard of Hearing People, Inc.

shift, Doppler. sometimes used in reference to sound to mean the same as Doppler effect. More accurately used to refer to a change in light rays rather than a change in sound frequency as a result of the movement of the source of the rays or waves.

shifting voice test. a test of malingering based on the shifting of speech intensities at each ear. It is a modification of the Stenger speech test.

shock wave. an intensely powerful wave of compressed air that may cause damage to the physical structure of the ear.

short increment sensitivity index. SISI. a test of the ability to recognize one decibel increases in intensity during a series of bursts of pure tone presented 20 dB above threshold.

short process. a comparatively short projection of bone; that is, short compared to other projections on the same bone, e.g., the short process of the malleus.

Shrapnell's membrane (Henry J. Shrapnell, English physician, 1761-1841). small thin triangular portion of the eardrum in the upper part of the membrane. Since it is not as tense as the rest of the eardrum, it is called the pars flaccida, the flaccid part, which fills the notch of Rivinus. *syn:* Rivinus's ligament.

shush *n.* a sibilant sound used to call for silence.

SI. sensitivity index. Speech interference.

sibilant *adj.* breathy or hissing as in making the sound of "s" or "sh."

sibilant *n.* consonant sound made by allowing air to escape between the teeth and palate.

sibilate *v.* to allow air to escape between the teeth and palate. To hiss.

sibilation *n.* word pronunciation in which "s" sounds predominate.

sibling *n.* one of the children of the same parentage.

sibship *n.* all the children in a family.

side band. the set of frequencies on either side of a carrier frequency.

side-tone. the auditory signal by which a speaker monitors his own voice.

side-tone, delayed. delayed auditory feedback (DAF). A system by which the speaker's own words are returned (feedback) through earphones after a time delay of a few milliseconds. A test of malingering.

Siebenmann's canals (Friedrich Sibenmann, German physician, 1852-1928). tiny blood vessels in the aqueduct of the cochlea.

Siglish. Signed English. A signing system designed to help with syntax.

sigma (sig'mah). the 18th letter of the Greek alphabet, when spelled out, indicates a millisecond or one-thousandth of a second. As a capital letter, Σ is the symbol for summation, the sum of. The lower case sigma σ or s, is often used as the symbol for standard deviation.

sigmoid sinus (sig'moid si'nus). an S-shaped hollow space (sinus) between the temporal bone and the occipital bone.

sign (sīn) *v.* to communicate by using sign language.

sign *n.* a gesture or symbol expressing a word or idea.

sign language. a system of conventional symbols or gestures made with the hands to help the deaf communicate. It is distinct from finger spelling. There are various systems, among them American Sign Language, ASL (AMESLAN); Linguistics of Visual English, LOVE or LVE; Seeing Essential English, SEE₁; Signed English, SE (Siglish); Signing Exact English, SEE₂; Systematic Sign Language, SSL.

sign, positive Schwartze. reddish color of the promonotory as seen through the intact tympanic membrane. An indication of otosclerosis.

signal (sig′nal) *n.* the message amplified or transmitted by an electronic system.

signal detection theory. the belief that the ability to hear a given type of sound despite a masking noise will be influenced by the wording of the instructions.

signal to noise ratio. S/N. the relationship between the intensity of the speech signal to the intensity of the background or environmental noise.

signature, acoustic. the different characteristics of each combination of sounds that make the signal distinctive.

Signed English SE (Siglish). a modification of American Sign Language (AMESLAN) developed by Harry Bornstein and associates at Gallaudet College. It is designed to present a formalized gesture system that will help children learn to communicate more easily with better syntax and grammar.

Signing Exact English SEE₂. developed by Dr. Gerilee Gustasan and associates as a modification of Seeing Essential English in an effort to simplify the signing system and make it easier for parents, teachers, and children.

SIL. speech interference level.

silica gel (sil′ĭ-kah jel). (dessicant). an absorbent material, resembling white sand in appearance, used as a drying agent. Valuable in preventing the accumulation of moisture in hearing aids in humid climates.

simple sound source. a source that radiates sound uniformly in all directions in free-field conditions; *syn*: point source.

simple tone. 1. one complete cycle of a pure tone. 2. the sound sensation of a single pitch.

simple wave. portion of a pure tone.

simplex, herpes (sim′pleks her′pēz). a communicable virus infection that may affect the lips, nose, and genital area. It is believed responsible for congenital deafness and other severe handicaps when the herpesvirus is present in the genital tract during birth.

simulated deafness. The deafness of a malingerer, e.g., one who feigns or pretends deafness for personal advantage to gain industrial loss compensation or to avoid military service. Children may simulate deafness to explain school deficiencies. *syn*: functional deafness.

simultaneous method. communication by means of the manual alphabet, signs, speech, speechreading, and hearing aids. Now called Total Communication.

SIN. abbreviation for sinusoid.

sine wave (sinusoidal wave form). pure tone. A tone that has only one frequency with no harmonics or overtones.

single frequency screening test. a screening test limited to 4000 Hz or any one other frequency.

single-phase *adj.* pertaining to a circuit powered by a single alternating electromotive force.

sinistral (sin′is-tral). concerning the left side (as opposed to dextral, the right side of the body).

sinistraural (sin″is-traw′ral) *adj.* pertaining to one in whom the left ear appears to be dominant.

sintered filter. small cylinders containing tiny stainless steel balls fused in such an exacting manner that the degree of acoustic attenuation can be closely controlled.

sinus (si′nus) *n.* a cavity or hollow space.

sinus, cavernous. a cavity that extends from the sphenoidal fissure to the top of petrous portion of the temporal bone.

sinus, ethmoid. a cavity in the ethmoid bone.

sinus, lateral. one of the two cavities in the inner side of the skull passing near the mastoid antrum.

sinusitis (si″nŭ-si′tis) *n.* inflammation of a sinus.

sinusoid *n.* a wave form that is smoothly proportional in all directions, e.g., such as that produced by a pure tone.

sinusoidal wave. a wave form having the characteristics of a sine wave.

SISI. short increment sensitivity index.

SISI-gram *n.* a graphic representation of the results of a SISI test.

skeleton earmold. consists of canal, complete concha rim, and bridge.

semi-skeleton consists of canal, bridge, and helix. No concha rim.

¾ **skeleton** is the same as the Skeleton but with the central portion of the concha rim removed.

skew *n.* a variation from the normal distribution curve. *adj*: skew.

skew *v.* to vary from the normal distribution curve.

skew distribution. a distribution curve that is not symmetrical and whose mode has a different value than that of the mean.

skewness *n.* lack of symmetry in a distribution curve.

skin galvanic response   SGR. more commonly known as galvanic (or psychogalvanic) skin response. A change in skin resistance (the Feré effect) that results from a stimulus to the nervous system.

skirt *n.* the gradually expanding width of a narrow band noise below its maximum intensity.

ski-slope curve audiogram. usually denotes nearly normal hearing in lower frequencies (sometimes as high as 2000 Hz) followed by a precipitous drop of 25 dB or more per octave.

"ski-slope" hearing loss. abrupt elevation of threshold sensitivity above 1000 Hz.

SL. sensation level (re: threshold). Sound level.

SLM. sound level meter.

SN. sensorineural.

S/N. signal to noise (ratio). The relative intensity of the meaningful sound or message when compared to a masking noise.

SNHL. sensorineural hearing loss.

Snijders-Ooman Nonverbal Scale. SONS. a nonverbal test of conceptual thinking that may be adapted for the deaf. It is more commonly used in Europe.

snorkel *n.* a tube cemented to the outside of a post-auricle hearing aid to convey sound waves from the front of the ear to a microphone opening at the rear.

social adequacy index. SAI. a measurement of the individual degree of handicap computed from a table whose two dimensions are the speech reception threshold and discrimination score.

socio- a prefix referring to society or social.

sociocusis *n.* a word coined by Aram Glorig, MD to include both the progressive loss of hearing due to the aging process (presbycusis) and the loss due to disease or noise exposure in modern society.

sociometry *n.* the study of the relationships within a group or between groups of people, e.g., the deaf within the community. *adj*: **sociometric.**

socket, earphone. a socket within an earmuff designed to hold an earphone to allow communication in extremely noisy surroundings.

soft palate. the muscular, rearward portion of the roof of the mouth. It helps to separate the nose, mouth, and throat.

soft peak clipping. phrase used to refer to any method of circuit limitation of the output of a hearing aid below the maximum acoustic capacity of its transducers.

SO and HHN. Society of Otorhinolaryngology and Head-Neck Nurses.

solar battery. device for converting energy from the sun into electrical energy.

solum tympani (so'lum tim'pa-ne). the base of the tympanic cavity.

SOM. serous otitis media.

somat, somato- prefix referring to the body.

somatic *adj.* 1. relating to the physical body. 2. relating to nonproductive cells or tissue. 3. relating to structures of the body wall or skeleton.

somatic muscle system. muscles attached to the skeleton more commonly known as voluntary muscles.

son-, soni-, sono- prefix referring to sound.

sonagram *n.* a photograph of the pressure waves of a particular sound—a spectrogram.

Sona-Graph. trade name for a sound spectrograph—a device designed to display the spectrum of a sound signal.

sonalator *n.* a device that displays the sound patterns of speech on the screen of a cathode ray tube.

sonant (so'nant) *n.* a speech sound that is voiced. An unvoiced speech sound is called a surd. *adj*: **sonant.**

sonar *n.* another name for an echometer, a manmade apparatus for locating distant or invisible objects by means of sound waves reflected back by objects.

sone *n.* the unit of a subjective loudness scale based on average human judgments of comparative loudness. By 1971 definition, one sone is the loudness heard by an average normal listener when presented with a 1000 Hz tone at an intensity of 40 dB re .0002 dynes/cm² (or 40 phons). While two sones expresses the sensation of a sound being twice as loud as one sone, the intensity change required will vary but will represent an increase in phons of about 9 dB.

sone scale. a scale of loudness based on the sone as the unit.

sonic *adj.* concerning a sound wave within the human audible range.

sonic boom. noise created by shock waves from a plane flying faster than the speed of sound.

sonitus (son'ī-tus) *n.* another name for tinnitus or head noises.

sonometer *n.* an early device for testing hearing (D.E. Hughes 1879). It was probably the first instrument to be called an audiometer.

sonority *n.* fullness or resonance in tone. *adj*: **sonorant, sonorous.**

sonovox *n.* an electronic device that may be used to help one who has no larynx to communicate.

SONS. Snijders-Ooman nonverbal scale.

sound *n.* 1. the sensation resulting from stimulation of the auditory mechanism by air waves or vibrations. 2. an instrument that may be inserted into a cavity or tube (e.g., eustachian) for diagnosis or treatment.

sound *v.* 1. to create a sound wave. 2. to explore a tube or canal by means of a sound. 3. to measure the depth of water.

sound absorption. property by which materials diminish sound energy in various degrees—usually by converting the energy to heat.

sound analyzer. instrument designed to measure the various frequency components of a sound wave.

sound, audible. range of pressure waves in terms of intensity and frequency that can be recognized by the so-called normal ear.

sound box. device consisting of a vibrating needle and thin diaphragm used to convert phonograph record groove variations into sound.

sound, complex. sound that results from a mixture of pressure waves.

sound, diffuse. results when sound pressure waves are equal in all directions.

sound dosimeter (do-sim'ĕ-ter). an instrument designed to measure and record time of exposure to various noise levels.

sound energy. the energy or power transmitted as the result of the movement of a vibrating body.

sound field. SF. an area or room in which sound waves originate from a loud speaker system.

sound-field test. a hearing test involving the use of loudspeakers rather than earphones. Often called free-field test.

sound, impulsive. momentary or explosive sound.

sound, inaudible. sound that is above the range of the human ear in frequency (a dog whistle, for example) or below the range of the individual ear in intensity.

sound intensity. the ratio between the sound being measured and a reference level of intensity. This ratio is expressed in logarithmic units called decibels.

sound level. shortened phrase for sound pressure level as used in sound level meter.

sound level meter. an electronic device made up of a microphone, an amplifying network, and a meter to indicate the rms. (root-mean-square) value of the sound pressure in a complex sound wave. In addition to a flat C scale, it usually includes two other scales—A and B—that attenuate the low frequencies in various degrees. In some instruments there is also a D weighting scale to measure the annoyance level of fly-over noise. The instrument is sometimes referred to as a pressure meter, or sound pressure meter.

sound medium. any material through which sound pressure waves may pass.

sound patterns. a pictorial display of the spectrum of a sound as revealed by a spectrograph.

sound, periodic. sounds that repeat themselves regularly as a function of time, e.g., musical sounds.

sound periodicity. the regular recurrence of wave forms in mathematical relationship to

the fundamental (harmonics) that makes sound musical.

sound perseveration (per-sev"er-a'shun). sensation of sound that may continue after the stimulus has ceased. Also known as "after" hearing, it is similar to the afterimage in vision.

sound picture. a spectrogram or photograph of the pressure waves of a particular sound.

sound pressure. changes in the molecular pattern of a medium caused by the energy or force of sound. Measurement is in dynes per square centimeter.

sound pressure level. SPL. sound pressure level, stated in decibels, is a logarithmic ratio of the measured sound pressure and a reference sound pressure. As commonly used, SPL indicates the decibels mentioned are referred to .0002 dynes/cm². That is, .0002 dynes/cm² is used as the reference pressure in the formula, which is stated as: The sound pressure level of a sound is 20 times the logarithm to the base 10 of the ratio of the sound to the reference pressure.

$$SPL =$$

$$20 \log_{10} \frac{P(\text{measured sound pressure})}{P_0(\text{reference sound pressure})}$$

$$SPL \ (\text{re } .0002 \ \text{dyne/cm}^2) =$$

$$20 \log_{10} \frac{P}{.0002 \ \text{dyne/cm}^2}$$

sound pressure, maximum. the greatest degree of intensity of any single wave or designated range of waves.

sound pressure meter. another name for sound level meter.

sound pressure unit. the microbar—one dyne per square centimeter—is the unit of sound pressure.

sound probe. a tiny microphone on a thin rod or cylinder designed to study sound waves in small confined spaces with a minimum of disturbance to the wave form.

sound probe microphone. a tiny microphone, on a thin rod or cylinder, designed to study sound waves in small confined spaces with a minimum of disturbance to the wave form.

soundproof *adj.* unable to transmit sound.

soundproof *v.* to use absorbent material in such a manner as to prevent the passage of sound.

soundproof room. a chamber built in a manner to prevent the passage of sound.

sound propagation. the creation of sound pressure waves.

sound quality. the psychological sensation of the quality of sound results from the difference in overtones generated with the fundamental through varying resonators.

sound reflection. the return of sound pressure waves toward their source.

131

sound room. usually refers to a chamber that is sound-isolated or has been sound-treated (with sound-absorbent material) to minimize the effect of ambient noise.

sound shadow. another term for head shadow effect.

sound spectra. the composition of a sound as revealed by analysis of its various component tones.

sound symbol. the phoneme, word, or object that is recognized rather than the various frequencies that are represented by the complex wave.

sound-treat v. to use absorbent material in such a manner as to minimize the passage of sound.

sound-treated rooms. chambers whose walls, ceilings, and floors have been covered with absorbent material to minimize the passage of sound.

sound, ultrasonic. sound pressure waves whose frequency is above the audible range. Sometimes called ultra-audible sound.

sound wave. a change in the arrangement of molecules in a medium into successive patterns of compression and rarefaction.

sound waves, power of. the power of a sound wave is proportional to the square of the pressure. It is also proportional to the square of the velocity.

sounder, echo. an instrument for measuring depths by timing the transmission and reflection of sound waves.

SP. summating potential. Speech pathology (one holding CCC in speech pathology from ASHA).

space, cupola. the space in the middle ear above the ossicles. The tympanic attic.

space nerve. a branch of the vestibular nerve that connects with the semicircular canals for orientation in space.

space, Nuel's. a cleft or intermediate tunnel between the inner and outer tunnels of the organ of Corti. These spaces provide a passageway for nerve fibers and the endolymph that bathes and nourishes the inner cells.

SPAR (test). sensitivity prediction for the acoustic reflex. Comparison of acoustic reflex threshold to pure tone to the acoustic reflex threshold to broadband noise.

spatial function. ability to orient oneself in space—better when both ears are used.

spatial misorientation. the loss of the power or adjustment to one's position in space—often resulting from a lesion involving the semicircular canals.

spatial summation. the totaling algebraically of excitatory and inhibitory inputs (slight stimuli) by a cell body until a critical point is reached that causes the discharge of a nerve impulse.

spatulate (spat'u-lāt) v. to mix ear impression material with a thin, flexible knife-shaped instrument.

speaker n. short term for loudspeaker.

speaking difficulty. dysphonia.

speaking tube. 1. ear trumpet—a device with a large opening at one end designed to gather sound waves and direct them through a smaller opening into the ear canal. 2. pipe to carry words into different places or rooms in a building.

spectral fusion (spek'tral fu'zhun). the blending into one sound in the central cortex, different bands of noise presented simultaneously to each ear.

spectral line. a portion of a line spectrum. One of the series of vertical lines that graphically represent the frequency components of a complex sound wave.

spectrogram (spek'tro-gram) n. a photograph of the pressure waves of a particular sound.

spectrograph (spek'tro-graf) n. 1. a device for separating the pressure waves of a particular sound and making them visible so they can be photographed. 2. an instrument that makes such photographs.

spectrometer (spek-trom'ĕ-ter) n. an instrument designed to measure sound pressure waves after they have been separated.

spectrum (spek'trum) pl. **spectra** n. the distribution of pure tones that make up an envelope of sound. adj: **spectral.**

spectrum, acoustic. the distribution of frequencies and pressure of waves within an envelope of sound.

spectrum, band. the sound pressure levels of each octave (or narrower) component of a complex noise are measured and presented in diagrammatic form to show comparative relationships.

spectrum, continuous. a spectrum that includes all the pure tones within a given frequency range.

spectrum, line. a graphic representation in a series of vertical lines of the frequency components of a complex sound wave.

spectrum, tonal. image of a complex tone displaying all its frequencies and intensities as seen on an oscilloscope.

speculum, ear (spek'u-lum). a short funnel-shaped tube to facilitate inspection of, or operating in, the external or middle ear.

speech audiometer. an audiometer utilizing an amplifying circuit capable of presenting speech levels in graduated steps. It is used to determine individual thresholds of speech understanding—the speech reception threshold (SRT). It is also used to determine the PB score, i.e., the percentage of words understood when a phonetically balanced word list (of monosyllables) is presented at a comfortable listening level.

speech audiometry. the technique of measuring ability to understand speech under various conditions of intensity and noise interference using sound field as well as earphones and bone oscillators.

speech awareness test. SAT. a test of the ability to recognize that speech is being heard. Sometimes the test is done in the presence of conflicting sounds when the hearing impairment is not so severe that individual words cannot be understood; *syn:* speech perception test.

speech, cold-running. continuous speech delivery on a topic that is informative in content and delivery, rather than emotional. It may be used to establish the speech reception threshold.

speech, cued. a method of using fingerspelling symbols to help in speechreading when words that look alike on the lips are involved, "men" and "pen", for example.

speech, dactyl. fingerspelling: use of the manual alphabet. *syn:* dactylology.

speech deafness. auditory aphasia—inability to understand spoken language.

speech, delayed. failure of speech to develop as expected with chronologic age. It may be due to hearing impairment or brain injury, as well as to slow maturation.

speech discrimination score. SDS. a rating of speech understanding as determined by any one of several speech tests. Phonetically balanced (PB) word lists are most commonly used.

speech detectablity threshold. SDT. the point at which sounds can be determined to be speech even though the words are not recognized; *syn:* speech awareness threshold; speech perception threshold.

speech discrimination test. a test of the ability to understand speech as determined by scoring the number of words in a phonetically balanced (PB) word list repeated correctly.

speech discrimination test, K.S.U. a test of speech understanding prepared by Kenneth W. Berger, PhD, of Kent (Ohio) State University. It is based on multiple-choice words in sentences.

speech, echo. involuntary repetition of words or phrases just spoken by someone else. More commonly referred to as echolalia, less often as echologia, echophasia, echophrasia, and mimic speech.

speech, filtered. speech that has been passed through filters to alter its characteristics.

speech frequencies. the most important frequencies involved in speech recognition are generally considered to be 500, 1000, 2000, and 3000 Hz.

speech interference. SI

speech interference level. SIL. the level of intensity at which noise interferes with the understanding of speech. It is based on the

average in decibels of the noise in the three octave bands: 600 to 1200, 1200 to 2400, and 2400 to 4800 Hz; *syn:* noise interference level. NIL.

speech noise. a wide band of noise utilizing the frequencies between 500 and 2000 Hz—sometimes used for masking during speech audiometry.

speech pathologist. one who practices speech pathology; *syn:* speech therapist.

speech pathology. an inclusive term covering all aspects of the study of speech defects and disorders. More importantly, it includes the study of methods of correction of those defects.

speech perception test. a seldom-used test to determine the level of intensity at which sounds can be perceived as words. It is between the threshold of detectability and the threshold of intelligibility; *syn:* speech awareness test.

speechreading. to understand by close observation of the speaker's lips, facial expression, and gestures; sometimes referred to as "visual hearing."

speech reception threshold. the lowest sound pressure level at which 50% or more of the spondaic test words (words of two syllables having equal stress) are repeated correctly. "Cold-running speech" may also be used but is not as acceptable.

speech reception threshold test. a test used to determine the speech reception threshold.

speech sounds, high frequency. speech sounds whose greatest intensity occurs above 1000 Hz; e.g., most of the consonants.

speech test, low-redundancy. a test to determine the ability to understand speech when most of the repetitive factors have been removed by the use of filters.

speech test (group), Meyerson. a number of children are screened simultaneously by having them point to the appropriate picture in response to the word.

speech tests, recorded. lists of words that have been reproduced on records or tapes for the purpose of determining speech reception thresholds or discrimination abilities.

speech therapist. a specialist in the treatment of speech and language disorders; *syn:* speech pathologist.

speech therapy. the treatment of speech disorders.

speech threshold. level of speech intensity at which spondaic words are recognizable 50% of the time.

speech with alternating masking index. SWAMI. a test of the ability to understand speech while a masking white noise at a 20 dB higher level is alternated between ears.

speed of sound. at sea level, sound waves travel through the air at a speed of about 1130 feet per second at 70°F. For convenience, this is usually rounded off to 1100 feet per second. Sound waves actually travel at varying speeds, governed by the density of the material through which they pass, as well as the prevailing temperature.

sphen-, spheno- prefix meaning a wedge.

sphenoid bone (sfe′noid). a wedgeshaped bone in front of the temporal bone and above the jaw.

spherical recess. indentation in the wall of the vestibule of the inner ear in which the saccule is situated. The saccular fossa.

sphygmophone (sfig′mo-fōn) *n.* an instrument designed to make the pulse beat more audible.

spillover *n.* term that refers to amplification from one room being heard in another when a magnetic loop system is used.

spiral canal of the modiolus (mo-di′o-lus). the minute channel within the modiolus where the spiral ganglion of the cochlear nerve lies.

spiral cochlear canal. commonly known as the spiral canal of the cochlea. A portion of the bony labyrinth of the inner ear about 30 mm long making about 2¾ turns about a central bony supporting structure known as the modiolus, containing the scala tympani, scala vestibuli, and the cochlear duct.

spiral crest. the fine-toothed ridge of the bony spiral at the edge of the cochlea. Fibers of the auditory nerve pass through these minute openings.

spiral fibers, internal. nerve fibers in the cochlea that are believed to be terminal to the efferent nervous system; i.e., from the brain to the ear.

spiral ganglion of the cochlea. the elongated collection of nerve cells from the cochlear branch of the auditory nerve that pass from the modiolus to the organ of Corti. Another name for Corti's ganglion.

spiral innervation. the nerve system within the spiral of the cochlea.

spiral lamina (osseous). the bony plate that extends outward from the modiolus. It is part of the structure that divides the cochlea into sections.

spiral ligament (of cochlea). the thickened portion of the lining of the bony cochlea that forms the outer wall of the cochlear duct.

spiral limbus (spi′ral lim′bus). the border of the spiral lamina.

spiral nerves. neurons that separate from the cochlear nerve and move along the perimeter of the cochlea and branch inward to serve some of the hair cells.

spiral prominence. a ridge in the cochlea on the inner surface of the spiral ligament that contains blood vessels.

spirant (spi′rant) *n.* a fricative consonant.

SPL. sound pressure level (re: .0002 dynes per cm²).

split band amplification. the presentation of lower frequencies to one ear and higher frequencies to the other ear through hearing aids. This system is advocated by Barbara Franklin, PhD, especially for children. Some adults with difficult hearing problems also benefit. It has usually been found that the higher frequencies should be applied to the right ear and lower frequencies to the left ear.

spoken-voice test. an older, ineffectual, test of hearing based on the ability to identify spoken words at a distance of 15 to 20 feet.

spondaic (spon-da′ik) *adj.* concerning spondees or words of two syllables pronounced with equal stress.

spondee *n.* a word containing two syllables that are pronounced with equal intensity.

spondee word test. a test to determine the speech reception threshold (SRT) using words containing two syllables pronounced with uniform intensity.

sporadic deafness. a type of hereditary deafness that results from a mutant or recessive gene becoming dominant irregularly among members of a family—compare familial deafness.

squamosa (skwa-mo′sah) *n.* the thin scalelike portion of the temporal bone.

squamous (skwa′mus) *adj.* 1. scaly. 2. a thin platelike bone.

square wave. a succession of identical acoustical or electrical pulses that start and end instantaneously with equally spaced on and off periods.

squeal *n.* a shrill noise that results from acoustic feedback.

squelch effect. the lessening of the speech interference level of background noise when binaural hearing aids are used.

SR. stapedius reflex. stimulus response.

SRS. Social and Rehabilitation Service.

SRT. speech reception threshold.

SSL. systematic sign language.

SSPL. saturation sound pressure level.

SSW. staggered spondaic word (test).

stage (stāj) *n.* a transistor (or vacuum tube) and its complementary components that make up a distinctive portion of an amplifier.

staggered spondaic word test. SSW. the first syllable of an equally stressed two-syllable word is presented to one ear, then the second syllable is presented to the other ear.

standard articulation test. SAT. this test involves the use of nonsense syllables designed to determine the ability to hear correctly.

standard deviation. SD or sd. the range of variation from the mean in a series of numbers or scores. By definition, the standard deviation is the square root of the variance in a series, i.e., the square root of the mean square of a sum of squared deviations from the mean.

standard reference. a value, expressed as a number, that serves as the base for a scale of comparison in regard to intensity or frequency, e.g., .0002 dynes per square centimeter is the standard reference level for sound pressures.

standard reference intensity. most common reference point in terms of pressure is .0002 dyne/cm^2 or in terms of power: 10^{16} watt/cm^2.

standard reference level. for sound pressures: .0002 dynes per cm^2.

standard reference zero. for pure tone audiometers—see audiometric zero. For speech audiometers it is expected to be 19 dB re .0002 dyne/cm^2.

standing wave. a wave pattern produced when sound pressure waves of the same frequency and amplitude are traveling in opposite directions. The resulting amplitude will be zero at some points and double at others.

Stanford achievement test. test of educational levels of deaf children.

stapedectomy (sta″pĕ-dek′to-me) *n.* an operation used in the treatment of otosclerosis. The stapes is replaced by a prosthesis of polyethylene or wire.

stapedectomy, partial. one leg of the stapes, with part of the footplate attached, is used instead of total replacement of the stapes by plastic or wire prosthesis.

stapedial (stah-pe′de-al) *adj.* pertaining to the stapes.

stapedial nerve. a branch of the facial nerve (VIIth) that connects with the stapedius, the muscle controlling the stapes.

stapedial reflex decay. an impedance meter is used to measure the ability of the stapedius muscle to remain tense. It is considered an objective tone decay test.

stapediomyringopexy (stah-pe″de-o-mĭ-rin-goh′pek-se) *n.* fixation of the head of the stapes to the tense portion of the eardrum; *syn*: myringostapediopexy.

stapediopexy (stah-pe′de-op″ek-se) *n.* surgical fixation of the stapes.

stapedioplasty (stah-pe″de-o-plas′te) *n.* a surgical technique for the relief of otosclerosis without the use of a prosthesis.

stapediotenotomy (stah-pe″de-o-tĕ-not′o-me) *n.* surgical sectioning of the tendon of the stapedius muscle.

stapediovestibular (stah-pe″de-o-ves-tib′u-lar) *adj.* referring to the area surrounding the stapes and vestibule of the ear.

stapedis, capitus (stah′pe-dis kap′ĭ-tus). head of the stapes. The knob of the stirrup that connects with the anvil (incus).

stapedis, capitulum (ka-pit′u-lum). the small rounded end of the stapes (stirrup) that fits into the lenticular process of the incus (the lentiform nodule of Sylvius) and moves with it at the stapedo-incudal joint.

stapedius (stah-pe′de-us) *n.* the smaller of the two muscles in the middle ear.

stapedius muscle. the tiny muscle connected to the neck of the stirrup (stapes) from the wall of the middle ear near the facial nerve.

stapedius reflex. SR. a contraction of the stapedius muscle in response to a loud sound.

stapedius tendon. the tendon that anchors the stapedius muscle to the pyramid on the posterior wall of the middle ear cavity.

stapes (sta′pēz) *pl.* **stapes, stapedes** *n.* also known as the stirrup, the stapes is the third and inner bone of the ossicular chain. Moved by the incus, the stapes vibrates in the oval window.

stapes, base of. the flat platform (footplate) fitting into the oval window that supports and is activated by the crura (legs) of the stapes.

stapes, footplate of. the base on which the legs (crura) of the stapes rest in the oval window.

stapes, leg of. crus (*pl.* **crura**). sometimes called the support of the stirrup.

stapes mobilization. a surgical procedure revived and perfected by Samuel Rosen, MD (1896-1980) in the early 1950s. It was designed to loosen the footplate of the stapes in the oval window. The procedure has been largely superseded by the stapedectomy.

staphylococcus (staf″ĭ-lo-kok′us) *n.* a type of bacteria that may cause various infections. *adj*: **staphylococcal, staphylococcic.**

staphyloplasty (staf′ĭ-lo-plas″te) *n.* surgical repair of cleft palate; *syn*: staphylorrhaphy.

staphylorrhaphy (staf″ĭ-lor′ah-fe) *n.* staphyloplasty.

startle or reflex response. the startle reaction to a stimulus. It is evidenced by any or all of various sudden grimacing or stiffening movements.

stasis (sta′sis) *pl.* **stases** *n.* stoppage or slowing of the flow of body fluids.

-stasis, -stases. suffix indicating a stoppage or slowing.

static, statical (stat′ik, stat′ik-al) *adj.* stopped, stable, or at rest.

static *n.* scratching or sparking sounds produced by electrical disturbances.

static pressure. constant and unchanging pressure.

stationary wave. another name for a standing wave; *syn*: stationary vibration.

statoacoustic nerve (stat″o-ah-koo′stik). the eighth cranial or auditory nerve.

statoconia (stat″o-ko′ne-ah) *sing.* **statoconium** *n.* minute crystalline particles of aragonite (a type of calcium carbonate, $CaCO_3$).

syn: otoconia, ear crystals, ear dust, or otoliths (ear stones). By pressure upon the hair cells of the semicircular canals, these particles help activate the sense of balance.

statocyst (stat′o-sist) *n.* a small sac, containing a ridge of sensory hairs, called statoliths, at the base of the antennae of the crayfish that makes its orientation in space possible.

statokinetic (stat″o-kĭ-net′ik) *adj.* pertaining to bodily reactions during movement.

statokinetic reflex. reaction that results from movements of the body or head; *syn*: kinetic or accelerator reflex.

statolith (stat′o-lith) *n.* a hair-like structure within the statocyst of the crayfish to which sand grains are attached by mucus. This helps the crayfish maintain its balance.

steep or sudden-drop audiogram. usually denotes nearly normal hearing in lower frequencies (sometimes as high as 2000 Hz) followed by a precipitous drop of 25 dB or more per octave. *syn*: ski-slope or precipitous audiogram.

stellate ganglion (stel′āt). a starshaped cell station (ganglion) in the sympathetic nervous system.

Stenger effect. when a pure tone is presented to both ears but at different sensation levels, the sound will appear to be heard only in the ear that has the higher sensation level (SL).

Stenger test. a test for malingering based on the auditory phenomenon of referral to the ear in which the sound appears loudest (the Stenger effect). A pure tone is presented to the normal ear at an intensity 5 or 10 dB above its threshold, then the same tone is presented to the deafened ear at an intensity above its reported threshold. The malingerer will deny hearing any tone at all because the louder tone will mask the fact that the lower tone is still being presented to his good ear.

stenosis (stĕ-no′sis) *n.* closure or narrowing of the ear canal. *adj*: **stenotic, stenosed.**

Stensen's duct (N. Stensen, Danish physician, 1638-1686). tube that conveys saliva from the parotid gland to the mouth. *syn*: parotid duct (ductus parotideus).

step up. to increase the voltage of a current.

stere-, stereo (ste′re-o). prefix referring to three dimensions.

stereo *adj.* shortened version of stereophonic. *n*: **stereo.**

stereocilia (ste″re-o-sil′e-ah) *n.* hairlike fibers rooted in the hair cells—also known as cilia.

stereophonic *adj.* three-dimensional sound effect. *n*: **stereophony.**

stethoscope *n.* instrument used to listen to body sounds.

stethoscope, binaural. the most common type of stethoscope, designed for use with both ears.

stimulation method. a system of speech correction in which major emphasis is placed on teaching the correct speech sounds by having the patient listen to them.

stimulus *pl.* **stimuli** *n.* anything that induces an action (or reaction).

stirrup, or stirrup bone *n.* the stapes—the third and inner bone of the ossicular chain.

stock earmold. an earmold that is one of several standard sizes used for demonstration or temporary use until a custom earmold can be made.

stoma (sto′mah) *n.* an opening.

-stomy (sto′me). suffix referring to a surgical operation that usually creates an opening.

stone-deaf *adj.* slang for totally deaf.

stone, ear. otolith or calcium compound. Also called ear calculus, ear crystals, ear dust, and otoconia.

stop *n.* consonant sound made by a sudden halting of the expiration of air, e.g., between tongue and palate for "d" and "t."

STP. standard temperature and pressure.

strep throat. a sore throat caused by a streptobacillus.

strepto- (strep′to). prefix meaning twisted or twisted chain.

streptobacillus (strep″to-bah-sil′us) *n.* a bacteria whose individual cells are joined in a chain.

streptococcal, streptococcic (strep″to-kok′al, strep″to-kok′sik) *adj.* referring to disease caused by streptococci.

streptococcus (strep-to-kok′us) *pl.* **streptococci** *n.* a bacteria occurring in chains.

streptomycin (sulfate) (strep′to-mi″sin) *n.* drug used in infectious diseases that often damages hearing.

streptothricin (strep″to-thri′sin) *n.* an antibiotic considered more toxic than streptomycin.

stress (stres) *n.* an emphasis given to a speech sound.

stress *v.* to emphasize in speaking.

stria (stri′ah) *pl.* **striae** *n.* a tiny channel or groove.

stria vascularis (vas″ku-lar′is). network of capillaries that forms the outer wall of the inner tube of the cochlea.

striate, striated (stri′āt, ed) *adj.* striped or grooved.

striate *v.* to mark with stripes or grooves. *n*: **striation.**

stridor (stri′dor) *n.* high-pitched, harsh sound (like that of sawing) during breathing due to partial obstruction of air passages.

stridulation (strid″u-la′shun) *n.* a high-pitched rasping sound—such as that made by a cricket. *adj*: **stridulant;** *v*: **stridulate.**

strip printer. a type of teletypewriter in which the message is printed on a narrow strip of paper.

stroke (strōk) *n.* bursting or clotting of a blood vessel in the brain (called a cerebral vascular accident, CVA) causes sudden loss or lowering of consciousness and loss of voluntary muscular control. More lasting physical problems and speech and language disorders may result. *syn:* apoplexy.

Struycken monochord. a tight wire struck by a hammer or stroked by a bow to test hearing.

styloid (sti'loid) *adj.* the process or portion of the temporal bone to which muscles and ligaments are attached.

stylomastoid artery (sti"lo-mas'toid). a branch of the posterior auricular arteries (emerging from the external carotid artery) that supplies the tympanic cavity.

stylomastoid foramen. an opening in the temporal bone that allows passage of the facial nerve and the stylomastoid artery into the tympanic cavity.

sub- (sub). prefix meaning under, below, or beneath.

subaural (sub-aw'ral) *adj.* under the ear.

subcortex (sub-kor'teks) *n.* the white part of the brain just below the cerebral cortex. *adj:* **subcortical.**

subcortical lesion. damage in the brain area beneath the cerebral cortex.

subharmonic frequency. a frequency that is a submultiple (or an even fraction) of the fundamental.

subjective (sub-jek'tive) *adj.* 1. responses that can be voluntarily controlled. *opp:* objective. 2. symptoms or sensations that are evident only to the subject or patient.

subjective idiopathic tinnitus (id"e-o-path'ik ti-ni'-tus). term referring to the consideration of subjective tinnitus as resulting from an unknown disease or cause.

subjective tinnitus. head noises that can be heard only by the patient. (See objective tinnitus). *syn:* nonvibratory tinnitus.

subliminal (sub-lim'i-nal) *adj.* below the level of consciousness. *syn:* subconscious.

subminiature (sub-min'e-ah-chur") *adj.* extra small—often said of electronic parts used in hearing aids.

submucosa (sub"mu-ko'sah) *n.* the layer of connective tissue beneath a mucous membrane. *adj:* **submucosal.**

subsonic (sub-son'ik) *adj.* 1. speed less than the speed of sound. 2. below the audible range—felt as vibrations if intense enough. More properly referred to as infrasonic.

subsonic frequencies (infrasonic frequencies). frequencies below the lower frequency limit of normal hearing; i.e., frequencies of fewer vibrations than 16 cycles per second. (Subsonic is currently used chiefly to designate speeds slower than the speed of sound—about 760 miles per hour at sea level.)

subsonic vibrations. frequencies below 16 cycles per second that are felt as vibrations if intense enough.

substrate (sub'strāt) *n.* the foundation layer for an integrated circuit.

subthreshold *adj.* below the level of intensity that would elicit a response.

subtympanic (sub-tim-pan'ik) *adj.* below the middle ear cavity.

suffix (suf'iks) *n.* a portion of a word—constant in its meaning (as: -itis, inflammation)—that is attached to the end of other words to influence their meaning. Endings that change tense, number, etc. are also considered suffixes.

sulcus (sul'kus) *n.* a groove or furrow—as in the brain.

sulcus tympanicus (tim-pan'i-kus). groove into which the tympanic membrane (eardrum) fits. *syn:* tympanic groove, tympanic sulcus.

summating potential. SP. an electrical response of the hair cells in the cochlea to a sound stimulus that is similar to, but differs from, the cochlear microphonic.

summation, binaural (sum-ma'shun, bin-aw'ral). the cumulative effect of sound reaching both ears that results in a threshold lower than that of the better ear alone.

summation tone. the tone that is heard as the combination of frequencies of two originating tones.

summing computer. a computer designed to collect and average or algebraically sum the evidences of random electrical activity of the brain so the direct result of auditory stimulation becomes more apparent.

super- (soo'per). prefix meaning over or above.

superior (soo-pe're-or) *adj.* located over or above.

superior canal. one of the semicircular canals—part of the human balance mechanism.

superior colliculus (kŏ-lik'u-lus). one of a pair of projections on the midbrain containing integration centers for optic reflexes.

superior olive. the superior olivary complex, an early junction point of the auditory nerve fibers as they pass from the cochlea to the brain.

superior olivary complex (soo-pe're-or ol'i-ver"e kom'pleks). an early junction point of the auditory nerve fibers as they pass from the cochlea to the brain. *syn:* superior olive.

supersonic (soo"per-son'ik) *adj.* faster than the speed of sound. (Ultrasonic refers to the frequencies above the range of human hearing.)

suppurate (sup'u-rāt) *v.* to create or give out pus.

137

suppuration (sup"u-ra'shun) *n.* the process of forming pus. *adj*: **suppurative.**

suppurative otitis media, chronic. continually running ears as a result of infections.

supra- (soo'prah). prefix meaning above or over.

supra-aural (soo"prah-aw'ral) *adj.* above the ear.

supra-auricular (soo"prah-aw-rĭk'u-lar) *adj.* above the external ear.

supraliminal (soo"prah-lim'ĭ-nal) *adj.* above the threshold of awareness.

supramastoid (soo"prah-mas'toid) *adj.* above the mastoid bone (or mastoid process).

suprameatal (soo"prah-me-a'tal) *adj.* above the external ear canal.

suprameatal triangle. a triangular indentation above and in back of the bony portion of the external ear canal. It is one of the landmarks in a mastoid operation. *syn*: Macewen's triangle.

suprasonic (soo"prah-son'ik) *adj.* usually used as synonymous with ultrasonic; i.e., sound with frequencies of vibration above 20,000 per second. (Supersonic indicates faster than the speed of sound.)

suprastapedial (soo"prah-stah-pe'de-al) *adj.* above the stapes.

suprathreshold *adj.* above threshold. Louder than barely audible.

surd (surd) *n.* 1. an unvoiced speech sound (the opposite of sonant). 2. a voiceless person. *adj*: **surd.**

surdimute (sur'dĭ-mūt) *n.* 1. a person without speech due to deafness. 2. a condition of being without speech because of deafness. *adj*: **surdimute.** *syn*: aneneia.

surdity (sur'dĭ-te) *n.* a seldom-used term for deafness.

surdophrenia (ser"do-fre'ne-ah) *n.* a term used to describe the reactions of some deaf people to everyday events as if they were continual emergencies.

surgery, aural. surgery involving the ear.

surgical auditory evaluation. SAE. audiological study of reactions to various acoustic stimuli to determine the site of lesion as a prelude to possible surgical intervention.

susceptance *n.* ratio of energy flow and pressure in the ear canal as measured by an impedance meter.

sustentacular cell (sus"-ten-tak'u-lar). a cell that serves as a support for other specialized cells.

susurrus aurium (ear whispers). noises originating in the ear itself. *syn*: tinnitus.

SWAMI. speech with alternating masking index.

sweep-check test. another term for sweep test.

sweep frequency audiometry. a screening test in which the examiner uses a fixed level of intensity and a limited number of frequencies.

sweep frequency test. a screening test in which the examiner uses a fixed level of intensity (usually 15 or 25 dB) and a limited number of discrete frequencies.

switch, interrupter. the switch that interrupts (or presents) the pure tones of an audiometer.

syllable, nonsense. a monosyllable that has no meaning. Used in difficult speech discrimination tests.

sylvian fissure (sil've-an fish'ŭr). the deep narrow cleft that separates the frontal, parietal, and temporal lobes of the brain. (Sulcus lateralis cerebri or fissura cerebri lateralis: the lateral cerebral fissure.)

sympathectomy (sim"pah-thek'to-me) *n.* interruption of the sympathetic nervous system by surgery or local anesthesia. (Sometimes used in cases of Meniere's at the stellate ganglion in an effort to relieve vertigo without adversely affecting hearing.)

sympathetic vibration. another name for the condition of natural resonance excited in a system or body.

symptom (simp'tum) *n.* a change from the normal body function—a sign that something abnormal is occurring—indicative of a disorder or disease.

symptom, Bezold's. inflamed fluid-filled swelling at the tip of the mastoid process.

syn- prefix indicating together or with. Variations of the prefix include syl-, sym-, and sys-.

synapse (sin'aps) *n.* a junction point between nerve cells (neurons).

synarthrosis (sin"ar-thro'sis) *n.* restricted or lack of movement in a joint.

synchondrosis (sin"kon-dro'sis) *n.* cartilaginous restriction of movement of a joint.

synchronous auditory feedback. SAF. the hearing (or feedback) of the speaker's own words as they are spoken.

syndesmosis (sin"des-mo'sis) *n.* restricted movement of a joint resulting from connective tissue attachments.

syndesmosis tympanostapedia (tim"pah-no-stă-pe'de-ah). the connection of the footplate of the stapes with the oval window.

syndrome (sin-drŏm) *n.* a running together. A collection of bodily signs and symptoms that typify a particular disorder. *adj*: **syndromic.**

syndrome, Alport's. deafness associated with hereditary kidney disease (nephropathy) and mental retardation.

syndrome, Apert's. an unusual congenital group of symptoms including a peaked head (associated with achondroplasia) and webbed fingers.

syndrome, auriculotemporal. sweating and flushing of the ear as a result of jaw movement while eating.

syndrome, Cockayne's. complex of associated symptoms including dwarfism, mental retardation, and ear and eye malformations.

syndrome, Cogan's. a disease involving connective tissue, characterized by tinnitus, deafness, vertigo, blurred vision, or blindness.

syndrome, Costen's. earache resulting from loss of (or bad fitting) teeth.

syndrome, D₁ (or D₁ trisomy). variable malformation of infants resulting from irregularities in chromosomes of group D, no. 13, 14, or 15. Malformed ears appear as one of the signs in all cases. *syn*: trisomy D₁ syndrome or trisomy 13-15 syndrome.

syndrome, Down's. (John Langdon Haydon Down, English physician, 1828-1896). mongolism. Mental retardation and hearing impairment as well as physical deformities are characteristic.

syndrome, first arch. a complex of symptoms similar to Treacher–Collins (incomplete development of the lower jaw and cheek bones, low-set ears, and misshaped lower eyelids) but more severe with additional facial malformations.

syndrome, Gradenigo's. a group of symptoms including earache (otalgia), ear discharge (suppurative otitis media), double vision (diplopia), and abscess of the temporal bone associated with localized meningitis involving the Vth and VIth cranial nerves.

syndrome, Klippel-Feil. a complex of symptoms that, in addition to deafness, includes a short neck, fused vertebrae, and abnormalities of the brain stem and cerebellum.

syndrome, Laurence-Biedl or **Laurence-Moon-Biedl.** a complex of hereditary and congenital symptoms including eye and ear defects.

syndrome, Marfan's. a complex of symptoms including ear, eye, skull, and finger defects.

syndrome, Meniere's. more commonly referred to as Meniere's disease.

syndrome, Michel's. a complex of symptoms that includes failure of development of the inner ear.

syndrome, Mondini's. symptoms include incomplete development or malformation of the inner ear.

syndrome, otomandibular (o″to-man-dib′u-lar). incomplete development of the lower jaw, accompanied by malformations of the ear; *syn*: otomandibular dysostosis.

syndrome, Pierre Robin (ro-ban′). a complex of symptoms including incomplete jaw development, cleft palate, tongue anomalies, and eye defects.

syndrome, Pendred's. a congenital glandular deficiency characterized by goiter. The accompanying deafness is sensorineural.

syndrome, Ramsay-Hunt. a complex of symptoms of a viral infection of the VIIth (facial) nerve. Among the symptoms are earaches followed by aural (otitis) herpes—a rash of tiny blisters in and around the ear.

syndrome, Refsum's. a complex of hereditary defects including progressive deafness. *syn*: heredopathia atactica polyneuritiformis.

syndrome, Treacher-Collins. a complex of symptoms including incomplete development of the lower jaw and cheek bones accompanied by low-set ears and misshaped lower eyelids.

syndrome, trisomy E. similar to trisomy D₁, except that the extra chromosome is of group E, No. 17 or 18.

syndrome, Usher's. a group of symptoms accompanying congenital deafness: degenerative eye disease (retinitis pigmentosa), balance problems, and ear canal abnormalities.

syndrome, Waardenburg. a combination of symptoms, described by Waardenburg, that may be associated wth hereditary deafness. The appearance of a broad nasal bridge resulting from a fold of skin at the inner angle of the eyes, the irises of which may differ in color, and a streak of white hair in the middle of the forehead.

synergism, synergy (sin′er-jizm, sin′er-je) *n*. combined or cooperative action; usually results in coordinated movement or response superior to that evidenced when only one receptor is stimulated. *adj*: **synergetic, synergic.**

synergistically *adv*. normally understanding better with two ears than with only one.

synesthesia *n*. a subjective sensation other than the one being stimulated; e.g., seeing a color or image every time a particular sound is heard.

synostosis (sin″os-to′sis) *n*. restricted or lack of movement in a joint resulting from a bony connection.

syntax *n*. arranged together—the relationship of words and phrases; sentence structure.

syphilis *n*. an infectious venereal disease. It may be congenital and is usually chronic. When hearing is affected the result is called luetic deafness. *adj or n*: **syphilitic.**

syphilitic deafness. hearing loss caused by syphilis. Sometimes called luetic deafness.

syphiloma (sif″i-lo′mah) *n*. a tumor caused by syphilis. *syn*: gumma *adj*: **syphilomatous.**

systemic (sis-tem′ik) *adj*. affecting the whole body.

system, hardware. an instrumental auditory training system that requires the teacher's microphone to be directly connected to the students' headset through desk-type amplifiers.

139

T

T. international hearing aid symbol for input from telephone pickup coil.

T & A. tonsillectomy and adenoidectomy.

T areas. associated areas that may cause earache when damaged or diseased: tongue, tonsil, throat, tubal area, thyroid, temporomandibular joint.

tachistoscope (tah-kis'to-skōp) *n.* an apparatus designed to project pictures or figures for very brief periods—one-fifth of a second or less.

tactaphone *n.* device designed to make possible communication with the deaf and blind at a distance. It utilizes the sense of touch for Morse code or other signals.

tactile (tak'til) *adj.* relating to touch. *syn*: tactual. *n*: **tactility.**

tactile cue. a signal or hint that results from a feeling of vibration rather than sound.

tactilegram, tactilogram *n.* a chart of sensitivity that results from stimulation of the sense of touch.

taction *n.* the sense of touch or contact especially referring to the help given the speech-reader by the vibration of sound from a hearing aid.

tactual *adj.* concerning the sense of touch. *syn*: tactile.

talk-back unit. an electronic amplifying system that allows two-way communication.

Tarchanoff effect. the change in the electrical potential of the skin as a result of an external stimulus.

Tarchanoff method (also Tarchanow). electrodes are attached to the skin to measure the changes in electrical potential of the sweat glands that results from a sound stimulus as in EDR audiometry (compare Feré method). The T effect is sometimes referred to as the galvanic skin response.

TARP. total aural reconstructive prosthesis.

TAT. thematic apperception test.

TD. threshold of discomfort.

TDD. telecommunications device for the deaf.

TDH-39. telephonic dynamic headphone, model #39.

TDI. Telecommunications for the Deaf, Inc.

technician, audiometric. a person who is trained and qualified to administer audiometric tests and usually works under the supervision of an audiologist or otologist.

tectorial membrane. gelatinous membrane, attached to the bony spiral lamina that overlies the hair-cells within the cochlea of the inner ear. Another name for Corti's membrane.

tectorium *n.* the tectorial membrane or Corti's membrane—the "roof" membrane into which the cilia of the hair-cells project. *adj*: tectorial.

teeth, auditory. minute toothlike projections along the free margin of the labium vestibulare of the cochlea. *syn*: Huschke's auditory teeth.

teeth, Corti's. minute toothlike projections along the free margin of the labium vestibulare of the cochlea. *syn*: auditory teeth, Huschke's teeth.

tegmen *n.* the roof of the tympanic cavity (epitympanic recess).

telephone coil. an induction coil placed in a hearing aid and designed to pick up electrical impulses directly from the telephone so that these impulses can be amplified without interference from sounds coming through the hearing aid microphone.

telephone theory of hearing. an oversimplified explanation of the hearing process that says the ear is like a microphone and the auditory nerve a transmission line to the brain.

telephone theory of Rutherford. a discounted belief that the basilar membrane vibrates as a whole like the diaphragm of a telephone. W. Rutherford said in 1886 that the entire organ of Corti would be stimulated by each sound wave, which would then be translated into a nerve impulse of corresponding frequency and amplitude.

telereceptor *n.* a sense organ that can respond to a stimulus originating at a distance from the body, e.g., the ear. It may also be known as a distance receptor.

teletactor. a device by which speech energies were first divided into five frequencies, then amplified, and introduced to each of the five fingers of the hand by vibrators. In this way vibrations and rhymthic patterns were learned by deaf subjects, and consequently speech discrimination was made possible.

temporal *adj.* concerning the temples and the sides of the skull behind the eye sockets.

temporal bone. the bone at the side of the skull. The petrous portion contains the inner ear.

Temporal Bone Banks. Donation of temporal bones, which include both normal and impaired ears, facilitates research in deafness and ear disorders. The regional centers in the National Temporal Bone Banks Program of the Deafness Research Foundation are located as follows:

1. Eastern (and National) NTBB Center, Massachusetts Eye & Ear Infirmary, Boston, MA 02114. (617) 523-7900, ext 777. Harold F. Schuknecht, MD, Director.

2. Midwestern NTBB Center, University of Minnesota, 2630 University Avenue, SE,

Minneapolis, MN 55414. (612) 373-5466. Michael M. Paparella, MD, Director.

3. Southern NTBB Center, Baylor College of Medicine, Neurosensory Center, Room A523, Houston, TX 77030. (713) 790-5470. Bobby R. Alford, MD, Director.

4. Western NTBB Center, UCLA School of Medicine, 31-24 Rehabilitation Center, Los Angeles, CA 90024. (213) 825-4710. Paul H. Ward, MD, Director.

temporal evannation. use of an analog computer to differentiate between types of electroencephalographic (EEG) activity.

temporal lobe. a rounded projection on the underside of each hemisphere of the brain containing the hearing centers.

temporal pole. the forward portion of the temporal lobe.

temporary hearing loss. see temporary threshold shift.

temporary threshold shift. TTS. a reversible elevation in the threshold of hearing that may result from continuous exposure to sound. It is expressed in dB per frequency and related to exposure time. *syn:* auditory fatigue.

temporoauricular (tem″po-ro-aw-rik′u-lar) *adj.* concerning the temporal region and the ear.

temporomandibular joint (tem″po-ro-man-dib′u-lar). TMJ. junction of jawbone with skull just in front of the external ear. Misfit at this point (malocclusion) may cause earaches and (infrequently) hearing problems.

temporomaxillary (tem″po-ro-mak′sĭ-ler″e) *adj.* concerning the temporal bone and the jawbone. *syn:* temporomandibular.

tensor (ten′sor) *n.* a muscle that tightens a membrane or part of the body. *adj:* tensorial.

tensor tympani. the larger of the two middle ear muscles. It is attached to the temporal bone near the eustachian tube and connected to the handle of the malleus. It is activated by the Vth nerve and controls the tenseness of the eardrum.

terminal arbor. the branching end system of a nerve cell.

terminal threshold. the lowest intensity of sound pressure which, when increased, will cause no further increase in the sensation of loudness. Also known as terminal limen and tolerance limit.

test, absolute bone conduction. ABC. 1. a test to establish levels of threshold sensitivity in response to the stimulus of a bone oscillator while the ears are occluded or closed. (Relative bone conduction tests call for the ears to be open or unoccluded). 2. a tuning fork test made by comparing the bone conduction of the patient with that of the examiner. The ear canal of the patient is closed by the finger of the exam-

iner and the base of the tuning fork is placed on the mastoid process. If the examiner can still hear the fork in the same manner after the patient has ceased to hear it, this "reduced absolute bone conduction" usually indicates a sensorineural impairment. See Schwabach test.

test, air-bone gap. a test for the difference in hearing sensitivity as measured by air conduction and bone conduction.

test, alternate binaural loudness balance. a test for recruitment in which the patient is asked to balance the sensation of loudness experienced in a normal ear and an impaired ear.

Using a dual-channel audiometer (or two balanced audiometers) a pure tone is introduced in the normal ear at a level above threshold, e.g., 20 dB. The patient is asked to indicate when the tone presented alternately to the affected ear is equally loud. This point is noted on a chart and the intensity of the tone in the normal ear is increased 10 or 20 dB and the first step is repeated. These steps are continued and a laddergram constructed until the points on the chart are even—complete recruitment—or pass each other—over-recruitment. If the differences remain constant there is said to be no recruitment.

test, articulation. hearing test designed to measure the intelligibility of speech or of speech sounds. There are tests for individual sound articulation, syllable articulation, vowel or consonant articulation, initial or final consonant articulation.

test, auropalpebral reflex. a test of hearing sensitivity based on observation of eyelid muscle reaction in response to a sound stimulus.

test, Barany's caloric (Robert Barany, Viennese otologist). water, either above or below body temperature, is used to irrigate the external auditory canal. This stimulates the vestibular portion of the ear and results in more or less rapid eye movements (nystagmus).

test, Bekesy. five types of results of automatic audiometry described under audiometry, Bekesy.

test, Bender Gestalt. a test for personality and possible brain damage among the deaf.

test, binaural. a test of the ability to integrate and understand speech sounds presented to each ear simultaneously through narrow-band-pass filters—high to one ear and low to the other. Only a normally-functioning auditory system can get a perfect score.

test, binaural group. a screening test of hearing for several persons at the same time. Pure tones are presented in varying number of pulses to either ear. The testee indicates the number of pulses heard in

141

both ears at each presentation series. This system is utilized in both the Reger-Newby and Glorig automatic group screening audiometers.

test, binaural loudness balance. a test for recruitment by comparing judgments of loudness between ears. In alternate binaural loudness balance testing, a pure tone is presented first to one normal (or nearly normal) ear—then the intensity is adjusted in the other ear until the tones in both ears are judged to be equally loud. The values are plotted at increasing levels of intensity to see if the differences decrease with the changes.

test, Binet-Simon scale. a test of intelligence originally designed for children and later extended in range.

test, Bing. a comparison of the response to a bone vibrator stimulus (or tuning fork) when the ear canal is left open and then closed. It is also known as an occlusion test.

test, bone conduction. a test conducted by placing a bone oscillator on the skull, usually the mastoid process, to determine the threshold of hearing sensitivity when the conductive mechanism of the ear is bypassed. The test is designed to determine how well the balance of the hearing sense is functioning.

test, California. the answers to questions are analyzed in a personality test used with deaf children.

test, central pathway involvement. a comparison of the speech discrimination results when monosyllables are given to each ear separately—then both together. If the discrimination score fails to improve binaurally, a lesion of the central auditory pathway is indicated.

test, coin-click. outdated and inadequate test of hearing based on the ability to hear the clicking of coins.

test, delayed auditory feedback. DAF. a system by which the speaker's own words are returned (feedback) through earphones after a time delay of a few milliseconds. A test of malingering also known as delayed side tone. *syn:* delayed speech feedback test.

test, delayed side tone. a test for malingering in which the patient reads aloud while wearing headphones from a special device that relays his speech to him about 1/10 of a second after he has uttered it. The malingerer will be unable to keep his speech from becoming slurred and confused. *syn:* delayed auditory feedback.

test, delayed speech feedback. delayed auditory feedback.

test, distorted speech. same as filtered speech test.

test, Doerfler-Stewart. a test of functional or nonorganic hearing loss, based on a

comparison of the ability to understand spondaic words in quiet and in noise.

test, Drever-Collins scale. an intelligence test that may be used with the deaf.

test, electric response audiometry. ERA. a form of electrophysiologic audiometry in which an analog computer is included in the circuit to average out ongoing or spontaneous brainwave activity. A characteristic pattern of response to a sound stimulus may then become evident. Also referred to as evoked response audiometry.

test, electrodermal audiometry. EDA. a method of determining hearing thresholds by measuring changes in skin resistance, associated with a conditioned response to sound stimuli.

test, electroencephalic audiometry. EEA. a type of electrophysiologic audiometry. The electroencephalic response (EER), resulting from sound stimulation, causes changes in the pattern of the encephalogram (EEG). These changes are measured and quantified. *syn:* electroencephalographic audiometry (EEG).

tests, electrophysiologic audiometry. an inclusive term covering many types of so-called objective tests designed to measure the individual's response to a sound stimulus without subject cooperation being necessary.

An instrument is used that records changes in brain waves, heart rate, or skin resistance to sound stimuli. The reponse may be preconditioned or reinforced by a mild electric shock that follows the sound stimulus at an interval of about 0.6 seconds. Tests included are: evoked (or electric) response audiometry (ERA), cardiac evoked response audiometry (CERA), electrocardiographic response (ECR), electrodermal audiometry (EDA), and electroencephalic audiometry (EEA).

test, everyday speech. a test of speech understanding based on the use of sentences especially prepared at the Central Institute for the Deaf which were designed to represent everday American speech.

test, evoked response audiometry. ERA. another name for electric response audiometry.

test, Ewing. test of infant hearing designed by the Ewings of England based on the quiet presentation of familiar sounds (e.g., cup and spoon).

test, eye blink. closure or blink of an eye (the auropalpebral reflex) resulting from stimulation by sudden sound at controlled levels.

test, fading-numbers. an almost obsolete group hearing test in which a phonograph record presents pairs of one-digit numbers at successively lower (3 dB) levels of intensity.

test, faint speech. a test of speech discrimination in which monosyllabic words (PB lists) are presented at 5 to 15 dB above threshold (SL—sensation level).

test, fast adaptation. less often used term for tone decay test.

test, filtered audiometric speech. a test of speech discrimination in which words are presented at a level that is comfortably loud but filters allow only controlled frequency bands to be heard.

test, filtered speech. same as filtered audiometric speech test.

test, 4-C. a test of hearing involving the use of the 4-C group audiometer. Two-digit numbers are given progressively more softly. The last number heard by each listener indicates his threshold.

test, Fowler. a test of recruitment involving loudness balancing.

test, free-field. another name for sound field test.

test, Gelle's (je-la') (Marie-Ernst Gelle, French otologist, 1834-1923). a test designed to determine the mobility of the ossicles and especially the stapes. A tuning fork is applied to the mastoid process while a rubber tube with an air bulb is used to compress the air in the ear canal. If the threshold does not change as the air is compressed, the problem is considered to be conductive in that the stapes is fixed.

test, group screening. a test designed to be administered to several people at the same time that will indicate any who may need further attention.

test, Hiskey. a test of hearing or understanding of verbal directions that is said to also indicate levels of intelligence. Also known as the Nebraska test.

test, house-tree-person. H-T-P. a personality test sometimes used with the hearing handicapped.

test, intracutaneous. a test of sensitivity by injection into the skin of a substance that may cause an allergic reaction.

test, Johnston (group). several children are screened simultaneously by having them keep their eyes closed and raise their hands as they hear pure tones that are presented randomly to various parts of the group at the same time.

test, K.S.U. speech discrimination. a test of speech understanding prepared by Kenneth W. Berger, Ph.D., of Kent (Ohio) State University. It is based on multiple-choice words in sentences.

test, lateralization. the Weber test. A bone oscillator or tuning fork is placed in the middle of the forehead and the difference in response between ears (lateralization) is noted. If the tone is heard in the poorer ear, a conductive loss is indicated. If the

loss is sensorineural, the tone will be heard in the better ear.

test, limited frequency screening. a screening test limited to 1, 2, or 3 frequencies at preset levels of intensity. It is sometimes referred to as reduced screening.

test, Lombard. a test for malingering in which the patient is asked to read aloud while wearing headphones. As he reads, continuous sound (usually white noise) is presented to the "deafened" ear or ears. Since the normally-hearing person unconsciously tries to talk above the background noise level (the Lombard effect), the malingerer will usually react in the same way, i.e., raise his voice while reading aloud.

test, loudness balance. a test for recruitment, by comparing judgments of loudness, which is performed either monaurally or binaurally.

test, low-redundancy speech. a test to determine the ability to understand speech when most of the repetitive factors have been removed by use of filters.

test, Luscher-Zwislocki. a test of the difference limen (DL) for intensity. A tone is presented that varies in intensity but centers around a sensation level (SL) of 40 dB. The variation in intensity (which the patient hears as beats) is gradually reduced until the beats seem to disappear. This point is the patient's DL for intensity (or jnd for loudness).

test, malingering. any one of a number of tests to determine if one is feigning a handicap.

test, Massachusetts (group). a number of children are screened simultaneously by having them indicate on a scoring sheet whether or not a pure tone is heard as it may or may not have been presented during a series of six bursts.

test, Metropolitan achievement. a reading test that has been revised for use with the deaf.

test, Metz recruitment. an acoustic impedance measurement that may indicate recruitment in a patient with a hearing impairment if a stapedius reflex is elicited by a stimulus smaller than 60 to 70 dB above threshold.

test, Meyerson group speech. a number of children are screened simultaneously by having them point to the appropriate picture in response to the word.

test, modified Rainville. M-R. the masking noise is introduced through the forehead rather than at the mastoid (as in the Rainville test).

test, modified rhyme. MRT. a multiple-choice speech test in which the listener is asked to circle the word spoken. The vowel nucleus in each set is the same, but the consonants differ.

test, modified Stenger. speech is used instead of pure tones for the Stenger test of malingering.

test, modified tone decay. MTDT. a pure tone is presented 5 dB above the threshold level. If and when the tone disappears, the intensity is increased 5 dB. The number of times this increase must be repeated (the shift in one minute, for example) is noted as an index of the degree of tone decay at that frequency.

test, monaural loudness balance. a test for recruitment by comparing judgments of loudness between frequencies in the same ear. A pure tone of a better (lower, preferably normal or nearly normal) frequency is presented at successively increasing levels above its threshold. A pure tone of a higher frequency is adjusted each time until the tones are judged to be equally loud. The values are plotted at the increasing levels of intensity to see if the differences decrease with the changes. *syn*: alternate monaural loudness balance test.

test, monochord. an early device for testing hearing, consisting of a taut wire activated by a hammer or a violin bow.

test, Moro reflex. the presentation of a sound stimulus to observe the reaction of a newborn.

test, Nebraska. another name for the Hiskey test.

test, Nielsen group. the hearing sensitivity of a number of children is determined at the same time by scoring their indicated responses as intensities decrease during the random presentation of a series of long and short tones.

test, nonlanguage scale. test that depends upon standardized pantomime and gestures to transmit instructions.

test, nystagmus (nis-tag′mus). water is used alternately above and below body temperatures to irrigate the external ear canal. The resulting involuntary eye movements are studied in relation to vestibular or labyrinthine function.

test, occlusion. a comparison of the response to a bone vibrator stimulus when the external ear canal is left open and then closed. Also known as the Bing test, the comparison of absolute and relative bone conduction thresholds is essentially an occlusion test.

test, physiological audiometry. test of hearing that depends upon the measurement of changes in electrical response from either the skin (electrodermal) or the brain (electroencephalic).

test, progressive matrices. a test of intelligence sometimes used with deaf and hard of hearing adults.

test, psychogalvanic skin response (or resistance). commonly known as PGSR or GSR test. An auditory stimulus is given (as a warning signal) followed by a mild shock. The change in electrical resistance of the skin is recorded automatically by a stylus on a moving roll of paper. After adequate conditioning, the shock is withheld and a response to an auditory stimulus alone may thus be measured. It is sometimes referred to as a psychogalvanometric test.

test, pulse-tone (group). another name for, or a variation of, the binaural group test.

test, pulsed tone threshold audiometry. the determination of thresholds of hearing sensitivity by means of short bursts of pure tones.

test, Rainville. a bone-conduction test devised by M. J. Rainville about 1955. It involves a comparison of the air and bone masking intensities required to mask an air-conducted pure tone threshold.

test, Randall's Island performance. a nonverbal test of intelligence suitable for preschool deaf and hard of hearing children. It involves performance and manipulative tasks.

test, recorded speech. list of words that have been reproduced on records or tapes for the purpose of determining speech reception thresholds or discrimination abilities.

test, reduced screening. also known as limited frequency screening test.

test, Reed's. a rhyming word-picture test of discrimination devised by Michael Reed.

test, reflex. a broad term that usually refers to the observation of physiological reactions to sudden sound stimuli—especially of babies and young children.

test, revised Beta. a nonlanguage test of intelligence suitable for use with deaf and hard of hearing adults.

test, Rinne. (rin′neh). primarily a tuning fork test. After being struck lightly, the fork is held alternately with its base on the mastoid process, then with its acoustic axis in line with the ear canal, until it is no longer heard in one position or the other. When the sound is heard longer by air it is described as a positive Rinne (symbol +R). When the sound is heard longer by bone it is known as a negative Rinne (symbol −R). A negative Rinne is also indicated by pure tone audiometry when there is an air-bone gap, i.e., when the bone oscillator produces a better threshold than by air. A negative Rinne may be indicative of a conductive hearing loss or a conductive component in a mixed loss.

test, Rorschach. a measurement of personality and intelligence based upon interpretation of the subject's explanation of or comments in regard to ink-blot design.

test, rotary. a test of equilibrium. The patient is seated in a Barany chair which can be turned rapidly in a circular motion and stopped suddenly.

test, Rudmose group. the use of the Rudmose audiometer with multiple attenuators and recorders to automatically test the hearing of several subjects at the same time.

test, running speech. a method of determining the speech reception threshold (SRT) by the use of unemotional connected discourse progressively reduced in intensity until it can no longer be understood.

test, SAL. a sensorineural acuity level or bone conduction test that involves introducing a masking noise through a bone oscillator placed on the forehead while pure tones are presented through the earphones of the audiometer. The results are compared with those obtained with normal ears.

test, Schwabach (shvah'bak). a bone conduction test using tuning forks. It is a comparison of the patient's bone conduction with that of a normally hearing person. The results are categorized as normal, increased, or decreased, and may be indicated in seconds of difference.

test, screening. a test of hearing sensitivity designed to pick out (or screen) individuals who may need more careful testing or medical attention.

test, Sheridan's. a screening test of infant hearing based on meaningful sounds, designed by Dr. Mary Sheridan.

test, single frequency screening. a screening test limited to 4000 Hz.

test, shifting voice. a test of malingering based on the shifting of speech intensities at each ear. It is a modification of the Stenger speech test.

test, SISI. short increment sensitivity index. A test of the ability to recognize one decibel increases in intensity during a series of bursts of pure tone presented 20 dB above threshold.

test, Snijders-Ooman nonverbal scale. SONS. a nonverbal test of conceptual thinking that may be adapted for the deaf. It is more often used in Europe.

test, sound-field. a hearing test involving the use of loudspeakers rather than earphones; *syn*: free-field test.

test, speech awareness. SAT. a test of the ability to recognize that speech is being heard in the presence of conflicting sounds or when the hearing impairment is so severe that individual words cannot be understood.

test, speech discrimination. a test of the ability to understand speech as determined by scoring the number of words in a phonetically balanced list repeated correctly.

test, speech perception. a seldom used test to determine the level of intensity at which sounds can be perceived as words. It is between the threshold of detectability and the threshold of intelligibility.

test, speech reception threshold. a test to determine the lowest intensity level at which 50 percent or more of the spondaic test words (words of two syllables having equal stress) can be repeated correctly. Cold running speech may also be used but is not as acceptable.

test, spoken-voice. an older, ineffectual test of hearing based on the ability to identify spoken words at a distance of 15 or 20 feet.

test, spondaic word. a test to determine the speech reception threshold (SRT) using words containing two syllables pronounced with uniform intensity.

test, staggered spondaic word. SSW. the first syllable of an equally stressed two-syllable word is presented to one ear, then as the second syllable of that word is presented to the same ear, the first syllable of another spondaic word is presented to the other ear followed by its second syllable in that ear while no sound is presented to the first ear.

test, Stanford achievement. a test of educational level that may be used with deaf children.

test, Stenger. a test for malingering based on the auditory phenomenon of referral to the ear in which the sound appears loudest (the Stenger effect). A pure tone is presented to the normal ear at an intensity 5 or 10 dB above its threshold, then the same tone is presented to the "deafened" ear at an intensity above its reported threshold. The malingerer will deny hearing any tone at all because the louder tone will mask the fact that the lower (in intensity) tone is still being presented to his "good" ear.

test, Struycken monochord. a tight wire struck by a hammer or stroked by a bow to test hearing.

test, SWAMI. speech with alternating masking index. A test of the ability to understand speech while a masking white noise at a 20 dB higher level is alternated between ears.

test, sweep. a screening test in which the examiner uses a fixed level of intensity (usually 15 or 25 dB) and a limited number of discrete frequencies.

test, sweep-check. another term for sweep test.

test, thematic apperception. TAT. a personality test adaptable to deaf and hard of hearing adults.

test, tone decay. the presentation of a continuous tone at successively higher (5 dB) levels of intensity to an impaired ear until the tone can be heard for one minute. Also see modified tone decay test.

test, tuning fork. a test of hearing sensitivity that utilizes a tuning fork. The bone oscillator of the pure tone audiometer can be effectively substituted.

test, two-frequency. a screening test of hearing sensitivity based on the use of 4000 Hz and one other frequency (usually 500 Hz, but sometimes 2000 Hz).

test, uncomfortable loudness level recruitment. if the subject can only tolerate a tone a few dB above his threshold, recruitment is present, according to J. L. Bangs and C. J. Mullins.

test, Vineland social maturity scale. a test of behavioral development.

test, voice-reflex. another term for Lombard test.

tests, W-1, W-2. thirty-six bisyllabic words with equal stress on each syllable used to determine the speech reception threshold. W-1 list was recorded at a constant level; the W-2 list was recorded with average attenuation of 1 dB per word.

test, W-22. a phonetically balanced word list used as a test of discrimination.

test, watch-tick. an obsolete test of hearing based on the ability to hear the ticking of a watch.

test, Weber. a bone conduction test used mainly in cases of unilateral deafness. The bone oscillator (or tuning fork) is placed on the midline of the forehead to determine the ear in which the sound is heard. An ear conductively affected will hear the tone better than the normal ear. On the other hand, in cases of unilateral perceptive deafness, the sound will be referred to (heard in) the normal ear.

test, Wechsler-Bellevue. W-B. a test of intelligence suitable for use with the deaf.

test, Wechsler intelligence scale for children. WISC. an intelligence test suitable for use with deaf children.

test, Wechsler performance scale. an intelligence test that may be adapted for use with deaf adults.

test, word intelligibility by picture identification. WIPI. simple pictures are used that the child can easily identify when he hears and recognizes the word spoken by the examiner. The child is scored on the number of pictures he points to correctly.

tetrotus (tet-ro'tus) *n.* an individual malformed by having four ears.

thalidomide (thah-lid'o-mīd) *n.* a drug, used primarily to calm nerves or induce sleep, that has been found to cause congenital defects.

thematic apperception test (them-at"ik ah"per-sep'shun). TAT. a personality test adaptable to deaf and hearing-impaired adults.

theory (the'or-e) *n.* an intellectual speculation as to the best solution to a problem or plausible explanation of a phenomenon.

theory of hearing, frequency. the generally discounted belief that pitch discrimination is dependent upon the number of times per second that impulses pass over the auditory nerve.

theory of Helmholtz. Helmholtz' resonance theory of hearing.

theory, lamina. an obsolete idea that portions of the bony lamina resonate in response to stimuli of different frequencies.

theory (phase) of binaural localization. difference in time of arrival of wave peaks to each ear make localization of sound possible—most effectively at frequencies below 1000 Hz.

theory, place. the belief that pitch discrimination is dependent upon the response to the stimulation of localized areas along the basilar membrane within the cochlea. The theory is often considered to extend to places within the brain.

theory, resonance. Helmholtz in 1857 advanced the theory that the hair cells within the organ of Corti act as resonators—each with its own natural period of vibration and each responding only to one tone of a particular frequency.

theory, selective resonance. an early version of the resonance theory of pitch perception involved various cavities thought to be behind the eardrum (Gaspard Bauhin, 1605). Later, in 1683, Joseph G. Du Verney theorized that the bony lamina resonated to different frequencies in accordance with its varying width.

theory of signal detectability. TSD. the belief that the ability to hear a given type of sound despite a masking noise, will be influenced by the wording of the instruction.

theory, telephone. an oversimplified explanation of the hearing process that says the ear is like a microphone and the auditory nerve a transmission line to the brain.

theory, traveling wave. Georg von Bekesy received the Nobel Prize in 1961 for his discovery of the traveling wave phenomenon which resulted in his theory: Movement of the footplate of the stapes causes a fluid wave to move along the basilar membrane with a rise and fall of amplitude. The point where the wave reaches its maximum amplitude is the point where the frequency of the sound is detected. Frequencies are highest toward the oval window and lowest toward the apex of the cochlea.

theory, volley. the belief that pitch discrimination in the lower frequencies is dependent upon nerve impulses firing in volleys; and in the higher frequencies it is dependent upon the response to the stimulation of localized areas along the basilar membrane in the cochlea.

theory, volley pitch perception. the theory that pitch is determined by the brain's interpretation of sequences (volleys) of electrical impulses carried by different groups of neurons within a nerve.

therapeutic (ther″ah-pu′tik) *adj.* concerning healing of disease or correction of disorders.

therapist, speech. a specialist in the treatment of speech and language disorders; *syn*: speech pathologist.

therapy (ther′ah-pe) *n.* treatment of physical or mental disorders.

therapy, audio. the application of therapeutic techniques to help an individual use his residual hearing to maximum advantage.

therapy, auricular. acupuncture at the pinna to affect other parts of the body or psychological problems (such as overeating or smoking).

therapy, speech. the treatment of speech and language disorders.

thermionic valve. an older British term for vacuum tube.

thermistor (ther′mis-tor) *n.* a semiconductor that varies in resistance with the temperature. It is used to control the effects of temperature changes in an electronic circuit.

third harmonic. the overtone that is three times the fundamental or lowest tone.

three-quarter skeleton earmold. same as the skeleton mold, but with the central portion of the concha rim removed.

3-dB rule. in calculating risk of possible damage to hearing from noise exposure: When the length of time of exposure is cut in half, an increase of 3 dBA (double the energy) is permissible without increasing the risk (ISO/TC43/SC-1).

threshold *n.* the point at which a listener can first determine that a sound is becoming audible.

threshold, absolute. the minimum level of intensity at which a sound can just be determined to be present.

threshold adaptation. another term for tone decay or fast adaptation.

threshold, aided. threshold obtained when an amplifier is used—usually a hearing aid.

threshold of audibility. the point on a sound pressure level scale at which 50% of the stimuli presented to the ear are heard; *syn*: threshold of detectability; auditory threshold of sensitivity.

threshold, auditory. the sound pressure level of the minimum acoustic signal that causes an auditory sensation for a specified percentage of the number of times the signal is presented to the ear. The auditory threshold for spondees, for example, is defined as the minimum sound pressure level at which a subject can repeat correctly 50% of the spondaic words presented to him. Auditory thresholds vary with different stimuli, and the particular stimulus must be specified.

threshold, bone conduction. level of intensity at which a pure tone can be recognized

through a bone oscillator pressed against the skull.

threshold of detectability. the threshold of sensitivity, i.e., the point at which 50% of the presentations of a pure tone can be heard.

threshold, differential. sometimes called "just noticeable difference" (jnd) or "difference limen" (DL). The smallest change in frequency or intensity that can be recognized.

threshold of discomfort. TD. the minimum level of intensity that will produce a sensation of discomfort. Considered to be about 120 dB or less.

threshold, elevated. a poorer threshold of sensitivity. This is indicated by marks at higher numbers on the audiogram. *syn*: higher threshold.

threshold of feeling. the minimum intensity level at which sound pressure produces a sensation of feeling distinct from the sensation of hearing. It may also be described as discomfort.

threshold of hearing. the minimum level of intensity at which sound pressure will produce the sensation of hearing.

threshold, higher. a poorer threshold of sensitivity, i.e., one reflecting higher numbers on an audiogram; *syn*: elevated threshold.

threshold of intelligibility. obsolete term for speech reception threshold—the intensity level at which 50% of the words presented can be repeated.

threshold, lowered. a better threshold of sensitivity, i.e., one reflecting lower numbers on an audiogram.

threshold, masked. the point at which a listener can first determine that a sound is audible in the presence of another or masking sound.

threshold of pain, tickle, or discomfort. the minimum level of intensity at which sound pressure will produce the sensation of pain, tickle, or discomfort.

threshold of perceptibility. a seldom-used term for the level of intensity at which sounds begin to be perceived as words. It is between the threshold of detectability and the threshold of intelligibility.

threshold, pure tone. level of intensity at which a pure tone is just recognizable during 50% of the presentations.

threshold, raised. an indication of lessened hearing sensitivity—the intensity of sound must be raised to be heard.

threshold of sensitivity. the faintest sound that can be heard at 50% of presentations. Formerly referred to as threshold of acuity.

threshold shift. a change in hearing sensitivity such as may be caused by exposure to noise. It may be either temporary (TTS) or permanent (PTS).

threshold shift, permanent. PTS. an irreversible loss of hearing sensitivity. The term usually relates to noise-induced hearing loss.

threshold shift, poststimulatory. the phenomenon by which a sound continues to be masked (not heard) for a brief period after the masking noise is discontinued. *syn:* forward or residual masking.

threshold shift, temporary. TTS. a reversible elevation in the threshold of hearing that may result from continuous exposure to sound. It is expressed in dB per frequency and related to exposure time. *syn:* auditory fatigue.

threshold, speech. more commonly known as speech reception threshold (SRT), it is the level at which spondaic words can be recognized 50% of the time.

threshold, terminal. · the lowest intensity of sound pressure that, when increased, will cause no further increase in the sensation of loudness; *syn:* terminal limen; tolerance limit.

threshold tone decay test. TTD. a test to determine if the subject can continue to hear a pure tone presented for one minute at his threshold of sensitivity.

throm-, thrombo- (throm). prefix indicating clotting of blood.

thrombase or **thrombin** (throm'bās, -bin) *n.* an enzyme that promotes blood clotting.

thrombocyte (throm'bo-sīt) *n.* a tiny disc-like blood component. A platelet. *adj:* **thrombocytic.**

thrombocytopenic purpura (throm"bo-si"to-pe'nik pur'pu-rah). a disorder characterized by bleeding into the skin and from mucous membranes. A defect in blood-forming organs causes a blood platelet deficiency. It is a suspected cause of sensorineural hearing loss—either gradual or sudden.

thromboembolism (throm"bo-em'bo-lizm) *n.* the blocking of a blood vessel caused by a blood clot that has broken away from another clot.

thrombosis (throm-bo'sis) *n.* a blood clot. When it occurs in an internal auditory artery it may cause sudden deafness. *adj:* **thrombotic.**

thrombus (throm'bus) *pl.* **thrombi** *n.* a blood clot that has not moved from where it was formed within a blood vessel. (An embolus circulates.)

thyroid stimulating hormone. TSH.

tile, acoustic. tile made of material designed to absorb sound waves.

timbre (tim'ber) *n.* characteristic tonal quality resulting from overtones of the fundamental.

TIN. tone in noise.

tin ear. slang for tone deafness—the inability to recognize musical tones or pitch differences.

tinnitus (tī-ni'tus) *n.* noises seeming to originate within the ear itself; *syn:* susurrus aurium, tinnitus cerebri, tinnitus aurium. (See tinnitus-related terms in Appendix X, Page 180.)

tinnitus, arterial or venous. head noises believed to result from blood-flow disturbances within the external or middle ear. A type of objective tinnitus.

tinnitus aurium (aw're-um). noise within the ear that may be localized to one or both ears and can be subjectively described. It may also be called either subjective or objective tinnitus; *syn:* tympanophonia.

tinnitus cerebri. a subjective sensation of sound in the head that is not localized to either or both ears. *syn:* tinnitus cranii.

tinnitus, clicking. a common name for Leudet's spasmodic head noises; *syn:* objective tinnitus.

tinnitus cranii. a subjective sensation of sound in the head that is not localized to either or both ears. *syn:* tinnitus cerebri.

tinnitus, hangover. as the name suggests, tinnitus that results from the intake of too much alcohol.

tinnitus instrument. a device that combines a hearing aid and tinnitus masker in one unit.

tinnitus, intractable. tinnitus that is resistant to any type of relief or treatment.

tinnitus, Leudet's. spasmodic clicking head noises arising from muscular spasms near the eustachian tube. *syn:* objective or clicking tinnitus.

tinnitus masker. an amplifying instrument shaped like a hearing aid but engineered to generate a band of white noise designed to mask out the individual's tinnitus.

tinnitus, nonvibratory. another term for subjective tinnitus—head noises that can be heard only by the patient.

tinnitus, objective. head noises arising from muscular spasms or blood-flow disturbances within the external or middle ear. Rare in occurrence, they may be audible to the examiner; *syn:* clicking tinnitus; Leudet's tinnitus.

tinnitus research audiometer. TRA. a term sometimes applied to an instrument designed to determine the pitch and intensity of the individual's tinnitus.

tinnitus, subjective. head noises that can be heard only by the patient; *syn:* nonvibratory tinnitus.

tinnitus, subjective idiopathic. a term referring to the consideration of subjective tinnitus as resulting from an unknown disease or cause.

tinnitus, vibrating or vibratory. better known as objective tinnitus, these noises can be heard by the examiner.

titer (ti'ter) *n.* standard of measurement of strength of a serum or vaccine.

TL. tolerance level.

TLC. tender loving care.

TMJ. temporomandibular joint.

toby-tester. an instrument designed by A. W. Henry, utilizing battery-powered toys as motivators in testing the hearing of young or retarded children.

toddler audiometry. a variation of behavioral audiometry reserved for younger children. It is dependent upon observation of the children's reaction (other than the infant startle response) to stimuli presented in sound field. A method devised by Anne Harrison.

tolerance level. TL. another term for threshold of discomfort (TD) or uncomfortable level.

tolerance limit. the lowest intensity of sound pressure that, when increased, will cause no further increase in the sensation of loudness. syn: terminal limen; terminal threshold.

tomogram (to'mo-gram) n. an x-ray picture taken of a particular layer of tissue by means of tomography.

tomography (to-mog'rah-fe) n. a method of x-ray photography that provides focus on a particular layer of tissue. syn: polytomography; planigraphy.

-tomy (to-me'). suffix indicating a surgical operation that either cuts into or severs a body part.

tonal gap (to'nal). a narrow band of frequencies that cannot be heard as well as the frequency bands on either side.

tonality n. the sensation that tones that are an octave apart sound more alike than tones separated by irregular intervals.

tonal island. a narrow band of frequencies that can be heard better than the frequency band on either side.

tonal spectrum (to'nal spek'trum). image of a complex tone displaying all its frequencies and intensities as seen on an oscilloscope.

tone (tōn) n. a sound that gives a definite sensation of pitch, loudness, and timbre. It may be either a pure or complex tone.

tone, combination or combined. the distinctive sound heard when two tones are presented at the same time. It may be heard differently in either intensity or pitch. syn: summation tone.

tone, complex. a sound wave made up of several combined pure tones.

tone control. a device designed to allow the user to alter the response of an amplifier by limiting the intensity of a portion of the frequency range.

tone deafness. inability to recognize musical tones or pitch differences. In extreme cases it is known as amusia.

tone decay. also known as fast adaptation, fast auditory fatigue, perstimulatory fatigue, or the Albrecht effect. This phenomenon is evidenced by the inability of an impaired ear to hear a continuous tone for a period of one minute until presented at higher levels on intensity.

tone decay test. the presentation of a continuous tone at successively higher (5 dB) levels of intensity to an impaired ear until the tone can be heard for one minute.

tone-decay test, modified. MTDT. a pure tone is presented 5 dB above the threshold level. If and when the tone disappears, the intensity is increased 5 dB. The number of times this increase must be repeated (the shift) in one minute is noted as an index of the degree of tone-decay at that frequency.

tone, delayed side. also known as delayed auditory feedback (DAF), a system by which the speaker's own words are returned (fedback) through earphones after a time delay of a few milliseconds. A test of malingering.

tone, difference. the distinctive sound heard as a pitch that represents the difference between the frequencies of two generating tones.

tone, fundamental. the lowest and loudest frequency of a complex tone; syn: fundamental frequency.

tone height. another term for pitch (as related to high or low frequency).

tone in noise. TIN. the measurement of the ability to recognize a tone in the presence of noise—a type of masking test.

tone-interrupter, pulse-tone technique. use of the tone interrupter to present pulsed tones through the audiometer.

tone, partial. a wave of a complex tone: the fundamental or each of its overtones.

tone, pure. a tone or note that has only one frequency with no harmonics or overtones; syn: sinusoidal wave; sine wave.

tone, simple. 1. one cycle of a pure tone. 2. the sound sensation of a single pitch.

tone, summation. the tone heard as the combination of the frequencies of two originating tones; syn: combination or combining tone.

tone, warble. a tone that results from rapid modulations of frequency within fixed limits around the basic pure tone frequency.

tonic accent. stress given a syllable or word by virtue of a change of the tone used in speaking.

tonometer (to-nom'ĕ-ter) n. an instrument used to measure the frequency of tones; adj: **tonometric.**

tonoscope (ton'o-skōp) n. device used to examine the interior of the skull and brain by means of the reflection of sound waves.

tonotopic (ton"o-top'ik) adj. the relationship of frequency to place along the organ of Corti.

tonsil, pharyngeal (ton'sil far-in-je-al). adenoid. Lymphoid tissue growing around the nasopharyngeal opening of the eustachian tube.

tonsillectomy (ton″sĭ-lek′to-me) *n.* surgical removal of tonsils.

topophone (top″o-fon′) *n.* a device consisting of two ear trumpets designed to assist in localizing sound.

TORP. total ossicular replacement prosthesis.

tortion swing test. a test of the effects of neck motion of the balance mechanism.

torus (to′rus) *n.* the bulge at the base of the eustachian tube.

torus tubarius (to′rus too-bah′re-us). a ridge of cartilage above and behind the pharyngeal opening of the eustachian tube; *syn:* eustachian cushion.

total communication. a new name for the simultaneous method, utilizing signs, finger spelling, electronic amplification (usually hearing aids), speech, and speech-reading in teaching the deaf. Facial expressions, gestures, and body English are also considered important.

total deafness. the extremely rare case in which there can be no sensation of sound because of damage to (or absence of) some portion of the hearing mechanism. Medically, it may be referred to as anacousis, anacusis, anakusis, orancusis, or orankusis.

total ossicular replacement prosthesis. TORP. An artificial strut placed between the eardrum and the oval window.

toxemia (tok-se′me-ah) *n.* disease caused by poisons in the blood. *adj:* toxemic.

toxic- or toxico- (tok-sik, ko). prefix referring to poison.

toxic *adj.* pertaining to a condition caused by a poison. *n:* toxicity.

toxic deafness. hearing loss resulting from the poisonous and damaging (toxic) effect of drugs such as kanamycin or quinine on the sensory mechanism. (See listing of toxic substances in Appendix XIII, Page 187)

toxicosis (tok″sĭ-ko′sis) *n.* a diseased condition caused by poison.

toxin (tok′sin) *n.* a poisonous substance produced by a living organism.

toxoplasmosis (tok″so-plaz-mo′sis) *n.* disease caused by microorganisms that may seriously damage the central nervous system, especially in infants.

Toynbee's Law (Joseph Toynbee, English physician, 1815-1866). when brain disease is due to otitis media, the cerebrum is involved in cases of inflammation of the tympanic attic, and the cerebellum and lateral sinus are involved in cases of mastoiditis.

Toynbee's maneuver. swallowing with the mouth and nose closed to draw air out of the middle ear. *syn:* valsalvation.

Toynbee tube. a tube designed for the examiner to listen to sounds within the patient's ear; e.g., in objective tinnitus. *syn:* Toynbee's otoscope.

TP. threshold pain.

TRA. tinnitus research audiometer.

tracings, continuous. C tracings. The graph that results when a continuous tone stimulus is used in automatic audiometry.

tracings, interrupted. I tracings. the tracings that result when pulsed tones are used in automatic audiometry.

tragal (tra′gal) *adj.* referring to the tragus.

tragi (tra′ji). 1. plural of tragus. 2. the hairs in the external auditory canal.

tragicus (tra′ji-kus) *n.* a vestigial vertical muscle on the outer surface of the tragus.

tragi lamina. the cartilage that shapes the tragus.

tragion (traj′e-on) *n.* a point in the anterior notch above the tragus used as an identification point in measurements.

tragus (tra′gus) *pl.* tragi *n.* 1. small stiff ridge in front of the external opening of the ear canal. Infrequently referred to as antilobium. 2. one of the hairs in the external auditory canal. *adj:* **tragal.**

trans- prefix meaning through, across, or beyond.

transcutaneous (trans″ku-ta′ne-us) *n.* through unbroken skin—as transcutaneous electroacupuncture; *syn:* percutaneous.

transdental (trans-den′tal) *adj.* pertaining to a method of amplification applied through the teeth.

transdermal (trans-der′mal) *adj.* pertaining to a method of stimulation through the skin.

transducer (trans-du′ser) *n.* a device designed to convert power from one system to another.

transducer, electroacoustic. a device designed to change electrical energy into acoustical energy and vice versa, e.g., hearing aid receivers and microphones.

transducer, electromechanical. a device designed to change electrical energy into mechanical energy and vice versa; e.g., a hearing aid bone oscillator.

transformer (trans-for′mer) *n.* an electronic device used to vary the voltage of an electric current between stages of a circuit.

transient (trans′e-ent) *n.* an acoustic signal that disappears rapidly.

transient distortion. inexact reproduction of a sound wave pattern resulting from sudden changes of voltage or load.

transient hearing loss. a temporary loss of hearing sensitivity usually considered more severe than a temporary threshold shift.

transilluminate (trans″ĭ-lu′mi-nāt) *v.* to shine a light through body tissues.

transistor (trans-is′tor) *n.* an electronic device that amplifies electric current by utilizing the semiconducting properties of an element such as germanium or silicon.

transistor, field-effect. FET. a semiconductor current path whose conductance is controlled by reverse-biasing a PN junction (positive-negative) to create an electric field perpendicular to the current.

transistor hearing aid. one designed to use transistors in its amplifying circuit.

transistorize *v.* to replace vacuum tubes with transistors.

transition region. the portion of a distribution curve where the performance measure along the response dimension changes from that obtainable by chance to a nearly maximum value.

transitional sounds. scarcely audible sounds that are made as the vocal cords change position from one speech sound to another.

translabyrinthine (trans"lab-ĭ-rin'thin) *adj.* through the inner ear.

translator (trans-la'ter) *n.* a hearing amplifier devised by Charles I. Berlin, PhD, to change low frequencies into ultrahigh frequencies (18,000 to 20,000 Hz) to benefit persons who can utilize those frequencies. See: transposer.

translator, frequency. a hearing aid designed to change the energy of low frequency phonemes into ultrahigh frequencies (18,000 to 20,000 Hz). It will also amplify those same frequencies when they occur naturally.

transmeatal tympanoplasty (trans-me-a'tal tim"pah-no-plas'te). surgical repair of the eardrum through the external ear canal.

transmission loss. the amount of energy lost as a sound is carried through walls or air passages.

transmission unit. early term for the bel.

transmitter (trans-mit'er) *n.* a device that sends out a signal by means of electronic or radio waves.

transonance (tran'so-nans) *n.* transmission of sounds arising in one body part through another, e.g., heart sounds through the lungs and chest wall.

transonic or **trans-sonic** (tran-sah'nik) *adj.* speed that nears the speed of sound—between subsonic and supersonic.

transplant, homograft (trans'plant ho'mo-graft"). a replacement of tissue or bones of the ear with natural tissue or bones.

transposer (trans-po'zer) *n.* a hearing aid designed to change high-frequency energy into low-frequency energy to benefit persons who have only a corner audiogram, those who hear only low frequencies. See: translator. *syn:* frequency transposer.

transudate (trans'u-dāt) *n.* fluid that may accumulate in the middle ear to cause serous otitis or mucous otitis.

transudates, otic. the fluids that pass through the mucous membrane lining the ear.

transudation (trans"u-da'shun) *n.* the act of passing through a membrane.

transude (trans-ūd) *v.* to pass through a membrane (e.g., capillary wall) as a fluid.

transverse (trans-vers') *adj.* crossing over or crosswise.

trapezoid body (trap'e-zoid). a group of nerve fibers that carry impulses to the contralateral (opposite) superior olivary complex.

trauma (traw'mah) *n.* 1. an injury to living tissue. 2. a mental disorder arising from emotional stress or physical injury.

trauma, acoustic. loss of hearing sensitivity as a result of relatively short exposure to noise—usually explosive.

trauma, auditory. injury to the ear or hearing.

trauma, iatrogenic (i-at"ro-jen'ik). damage unexpectedly occurring during the course of treatment.

trauma, mechanical. damage to the hearing mechanism as the result of a blow to the head—e.g., causing a break in the ossicular chain.

traumatism *n.* malformation or disorder resulting from injury.

traumatize *v.* to injure.

traveling-wave theory. movement of the footplate of the stapes causes a fluid wave to move along the basilar membrane with the rise and fall of amplitude. The point where the wave reaches its maximum amplitude is the point where the frequency of the sound is detected. Frequencies are highest toward the oval window and lowest toward the apex of the cochlea. Georg von Bekesy received the Nobel Prize in 1961 for his discovery of the traveling wave phenomenon that resulted in his theory.

Treacher-Collins syndrome. (Edward Treacher-Collins, English physician, 1862-1919). a complex of symptoms including incomplete development of the lower jaw and cheek bones accompanied by low-set ears and misshaped lower eyelids.

tremolo (tre'mo-lo) *n.* a vibrating or trembling sound.

triad, Bezold's. diminished perception of the low tones, better bone conduction, and negative Rinne—indicating otosclerosis.

triad, Hutchinson's. VIIIth nerve deafness, notched teeth, and chronic corneal inflammation. A syndrome associated with hereditary or prenatal syphilis.

triangle, suprameatal. a triangular indentation above and in back of the bony portion of the external ear canal. It is one of the landmarks in a mastoid operation. *syn:* Macewen's triangle.

triangular nucleus. the chief nucleus of the vestibular portion of the VIIIth cranial nerve. It is located in the pons—lower rear portion of the brain. *syn*: medial nucleus, Schwalbe's nucleus, Deiter's nucleus, nuclei vestibularis.

trichothecium roseum (trik″o-the′se-um). a species of mold sometimes found in cases of inflammation of the eardrum (mycomyringitis).

trigeminal nerve (tri-jem′in-al). the Vth cranial nerve that serves part of the head, jaws, and eyes. A branch connects with the tensor tympani.

trimester (tri-mes′ter) *n.* a period of three months. *adj*: **trimestral, trimestrial.**

triplacusis (tri″pla-ku′sis) *n.* the sensation of hearing a third pitch at the same time that different pure tones are presented simultaneously to each ear.

trisomy D₁ or **trisomy 13-15 syndrome** (tri′some). variable malformation of infants resulting from irregularities in chromosomes of group D, number 13, 14, or 15. Malformed ears appear as one of the signs in all cases. *syn*: D₁ or D₁ trisomy syndrome.

TROCA. tangible reinforcement operant conditioning audiometry. A type of behavioral audiometry that utilizes a signal light and a dispenser of treats such as jelly beans or mints.

trocar (tro′kar) *n.* an instrument designed to withdraw fluid from a cavity or to make an opening to allow insertion of a tube, e.g., through the eardrum.

Troltsch's pockets or **pouches** (Anton F. von Troltsch, German physician, 1829-1890). narrow slits in the wall of the tympanum forward (anterior) and behind (posterior) the handle of the malleus. More commonly

referred to respectively as the anterior and posterior tympanic recesses.

trough-shaped audiogram. denotes less hearing loss at the high and low frequencies than in the middle range.

trumpet, ear. a device with a large opening at one end designed to gather sound waves and direct them through a smaller opening into the outer ear canal.

TSD. theory of signal detectability.

TSH. thyroid stimulating hormone.

tsutsugamushi disease (soot″soo-gah-moosh′e). a disease resembling typhoid fever caused by a rickettsia transmitted by a laval mite. Tinnitus sometimes accompanies other symptoms.

TTD. threshold tone decay test.

TTS. temporary threshold shift.

TTS, exposure-equivalent rule. if a temporary threshold shift (TTS) already exists from one type of noise exposure, this time can be added to the time of exposure to the new noise.

TTY. teletypewriter.

TU. 1. transmission units. 2. terminal unit. (Part of a TDD—telecommunications device for the deaf). 3. toxic unit.

TU cradle. terminal unit cradle. The part of the acoustic coupling of the telecommunications device for the deaf in which the telephone handset rests.

tuba auditiva (too′bah aw″di-te′ vah). more commonly known as eustachian tube, and sometimes as auditory tube or pharyngotympanic tube.

tubal incompetency or **insufficiency.** lack of patency (ability to open) of the eustachian tube.

Table 6. NAEL Standardized Tube Size

Size	ID Decimal Inches	ID Millimeters	OD Decimal Inches	OD Millimeters
#9	.118	3	.158	4
#12	.085	2.15	.125	3.2
#13 (Standard)	.076	1.95	.116	2.9
#13 (Medium)	.076	1.95	.122	3.1
#13 (Heavy Wall)	.076	1.95	.130	3.3
#13 (Super Heavy Wall)	.076	1.95	.142	3.6
#14	.066	1.7	.116	2.9
#15	.059	1.5	.116	2.9
#15 (Heavy Wall)	.059	1.5	.140	3.6
#16	.054	1.35	.116	2.9

Another set of tubing sizes especially recommended for use in tube fittings of hearing aids is as follows:

Size	ID	OD
#11	.090	.160
#13	.074	.130
#15	.078	.130
#16	.044	.110

tube, auscultation. a tube designed for listening to sounds within the patient's ear.

tube, ventilating indwelling. a plastic tube inserted in the eardrum to provide pressure equalization in the middle ear when the eustachian tube is closed.

tubercle, bacillus. the microorganism that causes tuberculosis.

tubercle, Darwinian. a small projection from the upper part of the helix. It may appear simply as a thickening of the cartilage.

tubing. sizes for earmold tubing as standardized by the National Association of Earmold Laboratories, February, 1932 are given in Table 6, page 152.

tubotympanal (too″bo-tim-pah′nal) *adj.* concerning the eustachian tube and the eardrum.

tubotympanic canal. an embryonic stage in the development of the eustachian tube and tympanic cavity.

tubotympanitis (too″bo-tim″pah-ni′tis) *n.* inflammation involving both the middle ear and the eustachian tube.

Tulio effect (too′le-o). severe vertigo resulting from moderately high noise levels that affects people whose ears have been altered by disease or surgery so there is a direct pathway for sound pressure waves to the membranous labyrinth.

tumor (too′mor) *n.* an abnormal growth of tissue.

tumor, acoustic. a growth (either benign or malignant) on the sheath of the auditory (VIIIth) nerve; *syn:* acoustic neuroma.

tumor, glomus jugular. a painful tumor that may occur in the middle ear. It tends to be more painful with each pulsation of blood and may be involved in objective tinnitus.

tumor, vascular. a tumor involving blood vessels; *syn:* angioma.

tuning fork. a two-pronged metal fork that, when struck, vibrates in a fixed frequency to produce a pure tone. It may have an adjustable sliding bar to vary the frequency.

tuning fork test. a test of hearing sensitivity that utilizes a tuning fork. The bone oscillator of the pure tone audiometer can be substituted effectively.

tunnel cells. cells that line the inner tunnel of Corti. *syn:* pillar cells; rods of Corti.

tunnel, Corti. Corti's canal; a spiral canal within the organ of Corti between the outer and inner hair cells. Triangular in shape, it is bounded by the outer and inner pillar cells and is filled with endolymphatic fluid.

turgescent (tur-jes′ent) *adj.* swollen or beginning to swell.

tweeter *n.* a small loudspeaker that reproduces high-pitched sounds.

two-frequency test. a screening test of hearing sensitivity based on the use of 4000 Hz and one other frequency (usually 500 Hz, but sometimes 2000 Hz).

two-room testing. a method of determining response to sound stimuli. The subject is in a sound-treated room while the examiner observes reactions through a window as signals are introduced through headphones or loudspeakers.

TWX. teletypewriter.

tympanal (tim′pah-nal) *adj.* concerning the middle ear cavity; *syn:* tympanic, tympanitic.

tympanectomy (tim″pah-nek′to-me) *n.* surgical removal of the eardrum.

tympanic (tim-pan′ik) *adj.* concerning the middle ear cavity; *syn:* tympanal, tympanitic.

tympanic antrum. space in the temporal bone posterior to the tympanic cavity; *syn:* mastoid antrum.

tympanic attic. the space in the middle ear above the ossicles. *syn:* cupola space.

tympanic bone. the bone that encloses part of the middle ear and supports the eardrum.

tympanic bulla. bony cavity that encloses most of the middle ear cavity in some mammals. In the canoids it is undivided, while in the feloids it has a bony divider to form two cavities.

tympanic canal (canaliculus tympanicus). a bony tube containing Jacobson's (the tympanic) nerve. It runs from the tympanum to the lower surface of the petrous portion of the temporal bone.

tympanic cavity. middle ear cavity in the temporal bone. Its capacity is usually less than 2 cm³. Dimensions are: vertically about ½ inch (1.25 cm); diagonally about ⅓ inch (8 or 9 mm); narrowest point about 1/8 inch (2 mm).

tympanic cells. small groove-like depressions in the walls of the middle ear that connect with small cavities in the lower wall of the eustachian tube.

tympanic cord, tympanichord, or chordi tympani. a branch of the facial nerve that passes through the upper part of the middle ear. It conveys taste sensations and during middle ear operations it may be temporarily affected in such a way that food tastes unnatural.

tympanic fundus. the base or floor of the tympanic cavity.

tympanic gallery. the lower tube of the cochlea. The scala tympani or tympanic scala.

tympanic ganglion. the collection of nerve cells that separate from the glossopharyngeal nerve in the tympanic cavity.

tympanic groove. a shallow trench in the bottom of the inner bony portion of the outer ear canal into which the thickened ring (annulus) of the eardrum fits. *syn:* sulcus tympanicus.

tympanic membrane. the eardrum. Also called drum membrane and drumhead. It stretches across the inner end of the external ear canal and forms the outer boundary of the middle ear. It reacts to sound waves and starts the ossicular chain moving. It is about ⅓ inch (7 or 8 mm) in diameter.

tympanic membrane recess. tiny pocket in the wall of the tympanum, either forward (anterior) or behind (posterior) the handle of the malleus.

tympanic nerve. an afferent nerve that serves the eardrum and the middle ear. *syn*: Jacobson's nerve.

tympanic plexus. the network of nerves that serve the eardrum, eustachian tube, middle ear, and mastoid.

tympanic promontory. more commonly known simply as the promontory; a bony structure that protrudes into the middle ear cavity between the oval and round windows. It is formed by the first turn of the cochlea.

tympanic ring. 1. the tough fibrous ring that holds the eardrum in place. 2. an embryonic bony structure that develops into the tympanic plate of the temporal bone.

tympanic scala. the lower tube of the cochlea. More commonly known as the scala tympani.

tympanic sulcus. the tympanic groove into which the eardrum fits.

tympanicus, annulus or anulus*. the tympanic ring, a tough fibrous ring holding the eardrum in place. (*Nomina Anatomica (1960 revision) dropped one n, although it is not commonly used that way at present.)

tympanitis (tim″pah-ni′tis) *n*. 1. inflammation of the middle ear—otitis media. 2. inflammation of the eardrum—myringitis.

tympano- prefix referring to the eardrum or the middle ear.

tympanoeustachian (tim″pah-no-u-sta′ke-an) *adj*. concerning the tympanum and the eustachian tube.

tympanogram (tim-pan′o-gram″) *n*. a chart of the results of tympanometry—compliance measurements at the eardrum. The basic curves are described as:

A—peaks close to zero point.
A$_s$—(sub s)—shallower than normal.
A$_d$—(sub d)—deeper than normal.
A$_{dd}$—(sub dd)—doubly deep.
W—more commonly used term for doubly deep.
B—no peak.
C—negative peak.

tympanographic (tim″pah-no-graf′ik) *adj*. pertaining to charted results of eardrum measurements.

tympanomalleal (tim″pah-no-mal′e-al) *adj*. concerning the eardrum and malleus relationship.

tympanomastoid (tim″pah-no-mas′toid) *adj*. pertaining to the middle ear and the mastoid process.

tympanomastoiditis (tim″pah-no-mas″toidi′tis) *n*. inflammation in the middle ear and mastoid cells.

tympano-meatal flap (tim″pah-no-me-a′tal). flap of skin of the deeper portion of the auditory canal used to create a new oval window in the course of one type of fenestration operation.

tympanometry (tim″pah-nom′ĕ-tre) *n*. the measurement of the ability of the eardrum and ossicular chain to transmit sound pressure waves. An intact eardrum is subjected to air pressure changes to determine its stiffness (impedance) and compliance (admittance). The results may be charted on a tympanogram.

tympanophonia (tim″pah-no-fo′ne-ah) *n*. 1. tinnitus—noises within the ear. 2. autophony—ability of a person to hear his own voice louder than normally when the eustachian tube is unusually open; *syn*: tympanophony.

tympanophony (tim″pan-ah′fon-e) *n*. tympanophonia.

tympanoplasty (tim″pah-no-plas′te) *n*. 1. reconstructive surgery of the middle ear. 2. an opening designed to raise the level of hearing sensitivity either by creating a new tympanic membrane or separating acoustically the oval and round windows by means of a skin graft.

tympanoplasty, postauricular. repair of the eardrum by an approach from behind the pinna.

tympanosclerosis (tim″pah-no-sklee-ro′sis) *n*. a degeneration of connective tissue involving the eardrum. It is characterized by white chalky plaques of calcification that appear on the drumhead. *adj*: **tympanosclerotic.**

tympanostapedial (tim″pah-no-stă-pe′de-al) *adj*. pertaining to the tympanum and the stapes.

tympanostapediopexy *n*. surgical closure of the eardrum and the head of the stapes.

tympanostomy (tim″pah-nos′tah-me) *n*. alternative spelling for tympanotomy—surgical opening of the eardrum.

tympanotemporal (tim″pah-no-tem′po-ral) *adj*. pertaining to the eardrum and temporal bone relationship.

tympanotomy (tim″pah-not′o-me) *n*. surgical opening of the eardrum; *syn*: myringotomy.

tympanum (tim′pah-num) *pl*. **tympana, tympanums,** *n*. the middle ear.

tyrosine (ti-ro′sin) *n*. a chemical substance that fails to be formed from phenylalanine in the metabolic disorder known as phenylketonuria.

U

UCL. uncomfortable loudness, or uncomfortable loudness level.
UCS. unconditioned stimulus.
UF. undistorted faint.
UL. undistorted loud; uncomfortably loud.
ULL. uncomfortable loudness level.
ultra- (ul'trah). prefix meaning beyond usual limits; extreme or excessive.
ultra-audiometric (ul"trah-aw"de-o-met'rik). term used by Charles I. Berlin, PhD, to refer to the testing of pure tone frequencies that are above the limits available in standard commerical audiometers.
ultrasonic (ul"trah-son'ik) *adj.* pertaining to frequencies above 20,000 Hz.
ultrasonic sound. sound pressure waves whose frequency is above the audible range. Sometimes called ultra-audible sound.
ultrasonics *n.* science dealing with the use of frequencies above the audible range for therapeutic or diagnostic purposes.
ultrasound. ultrasonic sound.
ultrastructure (ul'trah-struk"chur) *n.* the ultramicroscopic composition of the inner ear cells.
UM. unmasked.
umbo (um'bo) *n.* the "navel" or depressed point on the eardrum that marks the end of the hammer's handle (the manubrium of the malleus).
un- prefix meaning not, no, the reverse, contrary, or negative.
uncomfortable loudness or **uncomfortable loudness level.** UCL or ULL. the intensity level at which a tone or sound becomes uncomfortably loud.
uncomfortable loudness level. ULL or UCL.
unconditioned stimulus. UCS. the use of sound (usually a pure tone) as a stimulus without a preconditioning electrical shock in electrophysiological audiometry.
undermasking. insufficient intensity of masking to prevent the better ear from participating in tests.
understanding *n.* the real meaning of hearing: comprehension or recognition and recall of sound.
uni- (u'ne). prefix meaning one.
uni-CROS. a type of CROS amplification involving the use of a microphone and receiver to the poorer ear and crossover of the signal to a receiver and open canal fitting in the better ear.
unilateral (u"nĭ-lat'er-al) *adj.* pertaining to one side only.
unimodal (u"ni-mo'dal) *adj.* a method of teaching that concentrates on one sense modality. *syn:* unisensory.

unioval, uniovular (u"ne-o'val, u"ne-ov'u-lar). twins from one egg.
unisensory approach. a method of teaching hearing-handicapped children by concentrating on only one sense modality, e.g., auditory teaching alone—without visual clues.
United States Pharmacopeia. USP. official list of drugs, chemicals, and medicinal preparations.
unit, phon (u'nit fōn). the unit for measuring the loudness level of a sound in comparison with a 1000 Hz tone. The loudness level in phons is numerically equal to the SPL of the 1000 Hz tone, but varies with frequency.
unit, power. the unit for measuring power is the watt.
unmasked hearing. 1. a hearing test without the use of masking. 2. modification of hearing aid response, by the use of special receivers or changes in circuitry, to reproduce only the frequencies above 1000 Hz. The purpose is to limit the tendency of the lower-pitched vowel elements to mask out and suppress the higher-pitched consonants.
upper partial. one of the overtones of the fundamental. *syn:* upper harmonic.
upper respiratory infection. URI. diseases of the nose and throat. These often affect hearing adversely.
upward masking. the phenomenon by which higher frequency sounds are made inaudible by the presence of lower frequency noises.
uraniscoplasty (u"rah-nis'ko-plas"te) *n.* surgical repair of cleft palate. *syn:* palatoplasty, uranoplasty.
uranoplasty (u'rah-no-plas"te) *n.* surgical repair of cleft palate. *syn:* palatoplasty, uraniscoplasty.
Urbantschitsch whistle. a whistle devised by Victor Urbantschitsch of Austria to test hearing.
URI. upper respiratory infection.
USASI. USA Standards Institute; formerly ASA and now ANSI.
U-shaped curve audiogram. denotes less hearing loss at the low and high frequencies than in the middle range. *syn:* trough-shaped audiogram.
Usher's syndrome. a group of symptoms accompanying congenital deafness: degenerative eye disease (retinitis pigmentosa), balance problems, and ear canal abnormalities.
USP. United States Pharmacopeia.
USPHS. United States Public Health Service.
utricle, utriculus (u'tre-k'l, u-trik'u-lus) *n.* the larger of the two sacs that occupy a portion of the membranous labyrinth of the vestibule of the inner ear. (The smaller sac is the saccule).

utricular fossa. elliptical recess. A small cavity in the upper part of the vestibule in which the utricle is lodged.

utriculitis (u-trik″u-li′tis) *n.* 1. inflammation involving the utricle of the vestibule. 2. inflammation of the inner ear.

utriculosaccular (u-trik″u-lo-sak′u-lar) *adj.* involving both the utricle and the saccule.

utriculosaccular duct. a tiny tube connecting the utricle and saccule.

V

VA. Veteran's Administration.

vacuum tube. a glass-enclosed device designed to regulate the flow of electric current. Free electrons emitted by a cathode are attracted to an anode while the flow is controlled by a grid.

vacuum tube hearing aid. one designed to use vacuum tubes—now obsolete.

Valsalva's ligaments (Antonio M. Valsalva, Italian physician, 1666-1723). the auricular ligaments.

Valsalva's maneuver. blowing forcibly to open the eustachian tube by holding nose and closing mouth. Named for its originator, Antonio Valsalva. Sometimes called Valsalva's experiment.

valsalvation *n.* swallowing with the mouth and nose closed to draw air out of the middle ear. *syn:* Toynbee's maneuver.

valve *n.* British term for vacuum tube. Transistors were originally called cold valves by the British.

valve, thermionic. an older British term for vacuum tube.

vancomycin *n.* an ototoxic drug in the streptomycin family.

van der Hoeve-de Kleyn triad. a syndrome in which familial deafness, resembling otosclerosis, is accompanied by fragile bones and blue-tinted whites of the eyes.

variable venting valve. VVV. a movable device inserted in an earmold ventng hole used to regulate the size of the opening of the vent.

varicella (var″ĭ-sel′ah) *n.* chickenpox.

vari-gain compression. a type of output control that changes with the input.

VARO. Veteran's Administration Regional Office.

vas-, vasi-, vaso- prefix meaning channel, duct, or vessel.

VASC. verbal auditory screening for children.

vascular (vas′ku-lar) *adj.* concerning blood vessels.

vascular sclerosis. arteriosclerosis. Thickening of the arterial walls—said to contribute to presbycusis, the loss of hearing as part of the aging process.

vascular stria. network of capillaries that forms the outer wall of the inner tube of the cochlea.

vascular tumor. a tumor involving blood vessels. A possible cause of tinnitus. *syn:* angioma.

vasodilation (vas″o-di-la′shun) *n.* widening of the inside diameter of blood vessels—usually by a drug (vasodilator).

vasodilator (vas″o-di-lāt′or) *n.* a drug used to dilate blood vessels; e.g., niacin, sodium nicotinate.

vasomotor (vas-o-mo′-tor) *adj.* concerning the nerves and nerve centers that control the size of the blood vessels; dilation or constriction.

vasospasm (vas′o-spazm) *n.* an abnormal contraction of a blood vessel that may produce sudden deafness.

vector (vek′tor) *n.* a carrier of a disease (usually an insect) between infected and noninfected individuals.

velocity of light waves. about 186,000 miles per second.

velocity, particle. the speed of movement of an individual particle of the medium through which a sound wave is passing, compared to the movement of the medium as a whole. The unit of measurement is the centimeter per second (cps).

velocity of sound waves. about 1100 feet per second in air at sea level, about 5000 feet per second in salt water, and about 15,000 feet per second in steel.

venation (ve-na′shun) *n.* the arrangement of veins in an organ. *adj:* **venational.**

venous or arterial tinnitus. head noises believed to result from blood-flow disturbances within the external or middle ear. A type of objective tinnitus.

vent *v.* to drill a hole in an earmold to relieve pressure or alter the acoustic response.

vent sizes for earmolds. $1/32″$ =small; $1/16″$ =medium; $1/8″$ =large.

ventilating indwelling tube. a plastic tube inserted in the eardrum to provide pressure equalization in the middle ear when the eustachian tube is closed.

ventral (ven′tral) *adj.* pertaining to, or toward the front. *opp:* dorsal.

ventral cochlear nuclei. the forward collective termination of the cochlear nerve fibers in the brain stem.

verbal alexia. inability to learn to read (e.g., by the phonics approach) due to failure to recognize differences and similarities in voiced sounds. *syn*: auditory alexia.

verbotonal method. a system of teaching the deaf devised by Peter Guberina of Yugoslavia, based on making maximum utilization of the child's optimal frequency range of residual hearing.

vermis, cerebellar. a narrow lobe of the brain between the two hemispheres of the cerebellum.

vertex (ver'teks) *n.* top or summit. Top of the head.

vertex potential. V-potential. electroencephalic response as revealed by an electrode placed on top of the head.

vertigo (ver'tĭ-go) *n.* dizziness or a sensation of whirling or irregular motion that arises from problems within the vestibular portion of the inner ear. Objective vertigo is the name given the sensation that the world is spinning about the patient. Subjective vertigo indicates the patient feels he is moving in space. *adj*: **vertiginous.**

vertigo, auditory, aural, or labyrinthine. dizziness due to ear disease. Meniere's disease.

vesicle *n.* a blister or small sac containing fluid.

vesicle, auditory. embryonic cell body from which the ear develops. *syn*: otocyst.

vesicle, otic. the embryonic cell structure that becomes the inner ear.

vesicular (vĕ-sik'u-lar) *adj.* concerning small sacs or blisters.

vestibular apparatus. the portion of the inner ear concerned with the body's position in space.

vestibular aqueduct (ves-tib'u-lar). a portion of the bony endolymphatic canal through which the membranous tube containing endolymph passes.

vestibular canal. the scala vestibuli. A tube that extends from the oval window to the tip of the cochlea (helicotrema).

vestibular cecum. the lower end of the cochlear duct in the vestibule.

vestibular crest. a ridge on the wall of the vestibule of the labyrinth. It contains minute holes through which nerve fibers pass.

vestibular fissure. a narrow groove in the lower part of the first turn of the cochlea.

vestibular ganglion. a collection of nerve cells within the internal auditory canal from the semicircular canals. *syn*: Scarpa's ganglion.

vestibular labyrinth. portion of inner ear containing semicircular canals, the utricle, and saccule.

vestibular membrane. Reissner's membrane, which separates the scala vestibuli from the scala media.

vestibular nerve. the branch of the VIIIth cranial nerve that serves the utricle, saccule, and the semicircular canals.

vestibular neuronitis (ves-tib'u-lar nu"ro-ni'tis). inflammation of the vestibular nerve cells of the ear. Dizziness is associated with the disorder in which there is no accompanying hearing loss; a possible cause of tinnitus.

vestibular nucleus. the point in the brain stem where fibers of the vestibular nerve join together.

vestibular sense. the sense of balance.

vestibular stairway. scala vestibuli, vestibular canal.

vestibular window. resting place for the footplate of the stapes, the vestibular window allows the mechanical action of the ossicles to be transmitted into fluid waves in the perilymph of the cochlea beginning in the scala vestibuli. *syn*: fenestra ovalis, oval window.

vestibule *n.* portion of inner ear between cochlea and semicircular canals. It contains the saccule and the utricle.

vestibule, bony. cavity in the temporal bone that contains the vestibule of the inner ear.

vestibulocochlear nerve (ves-tib'u-lo-kok"le-ar). the VIIIth cranial nerve. *syn*: acoustic or auditory nerve.

vestibulometry (ves-tib"u-lom'ĕ-tre) *n.* a test of vestibular function.

vestibulostapedial joint. the point of articulation (movement) of the footplate of the stapes (or the bony baseplate) that rests in the oval window. The legs (crura of the stapes) are imbedded in the footplate to complete the stirrup. Basis stapedis.

vestibulotomy *n.* surgical cut into the vestibule of the inner ear.

VI. volume indicator (meter). More commonly known as VU meter.

vibrating or vibratory tinnitus. better known as objective tinnitus, these noises in the ear can be heard by the examiner.

vibration *n.* oscillation—moving back and forth between two points.

vibration, double. one cycle of a sound wave. The older term, double vibrations (dv) was replaced by cycles per second (cps), which has been in turn replaced by hertz (Hz).

vibration meter. device for the measurement of displacement, velocity, or acceleration of a vibrating body.

vibration, subsonic. frequencies below 16 cycles per second which are felt as vibrations, if intense enough.

vibrato. fairly fast beat or variations in pitch or loudness.

vibrator, bone conduction. a device for conveying mechanical vibration to the mastoid process (or other parts of the head) in a bone conduction test.

vibrator, ossicle. an instrument designed to free the stapes in the oval window in the stapes mobilization operation.

vibrometer *n.* a device that was supposed to treat deafness by massaging the eardrum with rapid vibration.

vibrotactile sense. the feeling of vibration. A difficult point to distinguish in bone conduction testing—especially at low frequencies with children who have profound hearing losses.

Vineland social maturity scale test. a test of behavioral development.

viral (vi'ral) *adj.* pertaining to a virus.

viral otitis. inflammation attributed to a virus infection.

virulence (vir'u-lens) *n.* the power of microorganisms to cause disease. *adj*: **virulent.**

virus infection (vi'rus). bodily injurious effects of invasion by nonfilterable microorganisms.

visemes (vīz'eems) *n.* speech sounds that look alike on the lips. *syn*: homophenous words.

visible speech. 1. a system of symbols indicating the position of the various speech organs used in producing vocal sounds. Visible speech was developed by Alexander Melville Bell (father of A.G. Bell) to assist in teaching the deaf child to speak. 2. an electronic device that varies light in intensity and frequency patterns of colors which make speech understandably visible to the deaf. 3. combined use of speech and finger spelling—as in the Rochester Method.

visual hearing. speechreading; old term for lipreading.

vocal index. an obsolete attempt to standardize whispered and voiced tests of hearing by setting up a distance ratio between the two.

vocalization *n.* vibration of vocal cords in the larynx. The production of voiced sounds—phonation.

vocal resonance. the sounds of the voice as heard through a stethoscope held to the chest.

vocoder. instrument devised in 1936 to transmit speech patterns either visually or tactually; e.g., the stimuli may be presented to the fingers through bone conduction transducers.

voice prints. a picture of the spectrum of a voice as revealed by a spectrograph.

voice-reflex test. a test for malingering in which the patient is asked to read aloud while wearing headphones. As he reads, continuous sound (usually white noise) is presented to the deafened ear or ears. Since the normally-hearing person unconsciously tries to talk above the background noise

level (the Lombard effect), the malingerer will usually react in the same way; i.e., raise his voice while reading aloud. *syn*: Lombard test, Lombard voice-reflex test.

voices, verbal. hearing of imaginary voices—auditory hallucinations. Less often known as phonemes.

Voit's nerve (Max Voit, German physician, b:1876). the branch of the auditory nerve that serves the saccule.

volley pitch perception theory. the theory that pitch is determined by the brain's interpretation of sequences (volleys) of electrical impulses carried by different groups of neurons within a nerve.

volley principle. the basic rationale for the volley theory of hearing and pitch perception.

volley theory of hearing. the belief that pitch discrimination in the lower frequencies is dependent upon nerve impulses firing in volleys, and in the higher frequencies upon the response to the stimulation of localized areas along the basilar membrane in the cochlea.

volt *n.* the unit of measurement of electromotive force. Named for Alessandro Volta, Italian physicist, 1745-1827.

voltage *n.* according to Ohm's law, voltage is defined as current times resistance.

voltage pulse. an electrical signal of limited duration that begins and ends abruptly. When sent through a transducer, a voltage pulse produces an acoustic pulse.

Voltolini's disease (Fridericus E. R. Voltolini, German physician, 1819-1899). a disease of the labyrinth, which in young children may lead to deaf-mutism.

volume *n.* used interchangeably for either intensity or loudness.

volume control. device to regulate the gain of an amplifier. In a hearing aid it is designed to allow the user to adjust the amount by which the input signal is amplified.

volume control, automatic. AVC. in hearing aids, a special circuit designed to prevent sounds from being amplified too much for the impaired ear.

volume indicator. more commonly known as a VU meter, less often a volume-level indicator.

volume-level indicator. a device used to monitor voice or music intensity levels. More commonly known as a VU meter.

volume, reference. the strength or intensity of a speech signal that will cause a VU meter to register zero.

volume unit. VU. a unit of measurement of the intensity of a complex wave in terms of decibels in relation to a reference volume.

von Meyenburg's disease. a type of blood disease that may result in deformity of the cartilages of the ear and nose.

von Recklinghausen's disease. a disease characterized by numerous tumors involving nerve endings. *syn*: neurofibromatosis.

vowels *n.* continuous sounds made by varying the laryngeal tones through alteration of the shape of the mouth and changing the placement of the tongue and palate. They are complex tones of lower frequency.

V-potential. the vertex potential—electroencephalic response as revealed by an electrode placed on the top of the head.

VRA. Vocational Rehabilitation Administration. Visual reinforcement audiometry.

VU. volume unit.

VU-meter. volume-level indicator. A device used to monitor voice or music intensity levels.

VVV. variable venting valve.

W

W-1, W-2 tests. thirty-six bisyllabic words with equal stress on each syllable used to determine the speech reception threshold. W-1 list was recorded at a constant level; the W-2 list was recorded with attenuation of 1 dB per word.

W-22 test. a phonetically balanced word list used as a test of discrimination.

Waardenburg syndrome. a combination of symptoms described by P.J. Waardenburg that may be associated with hereditary deafness: the appearance of a broad nasal bridge resulting from a fold of skin at the inner angle of the eyes, the irises of which may differ in color, and a streak of white hair in the middle of the forehead.

WAIS. Weschsler (or Wechsler) adult intelligence scale.

Walsh-Healey Act of 1969. Federal legislation, of which one provision was to limit noise-exposure in order to protect workers from a cumulative hearing handicap.

waltzing guinea pigs. animals that exhibit hereditary degeneration of the organ of Corti.

warble tone. a tone resulting from rapid modulations of frequency within fixed limits around the basic pure tone frequency.

waterfall curve audiogram. usually denotes nearly normal hearing in lower frequencies (sometimes as high as 2000 Hz) followed by a precipitous drop of 25 dB or more per octave.

"waterfall" hearing loss. "ski-slope" loss.

watch tick test. obsolete test of hearing based on the ability to hear the ticking of a watch.

watt *n.* (James Watt, Scottish engineer, 1736-1819). The watt = 1/746 horsepower. The absolute meter-kilogram-second unit of power equal to the work done at the rate of one absolute joule per second. Electrically, the rate of work represented by a current of one ampere under pressure of one volt and taken as the standard in the U.S.

wave *n.* a disturbance of the molecules of a medium in a regular pattern of compression and rarefaction.

wave, alpha. a basic brainwave pattern of about 10 peaks per second on an electroencephalogram (EEG).

wave, aperiodic (ah″pe-rī-od′ik). a wave form that does not repeat itself in a regular pattern. *syn*: nonperiodic wave.

wave or rhythm, beta. a brainwave pattern of more than 10 peaks per second on an electroencephalogram (EEG).

wave, complex. sound made up of several combined pure tones.

wave crests. peaks of compression of successive waves.

wave, deflected. a wave diverted from its straight path. *syn*: diffracted wave.

wave or rhythm, delta. a very slow brain wave pattern on an EEG during normal sleep. It is abnormal if subject is awake.

wave, electromagnetic. a wave produced by periodic variations of intensity of an electric charge, e.g., light waves, radio waves.

wave filter. a device that separates wave forms on the basis of their frequencies.

waveform *n.* a graph showing the pattern of intensity, amplitude, or pressure at any moment of time.

wave, incident. a sound pressure wave moving away from the source. The opposite of reflected wave.

wavelength *n.* the distance of a wave from peak to peak. One complete cycle.

wave pattern, complex. sound made up of a number of pure tones.

wave, periodic. a waveform that repeats regularly in a time period.

wave, reflected. a sound pressure wave moving toward the source. The opposite of an incident wave.

wave, sound. a change in the arrangement of molecules in a medium into successive patterns of compression and rarefaction.

wave, square. a succession of identical acoustical or electrical pulses that start and end instantaneously with equally spaced on and off periods.

waves, hertzian. electromagnetic or radio waves. They are similar to light waves, but longer.

waves, pressure. successions of compressions and rarefactions of the air caused by a vibrating body.

wave train. a sequence of cycles of sound pressure.

wave train, damped. a sequence of cycles of sound pressure in which the amplitude of the successive cycles is diminished progressively.

wax, ear. cerumen.

W-B. Wechsler-Bellevue intelligence test.

Weber-Fechner law. (Gustave T. Fechner, German physicist, 1801-1887). generalization in neuropsychology that states that the just noticeable difference (jnd) in sensation resulting from a stimulus varies (arithmetically) in proportion to the intensity of the stimulus (logarithmic increase) by multiplication.

Weber's test. (Ernst H. Weber, German physician, 1795-1878). a bone conduction test used mainly in cases of unilateral deafness. The bone oscillator (or tuning fork) is placed on the midline of the forehead to determine the ear in which the sound is heard. An ear conductively affected will hear the tone better than the normal ear. On the other hand, in cases of unilateral perceptive deafness, the sound will be referred to (heard in) the normal ear.

Wechsler-Bellevue test. W-B. a test of intelligence suitable for use with the deaf.

Wechsler intelligence scale for children. WISC. A test of intelligence adapted for use with deaf children.

Wechsler performance scale test. intelligence test that may be adapted for use with deaf adults.

wedge box. an anechoic chamber—lined with wedges of soft material to absorb sound reflections.

weighting (wāt'ing). 1. adding or subtracting frequencies or intensities to influence results of tests or measurements. 2. varying numbers or percentages to reflect relative importance.

weighting network. a system of modifying—weighting—the circuitry of a sound level meter to simulate the reduced sensitivity of the ear as evidenced by equal loudness contours. The A scale is attenuated in reverse of the 40 phon equal loudness contour. The B scale is attenuated in reverse of the 70 phon equal loudness countour. The C scale is flat, as is the equal loudness contour at 100 phons in the low frequencies.

Wernicke's area (Karl Wernicke, German physician, 1848-1905), a region in the temporal lobe of the cerebrum of the brain that is the center for understanding speech.

Wever-Bray effect (Ernest G. Wever, American psychologist, C. W. Bray, American physician). coclear microphonic: the electrical voltage produced by the hair cells of the cochlea. The electrical response follows the wave form of the acoustic stimulus in a manner similar to the action of a microphone.

whisper test. an obsolete and inadequate method of testing hearing.

Whisperlite. trade name for a visible speech device.

whistle, Galton's (Francis Galton, English scientist, 1822-1911). a tubular whistle, usually activated by a bulb, with a screwadjustable pitch, formerly used to test the frequency range of hearing.

white forelock. a white patch of hair over the forehead. One of the characteristic features of the Waardenburg syndrome. Another is defective hearing.

white noise. a sound that contains equal amounts of energy in all frequencies. syn: Gaussian noise

white noise masking. masking by means of a broad band of noise that contains equal amounts of energy at all frequencies.

wide band. a broad range of frequencies set off by filters.

wide-band noise. a sound containing a broad range of frequencies.

wide range audiometer. one designed to test, both by air and bone conduction, most of the auditory range in regard to both frequency and sound pressure level.

Willis' paracusis. (Thomas Willis, English physician, 1621-1675). apparent ability to hear (understand) better in noisy surroundings.

window, acoustic. the range of frequencies necessary to make a particular speech sound intelligible.

window, cochlear. the round window.

window, oval. resting place for the footplate of the stapes, the oval window allows the mechanical action of the ossicles to be translated into fluid waves in the perilymph of the cochlea beginning in the scala vestibuli. syn: fenestra ovalis, fenestra vestibuli.

window, round. covered by flexible membrane, this opening in the bony casing of the cochlea allows movement of the perilymph in the scala tympani to compensate for movement caused by the stapes at the oval window. syn: cochlear window; fenestra cochleae; fenestra rotunda.

window, vestibular. resting place for the footplate of the stapes, the vestibular window allows the mechanical action of the ossicles to be transmitted into fluid waves in the perilymph of the cochlea beginning in the scala vestibuli. *syn*: fenestra ovalis, oval window.

Wing's symbols. numbers and letters coded by George Wing of the Minnesota School for the Deaf in 1883 to indicate parts of speech.

WINL. within normal limits.

WIPI. word intelligibility by picture identification.

WISC-R. Wechsler intelligence scale for children—revised.

word deafness. inability to understand the spoken word although the sound is heard. *syn*: auditory aphasia, aphemesthesia.

words, homophenous (ho-mah'fĭ-nus). words that look alike on the lips.

words, homophonous (ho-mo-fo'-nus). words that sound alike but are spelled differently; e.g., know, no.

word intelligibility by picture identification. WIPI. a test utilizing pictures to obtain discrimination scores when working with young hearing-impaired children who have limited vocabularies. The test was devised by Mark Ross, PhD and Jay Lerman, PhD.

X·Y·Z

x-ray. 1. radiation of an extremely short wave length. 2. picture made with x-rays.

xanthomatosis (zan"tho-mah-to'sis) *n.* a metabolic disorder marked by deposits of yellow or orange nodules in the skin. It is sometimes associated with tinnitus.

Y-cord. a hearing aid cord that divides the electrical impulse from one transmitter to two receivers. A modified form is known as a V-cord. *syn*: pseudobinaural.

zero, audiometric. see audiometric zero.

zona (zo'nah) *n.* 1. zone, belt, or girdle. 2. shingles. A communicable virus infection that may affect the spiral ganglion and cause sensorineural deafness. *syn*: herpes zoster.

zona arcuata (ark-u-a'tah). inner portion of the basilar membrane supporting the organ of Corti.

zona membranacea. basilar membrane. *syn*: membrana basilaris; lamina basilaris cochlea.

zona pectinata. outer portion of the basilar membrane.

zone of normal hearing. the range of thresholds for speech from 0 to 25 dB (ISO).

zoster. herpes zoster, zona.

zoster, auricularis. shingles that invades the ear.

zoster, herpes. shingles. A communicable virus infection that may affect the spiral ganglion and cause sensorineural deafness.

zosteriform (zos-ter'ĭ-form) *n.* having the appearance of herpes zoster. *syn*: zosteroid.

zosteroid *n.* zosteriform.

Zwislocki coupler. a device that incorporates four resonant acoustic chambers and a condenser microphone. It was designed by Jozef J. Zwislocki, Syracuse University, to replace the 2 cc coupler.

zygomatic arch (zi"go-mat'ik). a structure on each side of the cheek where the malar bone articulates with the zygomatic process of the temporal bone.

zygomaticoauricularis (zi"go-mat"ĭ-ko-aw"rik-u-la'ris). the muscle that pulls the pinna of the ear forward.

zygomaticum *n.* the cheek bone.

Appendix I

COMMON AND UNCOMMON ABBREVIATIONS

AA — auditory analysis
achievement age
Associate in Arts
AAOO — American Academy of Opthalmology and Otolaryngology (now separated into two academies)
AAO-HNS — American Academy of Otolaryngology-Head and Neck Surgery
AAPM — American Association of Physicists in Medicine
AAPT — American Association of Physics Teachers
AARP — American Association of Retired Persons
ABC — absolute bone conduction
ABESPA — American Boards of Examiners in Speech Pathology and Audiology
ABI — auditory behavior index
ABLB — alternate binaural loudness balance (test)
ABR — auditory brainstem response
AC — air conduction
ACLC — automatic curvilinear compression assessment of children's language comprehension
ACTH — adrenocorticotropic hormone
AD — auricula dexter or auris dextra (right ear)
ADA — Academy of Dispensing Audiologists
average daily attendance (school)
AF — audiofrequency
AGC — automatic gain control
AGE — adult growth examination
AHRF — American Hearing Research Foundation
AHS — American Hearing Society—now NAHSA
AI — articulation index
AIP — American Institute of Physics
AL — annoyance level
AM — amplitude modulation
AMA — American Medical Association
AMLB — alternate monaural loudness balance
AMR — acoustic muscle reflex
ANA — Acoustic Neuroma Association
ANS — autonomic nervous system
ANSI — American National Standards Institute—successor to United States of America Standards Institute
AOEHI — American Organization for the Education of the Hearing Impaired
AOR — auditory oculogyric reflex
AP — action potential
APA — American Psychological Association
APR — auropalpebral reflex
APS — American Physical Society

AQ — achievement quotient
accomplishment quotient
ART — acoustic reflex threshold
AS — auricula sinister or auris sinistra (left ear)
ASA — Acoustical Society of America
American Standards Association (now ANSI)
ASHA — American Speech and Hearing Association (now ASLHA)
ASL — American Sign Language
ASLHA — American Speech-Language-Hearing Association—successor to ASHA (it is still referred to as ASHA in common usage)
ASTM — American Society for Testing and Materials
ATA — American Tinnitus Association
AU — auris uterque (both ears)
AV — international hearing aid symbol for automatic volume control
AVC — automatic volume control
BAP — best audible pressure
BBA — best binaural average
BC — bone conduction
BE — behind ear (England)
BER — brainstem evoked response
BERA — brainstem evoked (or electric) response audiometry
BHI — Better Hearing Institute
BICROS — bilateral contralateral routing of signals
bilateral cros
BS — Bachelor of Science
BSER — brainstem electric (or evoked) audiometry
BTE — behind the ear
BTL — Bell Telephone Laboratories
CA — chronological age
CAT — computer averaged technique
computerized axial tomogram (CAT scan)
children's apperception test
CCC — Certificate of Clinical Competence
CCM — contralateral competing message
CCS — Crippled Children's Services
CEC — Council for Exceptional Children
CERA — cardiac evoked response audiometry
cortical evoked response audiometry
CGS or cgs — centimeter-gram-second
CHAA — certified hearing aid audiologist
CHABA — Committee on Hearing and Bio-Acoustics
CHAMPUS — Civilian Health and Medication Program of the Uniformed Services
CHE — Committee on Hearing and Equilibrium (of AAO-HNS)
CID — Central Institute for the Deaf
CLD — central language disorder

163

CLL — comfortable loudness level
CLR — comfortable loudness range
CM — cochlear microphonics
CMI — Cornell Medical Index
CNC — consonant-nucleus-consonant
CNE — could not establish
CNS — central nervous system
CNT — could not test
COHI — Consumers Organization for the Hearing Impaired, Inc.
COR — conditioned optical (or orientation) response
CORA — conditioned orientation reflex audiometry
COSD — Council of Organizations Serving the Deaf
COT — critical off time
CP — cerebral palsy
cleft palate
CPS, cps, or c/s — cycles per second
CR — conditioned response (or reflex)
conditional reflex
critical ratio
CROS — contralateral routing of signals
CS — conditioned stimulus
conditioning stimulus
CT — computerized tomogram
CV — cardiovascular
consonant-vowel
CVA — cerebral vascular accident
CVC — consonant-vowel-consonant
DAF — delayed auditory feedback
dB — decibel (replaces db)
dBA — decibels of sound pressure on A scale of sound pressure level meter
dBB— dB of sound presure on B scale
dBC— dB of sound pressure on C scale ("s" or "f" may be added to indicate slow or fast response circuit)
DBA — doing business as
DFA — delayed feedback audiometry
DL — difference limen
DLD — difference limen difference
DLF — difference limen for frequency
DLI — difference limen for intensity
DLST — difference loudness summation test
DNA — did not answer
deoxyribonucleic acid
DNR — did not respond
DNT — did not test
DR — dynamic range
District Representative
DRC — damage risk criteria
DRF — Deafness Research Foundation
DS — discrimination score
D-S — Doerfler-Stewart (test)
DSHL — decibel sum hearing levels (threshold)
dv — double vibrations: A term that preceded cycles per second (cps) and Hertz (Hz)
ECG — electrocardiogram (more commonly EKG)
ECR — electrocardiographic response
EDA — electrodermal audiometry

EDR — electrodermal response
EEA — electroencephalic audiometry
EEG — electroencephalography
electroencephalogram
EENT — eye, ear, nose, and throat
EER — electroencephalographic response
EKG — electrocardiogram
ELBA — ear level bilateral attachment
EMF, Emf, or emf — electromotive force
EMG — electromyograph
ENG — electronystagmography
ENT — ear, nose, throat
EP — evoked potential
EQ — educational quotient
ERA — evoked (or electric) response audiometry
ERI — Ear Research Institute (now House Ear Institute—HEI)
ESN — educationally subnormal
ESP — extrasensory perception
FACP — Fellow of the American College of Physicians
FACS — Fellow of the American College of Surgeons
FAST — filtered audiometric speech test
FCP — functional communication profile
FET — field effect transistor
FF — free field
FIT — fusion at inferred threshold
FM — frequency modulation
GSR — galvanic skin response—variant of PGSR
H — international hearing aid symbol for high frequency emphasis tone-control position
HAE — hearing aid evaluation
HAF — Hearing Aid Foundation
HAIC — Hearing Aid Industry Conference—now Hearing Industries Association—HIA
HCA — Hearing Conservation Associaton
HDN — hemolytic disease of the newborn (hyperbilirubinemia)
HEAR — hearing education through auditory research or rehabilitation
HEI — House Ear Institute—successor to Ear Research Institute
HEW — Health, Education, and Welfare
HIA — Hearing Industries Association—successor to HAIC
HL — hearing loss (re: audiometric zero)
HMO — health maintenance organization
HPI — hearing performance inventory
HSMHA — Health Services and Mental Health Administration
HTHA — Hearing and Tinnitus Help Association
HTL — hearing threshold level
HTP — house-tree-person test
Hz — Hertz (Hertzian Waves—electromagnetic cps)
I — international hearing aid symbol for on: "in operation," as opposed to "o", "out of operation"

IC — integrated circuit
ICM — ipsilateral competing message
ID — inside diameter
identification
IFROS — ipsilateral frontal routing of signals
IHC — inner hair cell
IL —ɹ intensity level
ILA — induction loop amplification
IMC — Instructional Materials Center (of Office of Education)
IOP — Institute of Physics
IPA — international phonetic alphabet
ips — inches per second
IQ — intelligence quotient
IRI — index of response irregularity
IROS — ipsilateral routing of signals
IRP — incus replacement prosthesis
ISO — International Standards Organization
ITA — initial teaching alphabet
ITE — in the ear
ITPA — Illinois Test of Psycholinguistic Abilities
jnd — just noticeable difference
kc — kilocycle
KEMAR — Knowles Electronic Manikin for Acoustic Research
L — international hearing aid symbol for low-frequency emphasis tone-control position
LAFO — Los Angeles Foundation of Otology—now HEI
LDC — logarithmic or linear dynamic compression
LDL — loudness discomfort level
LL — loudness level
LPFS — low-pass filtered signal
LSHSS — language, speech, and hearing services in schools
M — international hearing aid symbol for microphone input selector
MA — mental age
Master of Arts
MAC — minimum auditory capabilities battery
MAF — minimum audible field
MAO — maximum acoustic output
MAP — minimum audible pressure
MAPS — Make A Picture Story
MCL — most comfortable loudness
MCR — most comfortable range
MDP — maximum deliverable pressure
MEK — methyl ethyl ketone
MEM — minimum effective masking
MKS or mks — meter-kilogram-second
MLB — monaural loudness balance
MLV — monitored live voice
MMC — monday morning clubber
MML — minimum masking level
MMPI — Minnesota Multiphasic Personality Inventory
MPD — minimum perceptible difference
MPO — maximum power output

MR — mentally retarded
M-R — modified Rainville (test)
MRT — modified rhyme test
msec — millisecond
MTDT — modified tone decay test
MTP — maximum tolerable pressure
MUM — maximum usable masking
N — International hearing aid symbol for normal tone-control position
n — number (involved in test or report)
NAD — National Association of the Deaf
nothing abnormal detected
NAEL — National Association of Earmold Laboratories
NAHSA — National Association of Hearing and Speech Agencies
NAS — National Academy of Sciences
NASC — National Alliance of Senior Citizens
NBC — National Board for Certification (in Hearing Instrument Sciences)
NBN — narrow band noise
NBS — National Bureau of Standards
NCHCA — National Commission of Health Certifying Agencies
NCI — National Captioning Institute
NDT — noise detection threshold
NEL — noise exposure level (now PEL)
NHA — National Hearing Association
NHAS — National Hearing Aid Society (formerly SHAA)
NHS — National Health Service (UK)
NID — National Institute for the Deaf (UK)
NIH — National Institutes of Health
NIHL — noise-induced hearing loss
NIL — noise interference level
NIMH — National Institute of Mental Health
NINDB — National Institute for Neurological Diseases and Blindness
NIOSH — National Institute for Occupational Safety and Health
NP — neuropsychiatry, neuropsychiatric
NR — no response
NRA — National Rehabilitation Association
NRC — National Research Council
NRR — noise reduction rating
nsec — nanosecond
NSF — National Science Foundation
NTBB — National Temporal Bone Bank
NTID — National Technical Institute for the Deaf
O — international hearing aid symbol for off: "out of operation," as opposed to "I", "in operation"
OBA — octave band analyzer
OD — outside diameter
OEM — opposite ear masked
OHC — outer hair cell
OSHA — Occupational Safety and Health Administration
OUT — Organization for Use of the Telephone, Inc.

OVR — Office of Vocational Rehabilitation
PA — power amplifier
public address
PAL — Psycho-Acoustic Laboratory (Harvard University)
PAS — para-aminosalicylic acid
PB — phonetically balanced
PBF — phonetically balanced familiar word lists
PBK — phonetically balanced kindergarten word lists
PC — international hearing aid symbol for peak clipping
PD — potential difference
PDU — partially deaf units (UK)
PE — probable error
physical education
polyethylene
PEL — permissible exposure limit (replaces NEL)
PEM — predictable earmold modification
PGA — psychogalvanic audiometry
PGR — psychogalvanic reflex or response
PGSR — psychogalvanic skin reflex or response
PHS — Public Health Service
PICA — Porch Index of Communicative Ability
PK — psychokinesis
PKU — phenylketonuria
PMI — pressure measuring instrument
PNdB — perceived noise decibels
PNL — perceived noise level
pps — pulses per second
PRF — pulse recurrence frequency
pulse repetition frequency
psi — per square inch
PTA — pure tone audiogram
pure tone average
PTS — permanent threshold shift
PVR — psychovoltaic response
PVV — positive venting valve
PWL — power watt level
RAS — reticular activating system
RCL — range of comfortable loudness
RDP — relative delivered pressure
RF — recruitment factor
radiofrequency
Rh — Rhesus factor
RI — reference intensity
residual inhibition
rms — root mean square
RNA — ribonucleic acid
ROC — receiver operating characteristics
RP — retinitis pigmentosa
RSA — Rehabilitation Service Administration
RTL — reference threshold level
SAE — surgical auditory evaluation
SAF — synchronous auditory feedback
SAI — social adequacy index
SAL — sensorineural acuity level
speech awareness level

SAM — School of Aerospace (or Aviation) Medicine
SAT — speech awareness threshold
SBA — Small Business Administration
SCONII — Subcommittee on Noise in Industry (replaced by CHE)
SD, sd — standard deviation
SDS — speech discrimination score
SDT — speech detectability (or detection) threshold
SE — Signed English
SEE — Seeing Essential English
Signing Exact English
SF — sound field
SGR — skin galvanic response
SHAA — Society of Hearing Aid Audiologists (now NHAS)
SHHH — Self Help for Hard of Hearing People, Inc.
SI — speech interference
sensitivity index
SIL — speech interference level
SIN — sinusoid
SISI — short increment sensitivity index
SL — sensation level (re: threshold)
sound level
SLM — sound level meter
SN — sensorineural
S/N — signal to noise (ratio)
SNHL — sensorineural hearing loss
SOHNN — Society of Otorhinolaryngology and Head-Neck Nurses
SONS — Snijders-Ooman nonverbal scale
SP — summating potential
speech pathology
SPAR — sensitivity prediction for the acoustic reflex
SPL — sound pressure level
SR — stapedius reflex
stimulus response
SRS — Social and Rehabilitation Service
SRT — speech reception threshold
SSL — systematic signed language
SSPL — saturation sound pressure level
SSW — staggered spondaic word (test)
STP — standard temperature and pressure
SWAMI — speech with alternating masking index
T — international hearing aid symbol for input from telephone pickup coil
T & A — tonsillectomy and adenoidectomy
TARP — total aural reconstructive prosthesis
TAT — thematic apperception test
TD — threshold of discomfort
TDH-39 — telephonic dynamic headphone, model #39
TIN — tone in noise
TL — tolerance level
TLC — tender loving care
TMJ — temporomandibular joint
TORP — total ossicular replacement prosthesis
TP — threshold of pain

TRA — tinnitus research audiometer
TROCA — tangible reinforcement operant conditioning audiometry
TSD — threshold of signal detectability
TSH — thyroid stimulating hormone
TTD — threshold tone decay (test)
TTS — temporary threshold shift
UCL — uncomfortable loudness level
UCS — unconditioned stimulus
UF — undistorted faint
UL — undistorted loud
ULL — uncomfortable loudness level (UCL more common)
UM — unmasked
URI — upper respiratory infection
USASI — USA Standards Institute (now ANSI)
USP — United States Pharmacopeia

USPHS — U. S. Public Health Service
VA — Veterans Administration
VARO — Veterans Administration Regional Office
VASC — verbal auditory screening for children
VI — volume indicator (meter) (more commonly VU meter)
VRA — visual reinforcement audiometry
Vocational Rehabilitation Administration
VU — volume units (meter)
VVV — variable venting valve
WAIS — Wechsler adult intelligence scale
W-B — Wechsler-Bellevue (test)
WIPI — word intelligibilty by picture identification (word test)
WISC-R — Wechsler intelligence scale for children-revised

Appendix II

GUIDE FOR THE EVALUATION
OF HEARING HANDICAP

American Academy of Otolaryngology Committee on Hearing and Equilibrium, and the American
Council of Otolaryngology Committee on the Medical Aspects of Noise

The Guide for the Evaluation of Hearing Handicap has required periodic revisions as new infomation has become available. The last revision was in 1965. This communication represents a change in the previous formula and details the reasons for the modifications. This is the effort of the American Academy of Otolaryngology Committee on Hearing and Equilibrium and the American Council of Otolaryngology Committee on the Medical Aspects of Noise and represents approximately two years of work. Both committees unanimously endorse the new formula, and the Committee on Hearing and Equilibrium, particularly its Subcommittee on Conservation of Hearing, was responsible for writing and revising the text. The Board of Directors of both the American Academy of Otolaryngology and the American Council of Otolaryngology have approved this modified formula.

Impairment, Handicap, and Disability

It is important for all physicians to be aware of their role in the evaluation of permanent impairment, handicap, and disability under any private or public program for the disabled. It is equally important for them to have the necessary information to assist them in fulfilling their particular responsibility—the evaluation of permanent impairment and handicap.

In various statements approved by the Committee on Hearing and Equilibrium and its predecessor, the Committee on Conservation of Hearing of American Academy of Ophthalmology and Otolaryngology (AAOO), the terms "hearing impairment," "hearing handicap," and "hearing disability" have all been employed, often with the intention of conveying substantially the same meaning. However, some confusion has existed because of connotations attached to each of the terms. In this section the definitions are restated to coincide with those approved by the AAOO in 1965.[1]

Permanent Impairment.—A change for the worse in either structure or function, outside the

From the American Academy of Otolaryngology and the American Council of Otolaryngology. This article first appeared in the "Journal of the American Medical Association" 241:19, May 11, 1979 pp 2055-2059. Reprinted with permission.

This article may be purchased in manual form for a nominal charge from the American Academy of Otolaryngology, 15 Second Street, S.W., Rochester, Minn. 55901.

Table 1.—Monaural Hearing Impairment*			
DSHL†	**%**	**DSHL†**	**%**
100	0.0	240	52.5
105	1.9	245	54.4
110	3.8	250	56.2
115	5.6	255	58.1
120	7.5	260	60.0
125	9.4	265	61.9
130	11.2	270	63.8
135	13.1	275	65.6
140	15.0	280	67.5
145	16.9	285	69.3
150	18.8	290	71.2
155	20.6	295	73.1
160	22.5	300	75.0
165	24.4	305	76.9
170	26.2	310	78.8
175	28.1	315	80.6
180	30.0	320	82.5
185	31.9	325	84.4
190	33.8	330	86.2
195	35.6	335	88.1
200	37.5	340	90.0
205	39.4	345	90.9
210	41.2	350	93.8
215	43.1	355	95.6
220	45.0	360	97.5
225	46.9	365	99.4
230	48.9	370	100.0
235	50.6		(or greater)

*1. From the audiogram of numerical record of the audiometric test, find the decibel sum of the hearing threshold levels (DSHL) of 500, 1,000, 2,000, and 3,000 Hz. Example:

```
  500    20
1,000    25
2,000    35
3,000    40
```
Total 120 DSHL

2. Under the DSHL heading, 120 DSHL (column 1, line 5) equals 7.5%.

3. Computation of percent of hearing handicap: If the monaural percent figure is the same for both ears, that figure expresses the percent hearing handicap. If the percent monaural hearing impairments are not the same, apply the formula:

$$\frac{(5 \times \% \text{ [better ear]}) + (1 \times \% \text{ [poorer ear]})}{6} =$$

% hearing handicap

Audiometers are calibrated to ANSI 1969 standard reference levels.

†Decibel sum of hearing threshold levels at 500, 1,000, 2,000, and 3,000 Hz.

range of normal, is permanent impairment. The term is used here in a medical rather than a legal sense. Permanent impairment is due to any anatomic or functional abnormality that produces hearing loss. This loss should be evaluated after maximum rehabilitation has been achieved and when the impairment is nonprogressive at the time of evaluation. The determination of impairment is basic to the evaluation of permanent handicap and disability.

Permanent Handicap.—The disadvantage imposed by an impairment sufficient to affect a person's efficiency in the activities of daily living is permanent handicap. Handicap implies a material impairment.

Permanent Disability.—An actual or presumed inability to remain employed at full wages is a permanent disability. A person is permanently disabled or under permanent disability when the actual or presumed ability to engage in gainful activity is reduced because of handicap and when no appreciable improvement can be expected.

The aforementioned definition of handicap is essentially identical with the definition of "impairment" appearing in the American Medical Association's *Guides to the Evaluation of Permanent Impairment,*[2] namely, a "medical condition that affects one's personal efficiency in the activities of daily living." Disability remains defined as an actual or presumed reduction in ability to remain employed at full wages, and it involves nonmedical factors such as age, sex, education, and economic and social environment. A permanent impairment that is a handicap is, therefore, a contributing factor to, but not necessarily an indication of, the extent of a person's permanent disability under workmen's compensation laws. "Impairment" need not imply appreciable handicap and may be used in a more general sense to denote any deviation from normal. The term "handicap" is so useful in this broad sense that the 1965 guide departed from previous use by employing "handicap" to identify a material impairment sufficient to "affect one's personal efficiency in the activities of daily living."

Evaluation of Permanent Impairment.—Evaluation of permanent impairment is an appraisal of the nature and extent of a person's illness or injury as it affects structure or function, and it lies within the scope of medical responsibility preparatory to the assessment of permanent handicap and disability.

Evaluation of Permanent Handicap.—Evaluation of permanent handicap is an appraisal of the disadvantage imposed by an impairment on the person's efficiency in the activities of daily living.

Evaluation of Permanent Disability.—Evaluation of permanent disability is an administrative responsibility based, in part, on medical information. It is an appraisal of a person's present and probable future ability to engage in

gainful activity as it is affected not only by the medical factor (permanent handicap) but also by other factors such as age, sex, education, and economic and social environment. Since many nonmedical factors have proved difficult to measure, permanent handicap often becomes the principal criterion of permanent disability.

Determination of disability is an administrative decision as to the worker's entitlement to compensation that should be based on complete medical evaluation and accurate assessment of function using standards that are uniform nationwide and that apply regardless of the manner in which the handicap was acquired.

Historical Background Information

Sensorineural hearing impairment cannot be assessed in terms of the loss of sensory cells and neurons; instead, some change in function must be measured. The changes in function that are commonly measured are the threshold sensitivity for pure tones and some index of the ability to hear and understand speech. The determination of threshold sensitivity for pure tones in quiet is a standard procedure. However, methods for assessing the ability to understand speech have not been well standardized, because the understanding of speech is affected by such variables as vocabulary, education, intelligence, and nature of speech test material, in addition to hearing ability per se.[3]

In the early days of pure-tone audiometry, the degree of hearing loss was expressed in terms of the total range of the audiometer (120 dB). This led to the so-called 0.8 rule, since each decibel represented 0.8% of this range.[4] In a medicolegal context, the 0.8 rule was illogical. Normal hearing sensitivity is not a single value but a range of values around audiometric zero. For example, a hearing level of 10 dB is considered normal but would have been rated as corresponding to an 8% hearing handicap under the 0.8 rule. At the other extreme, persons with hearing thresholds considerably below 120 dB cannot hear or understand everyday speech and the severity of their hearing loss was underrated.

Subsequent efforts[5, 6] to find better methods for the evaluation of hearing loss in medicolegal applications led to complex schemes that differentially weighted hearing levels at various audiometric test frequencies according to their relative importance for the hearing of speech. The resulting AMA method proved to be unsatisfactory in practice because of its complexity and because it was less appropriate for sensorineural than for conductive hearing losses.

Further efforts to define hearing loss were divided into two stages. The first stage[7] was to define handicap in terms of hearing for speech: the ability to identify spoken words or sentences under everyday conditions of normal living. This statement anticipated that during the second stage, standardized tests for the hearing of everyday speech would be developed. Specific quantitative recommendations for the determi-

Table 2.—Computatio

ANSI 1969	100	105	110	115	120	125	130	135	140	145	150	155	160	165	170	175	180	185	190	195	200	205	210	215	220
100	0																								
105	.3	1.9																							
110	.6	2.2	3.8																						
115	.9	2.5	4.1	5.6																					
120	1.3	2.8	4.4	5.9	7.5*																				
125	1.6	3.1	4.7	6.3	7.8	9.4																			
130	1.9	3.4	5	6.6	8.1	9.7	11.3																		
135	2.2	3.8	5.3	6.9	8.4	10	11.6	13.1																	
140	2.5	4.1	5.6	7.2	8.8	10.3	11.9	13.4	15																
145	2.8	4.4	5.9	7.5	9.1	10.6	12.2	13.8	15.3	16.9															
150	3.1	4.7	6.3	7.8	9.4	10.9	12.5	14.1	15.6	17.2	18.8														
155	3.4	5	6.6	8.1	9.7	11.3	12.8	14.4	15.9	17.5	19.1	20.6													
160	3.8	5.3	6.9	8.4	10	11.6	13.1	14.7	16.3	17.8	19.4	20.9	22.5												
165	4.1	5.6	7.2	8.8	10.3	11.9	13.4	15	16.6	18.1	19.7	21.3	22.8	24.4											
170	4.4	5.9	7.5	9.1	10.6	12.2	13.8	15.3	16.9	18.4	20	21.6	23.1	24.7	26.3										
175	4.7	6.3	7.8	9.4	10.9	12.5	14.1	15.6	17.2	18.8	20.3	21.9	23.4	25	26.6	28.1									
180	5	6.6	8.1	9.7	11.3	12.8	14.4	15.9	17.5	19.1	20.6	22.2	23.8	25.3	26.9	28.4	30								
185	5.3	6.9	8.4	10	11.6	13.1	14.7	16.3	17.8	19.4	20.9	22.5	24.1	25.6	27.2	28.8	30.3	31.9							
190	5.6	7.2	8.8	10.3	11.9	13.4	15	16.6	18.1	19.7	21.3	22.8	24.4	25.9	27.5	29.1	30.6	32.2	33.8						
195	5.9	7.5	9.1	10.6	12.2	13.8	15.3	16.9	18.4	20	21.6	23.1	24.7	26.3	27.8	29.4	30.9	32.5	34.1	35.6					
200	6.3	7.8	9.4	10.9	12.5	14.1	15.6	17.2	18.8	20.3	21.9	23.4	25	26.6	28.1	29.7	31.3	32.8	34.4	35.9	37.5				
205	6.6	8.1	9.7	11.3	12.8	14.4	15.9	17.5	19.1	20.6	22.2	23.8	25.3	26.9	28.4	30	31.6	33.1	34.7	36.3	37.8	39.4			
210	6.9	8.4	10	11.6	13.1	14.7	16.3	17.8	19.4	20.9	22.5	24.1	25.6	27.2	28.8	30.3	31.9	33.4	35	36.6	38.1	39.7	41.3		
215	7.2	8.8	10.3	11.9	13.4	15	16.6	18.1	19.7	21.3	22.8	24.4	25.9	27.5	29.1	30.6	32.2	33.8	35.3	36.9	38.4	40	41.6	43.1	
220	7.5	9.1	10.6	12.2	13.8	15.3	16.9	18.4	20	21.6	23.1	24.7	26.3	27.8	29.4	30.9	32.5	34.1	35.6	37.2	38.8	40.3	41.9	43.4	45
225	7.8	9.4	10.9	12.5	14.1	15.6	17.2	18.8	20.3	21.9	23.4	25	26.6	28.1	29.7	31.3	32.8	34.4	35.9	37.5	39.1	40.6	42.2	43.8	45.3
230	8.1	9.7	11.3	12.8	14.4	15.9	17.5	19.1	20.6	22.2	23.8	25.3	26.9	28.4	30	31.6	33.1	34.7	36.3	37.8	39.4	40.9	42.5	44.1	45.6
235	8.4	10	11.6	13.1	14.7	16.3	17.8	19.4	20.9	22.5	24.1	25.6	27.2	28.8	30.3	31.9	33.4	35	36.6	38.1	39.7	41.3	42.8	44.4	45.9
240	8.8	10.3	11.9	13.4	15	16.6	18.1	19.7	21.3	22.8	24.4	25.9	27.5	29.1	30.6	32.2	33.8	35.3	36.9	38.4	40	41.6	43.1	44.7	46.3
245	9.1	10.6	12.2	13.8	15.3	16.9	18.4	20	21.6	23.1	24.7	26.3	27.8	29.4	30.9	32.5	34.1	35.6	37.2	38.8	40.3	41.9	43.4	45	46.6
250	9.4	10.9	12.5	14.1	15.6	17.2	18.8	20.3	21.9	23.4	25	26.6	28.1	29.7	31.3	32.8	34.4	35.9	37.5	39.1	40.6	42.2	43.8	45.3	46.9
255	9.7	11.3	12.8	14.4	15.9	17.5	19.1	20.6	22.2	23.8	25.3	26.9	28.4	30	31.6	33.1	34.7	36.3	37.8	39.4	40.9	42.5	44.1	45.6	47.2
260	10	11.6	13.1	14.7	16.3	17.8	19.4	20.9	22.5	24.1	25.6	27.2	28.8	30.3	31.9	33.4	35	36.6	38.1	39.7	41.3	42.8	44.4	45.9	47.5
265	10.3	11.9	13.4	15	16.6	18.1	19.7	21.3	22.8	24.4	25.9	27.5	29.1	30.6	32.2	33.8	35.3	36.9	38.4	40	41.6	43.1	44.7	46.3	47.8
270	10.6	12.2	13.8	15.3	16.9	18.4	20	21.6	23.1	24.7	26.3	27.8	29.4	30.9	32.5	34.1	35.6	37.2	38.8	40.3	41.9	43.4	45	46.6	48.1
275	10.9	12.5	14.1	15.6	17.2	18.8	20.3	21.9	23.4	25	26.6	28.1	29.7	31.3	32.8	34.4	35.9	37.5	39.1	40.6	42.2	43.8	45.3	46.9	48.4
280	11.3	12.8	14.4	15.9	17.5	19.1	20.6	22.2	23.8	25.3	26.9	28.4	30	31.6	33.1	34.7	36.3	37.8	39.4	40.9	42.5	44.1	45.6	47.2	48.8
285	11.6	13.1	14.7	16.3	17.8	19.4	20.9	22.5	24.1	25.6	27.2	28.8	30.3	31.9	33.4	35	36.6	38.1	39.7	41.3	42.8	44.4	45.9	47.5	49.1
290	11.9	13.4	15	16.6	18.1	19.7	21.3	22.8	24.4	25.9	27.5	29.1	30.6	32.2	33.8	35.3	36.9	38.4	40	41.6	43.1	44.7	46.3	47.8	49.4
295	12.2	13.8	15.3	16.9	18.4	20	21.6	23.1	24.7	26.3	27.8	29.4	30.9	32.5	34.1	35.6	37.2	38.8	40.3	41.9	43.4	45	46.6	48.1	49.7
300	12.5	14.1	15.6	17.2	18.8	20.3	21.9	23.4	25	26.6	28.1	29.7	31.3	32.8	34.4	35.9	37.5	39.1	40.6	42.2	43.8	45.3	46.9	48.4	50
305	12.8	14.4	15.9	17.5	19.1	20.6	22.2	23.8	25.3	26.9	28.4	30	31.6	33.1	34.7	36.3	37.8	39.4	40.9	42.5	44.1	45.6	47.2	48.8	50.3
310	13.1	14.7	16.3	17.8	19.4	20.9	22.5	24.1	25.6	27.2	28.8	30.3	31.9	33.4	35	36.6	38.1	39.7	41.3	42.8	44.4	45.9	47.5	49.1	50.6
315	13.4	15	16.6	18.1	19.7	21.3	22.8	24.4	25.9	27.5	29.1	30.6	32.2	33.8	35.3	36.9	38.4	40	41.6	43.1	44.7	46.3	47.8	49.4	50.9
320	13.8	15.3	16.9	18.4	20	21.6	23.1	24.7	26.3	27.8	29.4	30.9	32.5	34.1	35.6	37.2	38.8	40.3	41.9	43.4	45	46.6	48.1	49.7	51.3
325	14.1	15.6	17.2	18.8	20.3	21.9	23.4	25	26.6	28.1	29.7	31.3	32.8	34.4	35.9	37.5	39.1	40.6	42.2	43.8	45.3	46.9	48.4	50	51.6
330	14.4	15.9	17.5	19.1	20.6	22.2	23.8	25.3	26.9	28.4	30	31.6	33.1	34.7	36.3	37.8	39.4	40.9	42.5	44.1	45.6	47.2	48.8	50.3	51.9
335	14.7	16.3	17.8	19.4	20.9	22.5	24.1	25.6	27.2	28.8	30.3	31.9	33.4	35	36.6	38.1	39.7	41.3	42.8	44.4	45.9	47.5	49.1	50.6	52.2
340	15	16.6	18.1	19.7	21.3	22.8	24.4	25.9	27.5	29.1	30.6	32.2	33.8	35.3	36.9	38.4	40	41.6	43.1	44.7	46.3	47.8	49.4	50.9	52.5
345	15.3	16.9	18.4	20	21.6	23.1	24.7	26.3	27.8	29.4	30.9	32.5	34.1	35.6	37.2	38.8	40.3	41.9	43.4	45	46.6	48.1	49.7	51.3	52.8
350	15.6	17.2	18.8	20.3	21.9	23.4	25	26.6	28.1	29.7	31.3	32.8	34.4	35.9	37.5	39.1	40.6	42.2	43.8	45.3	46.9	48.4	50	51.6	53.1
355	15.9	17.5	19.1	20.6	22.2	23.8	25.3	26.9	28.4	30	31.6	33.1	34.7	36.3	37.8	39.4	40.9	42.5	44.1	45.6	47.2	48.8	50.3	51.9	53.4
360	16.3	17.8	19.4	20.9	22.5	24.1	25.6	27.2	28.8	30.3	31.9	33.4	35	36.6	38.1	39.7	41.3	42.8	44.4	45.9	47.5	49.1	50.6	52.2	53.8
365	16.6	18.1	19.7	21.3	22.8	24.4	25.9	27.5	29.1	30.6	32.2	33.8	35.3	36.9	38.4	40	41.6	43.1	44.7	46.3	47.8	49.4	50.9	52.5	54.1
368	16.8	18.3	19.9	21.4	23	24.6	26.2	27.7	29.3	30.8	32.4	33.9	35.5	37.1	38.6	40.2	41.8	43.3	44.9	46.4	48	49.6	51.1	52.7	54.3
ANSI 1969	100	105	110	115	120	125	130	135	140	145	150	155	160	165	170	175	180	185	190	195	200	205	210	215	220

Better Ear (sum 500, 1,000, 2,000, 3,000 Hz)

nation of handicap would then be proposed. We still do not have such tests.

Other attempts to define hearing loss included studies relating the hearing of one or more forms of speech to the audiometric threshold for pure tones.[8, 10] The relative intelligibility of different speech materials was also investigated.[11, 12] The AAOO Committee on Conservation of Hearing (now the Committee on Hearing and Equilibrium) and the AMA Committee on Medical Rating of Physical Impairment reviewed the available information and reached the specific recommendations published in guides for the evaluation of hearing impairment (now handicap).[1, 2, 13] The specific recommendations were built on the principles published earlier.[7] Handicap was rated in terms of the ability to hear everyday speech in quiet. In the absence of a good test for hearing speech in quiet, the thresholds for pure tones were used to predict the threshold of hearing for speech. The simplest method for achieving a reasonably accurate prediction of impairment of hearing for speech was to use the average of the hearing threshold levels at 500, 1,000, and 2,000 Hz.[8, 10, 12] Prediction did not seem to be improved by the inclusion of other frequencies such as 3,000 or 4,000 Hz. Impairment of hearing was calculated from the number of decibels by which the average hearing threshold level exceeded 15 dB American Standards Association (ASA) 1951.[14] Complete or total hearing impairment was set at 82 dB ASA 1951. This value was approximately correct and had the added advantage that percent of impairment could be calculated simply as 1.5% times

f Hearing Handicap*

*Values are based on the following formula:

$$\frac{5 \times \% \text{ impairment of better ear} + \% \text{ impairment of worse ear}}{6} = \text{hearing handicap}$$

The axes are the sum of hearing levels at 500, 1,000, 2,000, and 3,000 Hz. The sum for the worse ear is read at the side; the sum for the better ear is read at the bottom. At the intersection of the column for the worse ear and the column for the better ear is the hearing handicap.

225	230	235	240	245	250	255	260	265	270	275	280	285	290	295	300	305	310	315	320	325	330	335	340	345	350	355	360	365	368
46.9																													
47.2	48.8																												
47.5	49.1	50.6																											
47.8	49.4	50.9	52.5																										
48.1	49.7	51.3	52.8	54.4																									
48.4	50	51.6	53.1	54.7	56.3																								
48.8	50.3	51.9	53.4	55	56.6	58.1																							
49.1	50.6	52.2	53.8	55.3	56.9	58.4	60																						
49.4	50.9	52.5	54.1	55.6	57.2	58.8	60.3	61.9																					
49.7	51.3	52.8	54.4	55.9	57.5	59.1	60.6	62.2	63.8																				
50	51.6	53.1	54.7	56.3	57.8	59.4	60.9	62.5	64.1	65.6																			
50.3	51.9	53.4	55	56.6	58.1	59.7	61.3	62.8	64.4	65.9	67.5																		
50.6	52.2	53.8	55.3	56.9	58.4	60	61.6	63.1	64.7	66.3	67.8	69.4																	
50.9	52.5	54.1	55.6	57.2	58.8	60.3	61.9	63.4	65	66.6	68.1	69.7	71.3																
51.3	52.8	54.4	55.9	57.5	59.1	60.6	62.2	63.8	65.3	66.9	68.4	70	71.6	73.1															
51.6	53.1	54.7	56.3	57.8	59.4	60.9	62.5	64.1	65.6	67.2	68.8	70.3	71.9	73.4	75														
51.9	53.4	55	56.6	58.1	59.7	61.3	62.8	64.4	65.9	67.5	69.1	70.6	72.2	73.8	75.3	76.9													
52.2	53.8	55.3	56.9	58.4	60	61.6	63.1	64.7	66.3	67.8	69.4	70.9	72.5	74.1	75.6	77.2	78.8												
52.5	54.1	55.6	57.2	58.8	60.3	61.9	63.4	65	66.6	68.1	69.7	71.3	72.8	74.4	75.9	77.5	79.1	80.6											
52.8	54.4	55.9	57.5	59.1	60.6	62.2	63.8	65.3	66.9	68.4	70	71.6	73.1	74.7	76.3	77.8	79.4	80.9	82.5										
53.1	54.7	56.3	57.8	59.4	60.9	62.5	64.1	65.6	67.2	68.8	70.3	71.9	73.4	75	76.6	78.1	79.7	81.3	82.8	84.4									
53.4	55	56.6	58.1	59.7	61.3	62.8	64.4	65.9	67.5	69.1	70.6	72.2	73.8	75.3	76.9	78.4	80	81.6	83.1	84.7	86.3								
53.8	55.3	56.9	58.4	60	61.6	63.1	64.7	66.3	67.8	69.4	70.9	72.5	74.1	75.6	77.2	78.8	80.3	81.9	83.4	85	86.6	88.1							
54.1	55.6	57.2	58.8	60.3	61.9	63.4	65	66.6	68.1	69.7	71.3	72.8	74.4	75.9	77.5	79.1	80.6	82.2	83.8	85.3	86.9	88.4	90						
54.4	55.9	57.5	59.1	60.6	62.2	63.8	65.3	66.9	68.4	70	71.6	73.1	74.7	76.3	77.8	79.4	80.9	82.5	84.1	85.6	87.2	88.8	90.3	91.9					
54.7	56.3	57.8	59.4	60.9	62.5	64.1	65.6	67.2	68.8	70.3	71.9	73.4	75	76.6	78.1	79.7	81.3	82.8	84.4	85.9	87.5	89.1	90.6	92.2	93.8				
55	56.6	58.1	59.7	61.3	62.8	64.4	65.9	67.5	69.1	70.6	72.2	73.8	75.3	76.9	78.4	80	81.6	83.1	84.7	86.3	87.8	89.4	90.9	92.5	94.1	95.6			
55.3	56.9	58.4	60	61.6	63.1	64.7	66.3	67.8	69.4	70.9	72.5	74.1	75.6	77.2	78.8	80.3	81.9	83.4	85	86.6	88.1	89.7	91.3	92.8	94.4	95.9	97.5		
55.6	57.2	58.8	60.3	61.9	63.4	65	66.6	68.1	69.7	71.3	72.8	74.4	75.9	77.5	79.1	80.6	82.2	83.8	85.3	86.9	88.4	90	91.6	93.1	94.7	96.3	97.8	99.4	
55.8	57.4	58.9	60.5	62.1	63.6	65.2	66.8	68.3	69.9	71.4	73	74.6	76.1	77.7	79.3	80.8	82.4	83.9	85.5	87.1	88.6	90.2	91.8	93.3	94.9	96.4	98	99.6	100

the number of decibels by which the average hearing threshold levels exceeded 15 dB ASA 1951.

In June 1971 new levels were adopted by the AMA to reflect the change in audiometric zero American National Standards Institute (ANSI) S3.6-1969.[15] The old threshold for hearing impairment of 15 dB ASA 1951 became 25 dB ANSI 1969, and the level for total impairment of 82 dB ASA 1951 became 92 dB ANSI 1969.

The Committee on Hearing and Equilibrium and its Subcommittee on the Conservation of Hearing have periodically reviewed the accuracy of the 1959 guidelines for the hearing of speech and found them appropriate as long as a quiet environment was considered the proper test background. These guidelines do not necessarily apply to the hearing of speech in noisy environments. Quiet was chosen originally for that purpose because it was easier to agree on its definition than on that of a standard noise environment that would simulate an everyday listening situation. However, when the noise level begins to approach the level of the speech signals, as occurs in many everyday listening situations, the 1959 guidelines no longer provide an accurate measure of handicap.[16-18]

The Committee believes that the basis for the calculation of hearing handicap should be altered to reflect a more realistic degree of the understanding of speech, not only in the quiet but also in the presence of some noise. Although a decrease in hearing sensitivity at 3,000 Hz has little effect on hearing speech in quiet,[8-10] it produces a handicap in the presence of noise[16-18] or when speech is distorted.[19-21]

The Committee believes that the hearing threshold level at 3,000 Hz should be included in the calculation of hearing handicap to provide a more accurate assessment of hearing handicap in a greater variety of everyday listening conditions.

Recommendations

The Committee on Hearing and Equilibrium of the American Academy of Ophthalmology and Otolaryngology recommends that the calculation of hearing handicap for adults be derived from the pure-tone audiogram obtained with an audiometer calibrated to ANSI S3.6-1969 standards (Tables 1 and 2). This computation does not apply to children who have not yet acquired language. Hearing handicap is always based on the functional state of both ears.

1. The average of the hearing threshold levels at 500, 1,000, 2,000, and 3,000 Hz should be calculated for each ear.

2. The percent impairment for each ear should be calculated by multiplying by 1.5% the amount by which the aforementioned average hearing threshold level exceeds 25 dB (low fence) up to a maximum of 100%, which is reached at 92 dB (high fence).

3. The hearing handicap, a binaural assessment, should then be calculated by multiplying the smaller percentage (better ear) by 5, adding this figure to the larger percentage (poorer ear), and dividing the total by 6.

Following are examples of the recommended calculation of hearing handicap:

A. Mild to Marked Bilateral Sensorineural Hearing Loss

	500 Hz	1,000 Hz	2,000 Hz	3,000 Hz
Right ear	15	25	45	55
Left ear	30	45	60	85

1. Calculation of the average hearing threshold level:
Right ear:

$$\frac{15 + 25 + 45 + 55}{4} = \frac{140}{4} = 35 \text{ dB}$$

Left ear:

$$\frac{30 + 45 + 60 + 85}{4} = \frac{220}{4} = 55 \text{ dB}$$

2. Calculation of monaural impairment:
Right ear:
35 dB − 25 dB = 10 dB; 10 × 1.5% = 15%
Left ear:
55 dB − 25 dB = 30 dB; 30 × 1.5% = 45%

3. Calculation of hearing handicap:
Smaller number (better ear)
15% × 5 = 75
Larger number (poorer ear)
45% × 1 = 45

Total, 120 ÷ 6 = 20%

Therefore, a person with the hearing threshold levels shown in this audiogram would have a 20% hearing handicap.

B. Slight Bilateral Sensorineural Hearing Loss

	500 Hz	1,000 Hz	2,000 Hz	3,000 Hz
Right ear	15	15	20	30
Left ear	20	20	30	40

1. Average hearing threshold level:
Right ear:

$$\frac{15 + 15 + 20 + 30}{4} = \frac{80}{4} = 20 \text{ dB}$$

Left ear:

$$\frac{20 + 20 + 30 + 40}{4} = \frac{110}{4} = 27.5 \text{ dB}$$

2. Monaural impairment:
Right ear:
20 dB − 25 dB = − 5 dB; 0 × 1.5% = 0%
Left ear:
27.5 dB − 25 dB = 2.5 dB;
2.5 × 1.5% = 3.75%

3. Hearing handicap:
Smaller number (better ear)
0% × 5 = 0.00
Larger number (poorer ear)
3.75% × 1 = 3.75

Total, 3.75 ÷ 6 = 1% (rounded off)

Therefore, the hearing handicap is 1%.

C. Severe to Extreme Bilateral Sensorineural Hearing Loss

	500 Hz	1,000 Hz	2,000 Hz	3,000 Hz
Right ear	80	90	100	110
Left ear	75	80	90	95

1. Average hearing threshold level
(use 92 dB maximal value):
Right ear:

$$\frac{80 + 90 + 100 + 110}{4} = \frac{380}{4} = 95 \text{ dB}$$

Left ear:

$$\frac{75 + 80 + 90 + 95}{4} = \frac{340}{4} = 85 \text{ dB}$$

2. Monaural impairment:
Right ear:
92 dB (maximum) − 25 dB = 67 dB;
67 × 1.5% = 100%
Left ear:
85 dB − 25 dB = 60 dB; 60 × 1.5% = 90%

3. Hearing handicap:
Smaller number (better ear)
90% × 5 = 450
Larger number (poorer ear)
100% × 1 = 100

Total, 550 ÷ 6 = 92%

Therefore, the hearing handicap is 92%.

American Academy of Otolaryngology Committee on Hearing and Equilibrium: *Chairman:* Francis I. Catlin, MD. *Committee Members:* Hugh O. Barber, MD; Derald E. Brackmann, MD; Robert W. Cantrell, MD; Richard R. Gacek, MD; Ralph V. Ganser, MD; George A. Gates, MD; F. Blair Simmons, MD; George H. Williams, MD. *Consultants:* Leo G. Doerfler, PhD; Donald H. Eldredge, MD; Joseph E. Hawkins, Jr. PhD; James F. Jerger, PhD; Ralph F. Naunton, MD; Juergen Tonndorf, MD; W. Dixon Ward, PhD.
American Council of Otolaryngology Committee on the Medical Aspects of Noise: *Chairman:* Robert W. Cantrell, MD. *Committee Members:* Meyer S. Fox, MD; Aram Glorig, MD; Donald J. Joseph, MD; William C. Morgan, Jr. MD; Maurice Schiff, MD; George H. Williams, MD. *Consultant:* Francis I. Catlin, MD.

References

1. David H: Guide for the classification and evaluation of hearing handicap in relation to the International Audiometric Zero. *Trans Am Acad Opthalmol Otolaryngol* 69:740-751, 1965.
2. Guide to the Evaluation of permanent impairment: Ear, nose, throat, and related structures. AMA Committee on Medical Rating of Physical Impairment. *JAMA* 177:489-501, 1961.
3. Silverman SR, Hirsh IJ: Problems related to the use of speech in clinical audiometry. *Ann Otol Rhinol Laryngol* 64:1234-1248, 1955.
4. Fletcher H: *Speech and Hearing.* New York, van Nostrand Co., 1929.
5. Tentative standard procedure for evaluating the percentage of useful hearing loss in medicolegal cases. Council on Physical Therapy. *JAMA* 119:1108-1109, 1942.
6. Tentative standard procedure for evaluating the percentage loss of hearing in medicolegal cases. Council on Physical Medicine. *JAMA* 133:396-397, 1947.
7. Principles for evaluating hearing loss. Council on Physical Medicine and Rehabilitation, abstracted. *JAMA* 157:1408-1409, 1955.
8. Carhart R: Speech reception in relation to pattern of pure tone loss. *J Speech Disord* 11:97-108, 1946.
9. Harris JD, Haines HL, Myers CK: A new formula for using the audiogram to predict speech hearing loss. *Arch Otolaryngol* 63:158-176, 1956.
10. Quizzle RR, Glorig A, Delk JH, et al: Predicting hearing loss for speech from pure tone audiograms. *Laryngoscope* 67:1-15, 1957.
11. French NR, Steinberg JC: Factors governing the intelligibility of speech sounds. *J Acoust Soc Am* 19:90-119, 1947.
12. Hirsh IJ, Reynolds EG, Joseph M: Intelligibility of different speech materials. *J Acoust Soc Am* 26:530-538, 1954.
13. Guide for the evaluation of hearing impairment: Report of the AAOO Committee on Conservation of Hearing (Subcommittee on Noise in Industry). *Trans Am Acad Ophthalmol Otolaryngol* 63:236-238, 1959.
14. *American Standard Specification for Audiometers for General Diagnostic Purposes. Z24.5-1951.* New York, American Standards Association, 1951.
15. *American National Standard Specifications for Audiometers. ANSI S3.6-1969.* New York, American National Standards Institute Inc, 1970.
16. Kryter KD, Williams C, Green DM: Auditory acuity and the perception of speech. *J Acoust Soc Am* 34:1217-1223, 1962.
17. Suter AH: The ability of mildly hearing-impaired individuals to discriminate speech in noise. EPA 550/9-78-100. AMRL-TR-78-4. US Environmental Protection Agency, 1978.
18. Aniansson G: Methods for assessing high frequency hearing loss in everyday listening situations. *Acta Otolaryngol* 320 (suppl): chapters 3 and 5, 1974.
19. Harris JD: Combinations of distortion in speech. The 25% safety factor by multiple-cueing. *Arch Otolaryngol* 72:227-232, 1960.
20. Harris JD, Haines JD, Myers CK: The importance of hearing at 3 kc for understanding speeded speech. *Laryngoscope* 70:131-146, 1960.
21. Harris JD: Pure-tone acuity and the intelligibility of everyday speech. *J Acoust Soc Am* 37:821-830, 1965.

GUIDELINES FOR AUDIOMETRIC SYMBOLS

Editor's Note: *The "Guidelines for Audiometric Symbols" was approved by the American Speech and Hearing Association Executive Board in December 1973. Members of the ASHA Committee on Audiometric Evaluation, which developed the guidelines, are F. L. Sonday, W. R. Wilson, J. B. Chaiklin, J. T. Graham, Z. G. Schoeny, and N. T. Hopkinson, Chairman. ASHA encourages the professional community to use these guidelines in clinical practice and in publications.*

The set of "Guidelines for Audiometric Symbols" is the first of a series developed by the Committee on Audiometric Evaluation under the Vice-President for Clinical Affairs of the American Speech and Hearing Association.

Each of the guidelines presents a recommended set of procedures based on existing clinical practice and research findings. The spirit of these guidelines is not to mandate a single way of accomplishing the clinical process; rather, the intent is to suggest standard procedures, that, in the final analysis, will benefit the patients we serve. The intention is to allow for a more efficient and uniform transfer of information.

Audiometric symbols used to record the results of conventional pure-tone threshold audiometry have never been standardized by the American Speech and Hearing Association. A wide variety of symbols and symbol systems is in use for recording data on audiograms, as has been demonstrated most recently by Martin and Kopra (1970) and by Sweetman and Miller in an ASHA convention paper (Chicago, 1969). Although certain audiometric symbols are in almost universal use, others are employed in widely disparate ways by different clinicians. Widespread use of unstandardized, idiosyncratic symbol systems increases the possibility of a misinterpretation of data when records are exchanged between clinical services. In addition, such use impedes the orderly exchange of information with other professions, in both clinical practice and published reports.

The purpose of these guidelines is to detail a set of standard audiometric symbols for recording graphically the results of pure-tone audiometry. From this set of symbols the clinician may select those necessary to record the information collected. Presentation of these guidelines does not imply that the audiogram is the only appropriate means of recording audiometric results[1]; however, when an audiogram is used, these symbols should be used.

The Audiogram

As recommended in the ANSI S3.6-1969 *Specifications for Audiometers,* the audiogram shall be shown as a grid with test frequencies, in Hertz (Hz), represented on the abscissa by means of a logarithmic scale and the hearing

level (HL), in decibels (dB), represented on the ordinate by a linear scale. One octave on the frequency scale shall be equivalent in span to 20 dB on the HL scale. The horizontal scale shall be labeled *Frequency in Hertz* and the vertical scale shall be labeled *Hearing Level in dB*. The zero reference threshold level should be shown prominently.

Grid lines of equal darkness and thickness are recommended at octave intervals on the frequency scale and at 10-dB intervals on the IIL scale. Grid lines used for interoctave frequencies should be finer and lighter in hue than those for octave frequencies.

The audiogram form is illustrated in Figure 1. Specific recommendations on the type and amount of additional information to be included on the audiogram form, such as client identification, tester identification, results of speech audiometry, and results of tuning fork tests, are not included in these guidelines since they more appropriately are specified by individual clinics.

The Audiometric Symbols

Any effort to modify behavior through the establishment of guidelines must consider current practices. One of the most recent sources used by the Committee on Audiometric Evaluation is Martin and Kopra's (1970) survey of audiometric symbols used by ASHA-certified audiologists. Although the Committee considered the apparent popularity of certain symbols, all symbols considered had to meet four basic criteria. Each symbol had to be

1. Simple in design, easily drawn, and sharply reproducible by xerography or other reproduction methods.

---

[1]In many clinics numerals are used to record the results of air-conduction and bone-conduction measurements. Examples of this form of reporting data are included in Newby (1972). Some clinicians choose to collect their data in numerical form and then transfer the results to an audiogram, using symbols for their reports. Others collect the raw data on audiogram forms, using symbols, and transfer numbers to a block form for reports. Still others collect and report clinical data consistently using either symbols or numbers.

2. Mutually exclusive from and internally consistent with other symbols in the system.
3. Capable of delineating, without recourse to color coding, the following distinctions:
   a. left ear from right ear,
   b. air conduction from bone conduction,
   c. unmasked from masked results,
   d. response from no response, and
   e. the transducer (phone, vibrator, or speaker) used to present signals.
4. Designed to permit multiple notation at a single level on the audiogram.

Based on these four criteria, the Committee on Audiometric Evaluation recommends the set of symbols presented in Table 1.

Further Specifications
Air-Conduction Symbols. The air-conduction symbols should be drawn on the audiogram so that the midpoint of the symbol centers on the intersection of the vertical and horizontal axes at the appropriate HL (shown in Figures 2 through 8).
Bone-Conduction Symbols. The bone-conduction symbols, with one exception, should be placed adjacent to, but not touching, the frequency axis and centered vertically at the appropriate HL. The symbol for the left ear should be placed to the right of the frequency axis and that for the right ear to the left of the frequency axis (Figures 2, 3, 5, 7, and 8).[2] The symbol for unmasked forehead bone conduction should be centered on the vertical axis at the appropriate HL (Figure 5).
Multiple Notation. When the left ear unmasked air-conduction threshold is the same as the right air-conduction threshold, the left air-conduction symbol should be placed inside the right air-conduction symbol (Figures 3, 4, 5, 7 and 8). When bone-conduction thresholds (except unmasked forehead bone conduction) occur at the same HL as air-conduction thresholds, the bone-conduction symbols should be placed adjacent to, but not touching the air-conduction symbols (Figures 2, 3, and 8). The midline bone-conduction symbol in this circum-

stance should be placed with the point of the carat barely entering the region of the air conduction symbols (Figure 5).

When bone conduction is measured at the mastoid with unmasked and masked thresholds occurring at the same HL, the unmasked symbol should be placed closest to the frequency axis. The masked symbol should surround, but not touch, the unmasked symbol (Figures 2 and 3).

MODALITY	EAR*		
	RIGHT	BOTH	LEFT
AIR CONDUCTION - EARPHONES UNMASKED	O		X
MASKED	△		▢
BONE CONDUCTION - MASTOID UNMASKED	<		>
MASKED	[		]
BONE CONDUCTION - FOREHEAD UNMASKED		∨	
MASKED	˥		˻
AIR CONDUCTION - SOUND FIELD		S	

*The fine vertical lines represent the vertical axis of an audiogram.

TABLE 1. Recommended symbols for threshold audiometry. Unless otherwise specified, symbols are to indicate that test signals used were pure tones. The same symbols may be used for warble tones and narrow-band noise, if so noted on the audiogram.

MODALITY	EAR*		
	RIGHT	BOTH	LEFT
AIR CONDUCTION - EARPHONES UNMASKED	O̷		X̷
MASKED	△̷		▢̷
BONE CONDUCTION - MASTOID UNMASKED	<̷		>̷
MASKED	[̷		]̷
BONE CONDUCTION - FOREHEAD UNMASKED		∨̷	
MASKED	˥̷		˻̷
AIR CONDUCTION - SOUND FIELD		S̷	

*The fine vertical lines represent the vertical axis of an audiogram.

TABLE 2. Recommended "no response" symbols for threshold audiometry.

[2]Although the Committee favored placing the bone-conduction symbols to the right of the frequency axis to indicate the right ear and to the left to indicate the left ear, which was the most common preference reported by the Kopra and Martin (1970) survey, it adopted the reverse format, which is right of the frequency axis for the left ear and left of the frequency axis for the right ear. This decision was made, partly, on arbitrary bases and, partly, in deference to the preferences expressed by representatives of the American Academy of Ophthalmology and Otolaryngology (AAOO). The rationale for the second most common system reported by Martin and Kopra is that the BC symbol should represent the patient's ears from perspective of the otolaryngologist facing the patient (Fowler, 1951) and the prevalence of similar notation systems depicting the human form found in medical records and medical examination forms.

Audiogram Key

for the

Charts Below

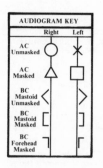

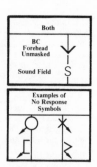

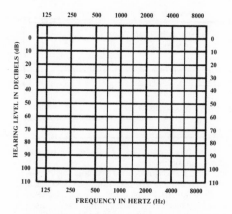

Figure 1. The audiogram form, showing appropriate dimensions. Note 20 dB on the ordinate equals an octave on the abscissa.

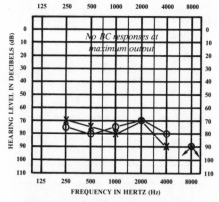

Figure 3. The use of masked bone-conduction (BC) symbols for the left and right ears and masked air-conduction (AC) symbols for the left ear. Note that the left ear BC symbols are to the right of the ordinates and the right ear BC symbols are to the left of the ordinates.

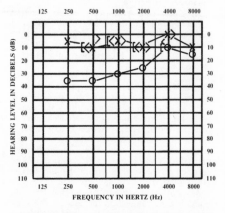

Figure 2. The use of symbols for masked bone-conduction (BC) thresholds for the right ear at 500 Hz, 1000 Hz, and 2000 Hz. Note that the BC brackets for the right ear are to the left of the ordinates and that the masked BC symbols are to the left of the unmasked symbol.

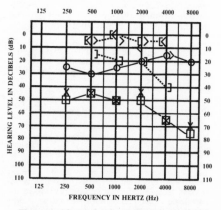

Figure 4. Air-conduction (AC) "no response" symbols (8000 Hz) and use of written "no response" notation.

176

**Audiogram Key
for the
Charts Below**

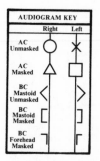

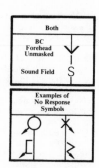

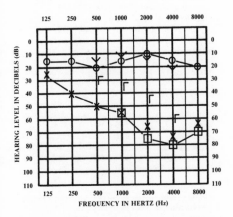

Figure 5. The use of masked and unmasked forehead bone-conduction (BC) symbols.

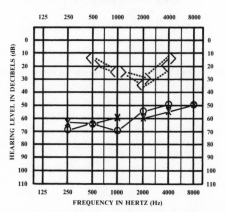

Figure 7. Air- and bone-conduction (AC and BC) symbols when bone-conduction thresholds were lower than air conduction.

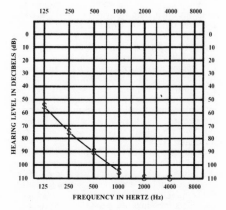

Figure 6. The use of air-conduction (AC) sound field symbols.

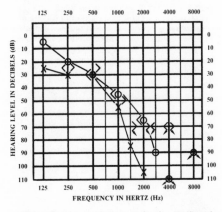

Figure 8. Air- and bone-conduction (AC and BC) symbols when thresholds were similar. The option was taken not to connect bone-conduction symbols because of the similarity. Symbols are shown for AC and BC when no response was obtained at high frequencies.

No Response. To indicate "no response" at the maximum output of the audiometer, an arrow should be attached to the lower outside corner of the appropriate symbol and drawn downward and at about 45° outward from the frequency axis—to the right for left-ear symbols and to the left for right-ear symbols. The arrow for sound-field or unmasked forehead bone-conduction symbol should be attached at the bottom and drawn straight downward.

The "no response" symbol should be placed on the audiogram at the HL representing the maximum output limit for the particular test frequency, test modality, and audiometer. Each of the "no response" symbols is shown in Table 2. Appropriate usage is illustrated in Figures 4, 6, and 8.

When a patient has many "no responses," notation other than by symbol may be used to conserve time and to avoid unnecessary cluttering of the audiogram, as shown in Figure 4. For example, when a patient fails to hear by bone conduction at maximum audiometric output, this finding may be expressed on the audiogram by writing "No BC responses at maximum output," rather than drawing a series of "no response" symbols on the audiogram. Another example is the patient who responds only at low frequencies. This may be summarized by writing "No responses obtained above 500 Hz at maximum output."

Responses to tactile sensation should not be plotted on an audiogram. If it is not possible to determine whether the patient's responses reflect tactile sensation or auditory sensation (or both), the examiner should make a prominent notation on the audiogram to alert the viewer to the possibility that the responses were confounded with vibrotactile sensation (Nober, 1964; 1967).

Lines Connecting Symbols. Lines may be used to connect the symbols on an audiogram. When used, a solid line should connect the air-conduction threshold values (Figures 2 through 8). Bone-conduction symbols may be connected by a dashed line when an air-bone gap exists (Figures 3 and 7). Otherwise, bone-conduction symbols should not be connected (Figures 2 and 8). The clarity of the audiogram will be improved if connecting lines approach, but do not touch or pass through symbols.

Symbols representing "no response" for air conduction or bone conduction should not be connected to each other or to any of the response symbols (Figures 4, 6, and 8).

Color Coding. Color coding is not necessary to transmit information about sidedness in this symbol system. In practice it may be desirable to avoid color coding because of the increasing use of multiple-copy audiograms and photoduplication of audiograms. However, if color is employed, red should be used for the right-ear symbols and connecting lines and blue for the left-ear symbols and connecting lines, with a third color used for the "both ears" symbols.

References

American National Standard Specifications for Audiometers (ANSI S3.6-1969). New York: American National Standards Institute, Inc. (1970).

Fowler, E. P., Signs, emblems and symbols of choice in plotting threshold audiograms. *Arch. Otolaryng,* 53, 129–133 (1951).

Martin, F. N., and Kopra, L. L., Symbols in pure-tone audiometry. *Asha,* 12, 182–185 (1970).

Newby, H. A., *Audiology.* (3rd ed.) New York: Appleton-Century-Crofts, 71–115 (1972).

Nober, E. H., Pseudoauditory bone conduction thresholds. *J. Speech Hearing Dis.,* 29, 469–476 (1964).

Nober, E. H., Vibrotactile sensitivity of deaf children to high intensity sound. *Laryngoscope,* 77, 2128–2146 (1967).

Sweetman, R. H., and Miller, M. L., What's the symbol? Paper presented at the Annual Convention of the American Speech and Hearing Association, Chicago (1969).

Norma S. Rees is Associate Editor of SPECIAL REPORTS. She is assisted in the review of SPECIAL REPORTS for the journal by the following editorial consultants: Irving Hochberg, Mary B. Mann, Michael I. Rolnick, James Yates, and Joanne Yates. Readers who wish to submit material or make suggestions for this department are urged to contact her at the City University of New York, Doctoral Program in Speech and Hearing Sciences, 33 West 42nd St., New York, New York 10036.

Appendix IV

GLOSSARY OF TINNITUS TERMS

acousma (ah-kooz'mah) *n.* tinnitus, head noises, esp. when considered an auditory hallucination.

acuphenes (ah-ku-fe'nus) *n.* tinnitus.

angioma (an"je-o'mah) *n.* a tumor involving blood vessels. A possible cause of tinnitus.

arterial tinnitus. head noises believed to result from blood-flow disturbances within the external or middle ear. Type of objective tinnitus. Also called venous tinnitus.

arthritis (ar-thri'tis) *n.* inflammation of a joint. Tinnitus may accompany this disease.

aspirin (as'pĭ-rin) *n.* salicylic acid. Drug used for the relief of pain. It is ototoxic for some individuals. Tinnitus may be the first indication of sensitivity.

ATA. American Tinnitus Association.

auditory hallucination. sensation of hearing something when there is no external auditory stimulus. Sometimes considered a form of tinnitus.

aural murmurs. tinnitus. Noises originating within the ear.

autogenesis (aw"to-jen'ĕ-sis) *n.* self-produced. This phenomenon forms the basis for biofeedback—sometimes used in the treatment of tinnitus. *adj*: **autogenic.**

biofeedback. electronic instruments are used to detect and amplify signals from the body, which the individual is trained to use in modifying specific physiological functions and emotional reactions. One application is in the management of tinnitus.

ceruminosis (sĕ-roo"mĭ-no'sis) *n.* excessive formation of ear wax. May cause objective tinnitus.

cholesteatoma (ko"le-ste"ah-to'mah) *n.* tumor or cyst that forms in the middle ear or deeper portion of the external auditory canal. Considered in tinnitus problems.

chondroma (kon-dro'mah) *n.* benign cartilaginous tumor: a possible cause of tinnitus.

cinchonism (sin'co-nizm) *n.* temporary deafness, ringing in the ears, headaches, etc., caused by the use of cinchona or its alkaloid derivatives (such as quinine).

clicking tinnitus. another name for Leudet's spasmodic head noises or Leudet's tinnitus. *syn*: objective tinnitus.

clonus (klo'nus) *n.* muscular spasm characterized by rapid alternation of contraction and relaxation. Possible cause of objective tinnitus.

cochlear hydrops (hi'drops). accumulation of fluid in the cochlea; a possible cause of tinnitus.

cochlear implant. electronic device designed to stimulate the hearing mechanism. It utilizes a coil of wire embedded under the skin behind the ear with an extension of wire into the fluid of the inner ear (cochlea). It is activated by an amplifier, similar to a body-type hearing aid, carried in a pocket. There is sometimes a side benefit in that tinnitus is reduced.

Cogan's syndrome. disease involving connective tissue; characterized by tinnitus, vertigo, deafness, blurred vision, or blindness.

deafferentation (de-af"er-en-ta'shun) *n.* severance of an afferent nerve. Sometimes tried for relief of tinnitus.

endolymphatic hydrops. malfunction of hearing and balance caused by excessive inner ear fluids. Often accompanied by tinnitus. *syn*: Meniere's disease or syndrome; labyrinthine hydrops.

glomus jugular tumor. a painful tumor that may occur in the middle ear. It tends to be more painful with each pulsation of blood and may be involved in objective tinnitus.

glomus tympanicum. glomus jugular tumor.

hallucinosis (hah-lu"sĭ-no'sis) *n.* the condition of having auditory hallucinations.

hangover tinnitus. as the name suggests, tinnitus that results from the intake of too much alcohol.

head noises. tinnitus, especially when considered an auditory hallucination.

hysterical deafness. nonorganic or functional hearing loss sometimes unconsciously developed as a result of subjective tinnitus.

intractable tinnitus. tinnitus that is resistant to any type of relief or treatment.

labyrinthine hydrops. endolymphatic hydrops. Meniere's disease.

labyrinthitis (lab"ĭ-rin-thi'tis) *n.* inflammation of the labyrinth. A suspect in tinnitus.

Leudet's tinnitus (Theodore E. Leudet, French physician, 1825-1887). spasmodic clicking head noises arising from muscular spasms near the eustachian tube. *syn*: objective tinnitus.

maskability (mask"ah-bil'ĭ-te) *n.* capable of being masked. Most often used to refer to the possibility of masking out annoying tinnitus.

Meniere's disease or **syndrome** (men"e-arz') (Prosper Meniere, French physician, 1799-1862). endolymphatic hydrops—the malfunction of hearing and balance caused by excessive inner ear fluids. Intermittent symptoms include tinnitus, dizziness, nausea, and progressive deafness. *syn*: labyrinthine hydrops.

179

minimum masking level. MML. as used in tinnitus studies, the lowest level of intensity of the selected band or bands of noise that will effectively mask out the tinnitus.

myringitis (mir″in-ji′tis) *n.* inflammation of the eardrum. Sometimes suspected in tinnitus.

myxedema (mik″sĕ-de′mah) *n.* disorder caused by thyroid deficiency. Symptoms include subcutaneous edema, drying of skin, loss of hair, and muscular weakness. A possible cause of tinnitus.

niacin (ni′ah-sin) *n.* nicotinic acid—an acid of the vitamin-B complex. Used in some cases of deafness, tinnitus, and Meniere's syndrome.

niacinamide (ni″ah-sin′am-īd) *n.* a nicotinic acid similar to niacin but causes less flushing.

nicotinamide (ni″ko-tin′ah-mīd) *n.* one of the vitamin-B complexes used in the same manner as nicotinic acid.

nicotinic acid (nik″o-tin′ik). an acid of the vitamin-B complex. A vasodilator sometimes used in cases of deafness, tinnitus, and Meniere's syndrome.

nonvibratory tinnitus. subjective tinnitus—head noises that can be heard only by the patient.

objective tinnitus. head noises arising from muscular spasms or blood-flow disturbances within the external or middle ear. Rare in occurrence, they may be audible to the examiner through the use of a stethoscope. *syn:* clicking tinnitus, Leudet's tinnitus, or vibrating tinnitus.

osteosarcoma (os″te-o-sar-ko′mah) *n.* a malignant bony growth. A tinnitus suspect.

otitis media (o-ti′tis me′de-ah). inflammation involving the middle ear.

otosclerosis (o″to-skle-ro′sis) *n.* bony disease involving the middle ear, with progressive loss of hearing; characterized by the growth of spongy bone around the stapes and oval window. *adj:* **otosclerotic.**

palatal myoclonus. muscular spasm of the soft palate. It may be heard through an ear to ear tube as a click within the patient's ear and may be a symptom of a brain stem lesion. A type of objective tinnitus.

paracusia imaginaria (par-ah-ku′se-ah ī-maj-ī-nar′e-ah). head noises; tinnitus.

residual inhibition. term coined by Jack A. Vernon, PhD, to describe a phenomenon that may or may not occur after removal of a sound used to mask tinnitus: A partial attenuation or complete absence of tinnitus for periods of time that may vary with the individual.

salicylate (sal′ī-sil″āt, sah-lis′ī-lāt) *n.* a salt of salicylic acid.

salicylic acid (sal″ī-sil′ik as′id). as a water-soluble white powder, it is the base for aspirin.

salicylism (sal′ī-sil″izm) *n.* poisoning caused by salicylic acid or one of its derivatives or salicylates. One symptom is tinnitus, others are nausea and vomiting.

schwannoma (schwon-no′mah) *n.* a small tumor involving a nerve sheath.

sonitus (son′ī-tus) *n.* another name for tinnitus.

subjective idiopathic tinnitus. term referring to the consideration of subjective tinnitus as resulting from an unknown disease or cause.

subjective tinnitus. head noises that can be heard only by the patient. Compare with objective tinnitus. *syn:* nonvibratory tinnitus.

susurrus arium (su-sur′us aw′re-um). ear whispers. Noises originating within the ear itself. Tinnitus.

tinnitus (tĭ-ni′tus) *n.* noises originating within the ear itself. One or both ears may be involved. If it can be heard by the examiner through an ear-to-ear tube or stethoscope, it is known as "objective" tinnitus; if it can only be heard by the patient, it is known as "subjective" tinnitus.

tinnitus aurium. little bells in the ear.

tinnitus cerebri (ser′ĕ-bre). subjective tinnitus not localized to either or both ears.

tinnitus cranii (kra′ne-i). tinnitus cerebri.

tinnitus instrument. a device that combines a hearing aid and tinnitus masker in one unit.

tinnitus masker. an amplifying instrument shaped like a hearing aid but engineered to generate a band of white noise designed to mask out an individual's tinnitus. Also sometimes used to help a stutterer attain fluency.

tinnitus research audiometer. TRA. a term sometimes applied to an instrument designed to determine the pitch and intensity of the individual's tinnitus.

tsutsugamushi disease (soot″soo-gah-moosh′e). a disease resembling typhoid fever caused by a rickettsia transmitted by a larval mite. Tinnitus sometimes accompanies other symptoms.

tympanophonia (tim″pah-no-fo′ne-ah) *n.* 1. tinnitus—noises within the ear. 2. autophony—ability of a person to hear his own voice louder than normally when the eustachian tube is unusually open; *syn:* tympanophony.

tympanophony (tim″pan-ah′fon-e) *n.* tympanophonia.

vascular tumor. a tumor involving blood vessels. A possible cause of tinnitus. *syn:* angioma.

venous tinnitus. head noises believed to result from blood-flow disturbances within the external or middle ear. A type of objective tinnitus. *syn:* arterial tinnitus.

vestibular neuronitis (ves-tib'u-lar nu"ro-ni'tis). inflammation of the vestibular nerve cells of the ear. A possible cause of tinnitus.

vibrating or vibratory tinnitus. better known as objective tinnitus, these noises in the ear can be heard by the examiner through an ear-to-ear tube.

xanthomatosis (zan"tho-mah-to'sis) n. a metabolic disorder marked by deposits of yellow or orange nodules in the skin. It is sometimes associated with tinnitus.

Appendix V

OTOTOXIC SUBSTANCES

Certain drugs and other substances are often suspected of being the cause of mild-to-severe hearing impairments, tinnitus, or both. Some drugs are said to cause problems when injected but not when taken orally. Some persons are more susceptible than others to a particular substance. Some items on the following list are not generally considered as drugs, but still may affect or cause tinnitus: e.g., alcohol, nicotine, caffeine. The aminoglycoside antibiotics are especially dangerous in combination with certain diuretics.

An asterisk (*) indicates drugs suspected of causing prenatal damage during the sixth and seventh weeks of pregnancy. Others may cause problems if used within the first trimester of pregnancy, especially during the sixth and seventh weeks: meprobamates [Miltown, Equanil]; chlordiazepoxides [Librax, Librium]; antinausea preparations [Antivert, Bonine, Marezine].

alcohol
amikacin
aniline dyes
antipyrene
aspirin
barbiturates
benzene
caffeine (coffee, tea, many soft drinks)
camphor
carbon disulfide
carbon monoxide
cephaloridine
chloramphenicol
chloroform
chloroquinine
*dihydrostreptomycin
ethacrynic acid
ergot
furosemide
*gentamycin
hydrochlorothiazide
iodine

iodoform
*kanamycin
lead
mannitol
mercaptomerin sodium
mercuhydrin
mercury
morphine
*neomycin
nicotine (tobacco)
nitrobenzol
novocain
*paromomycin
polymyxin B
polymyxin E
*quinine
salicylates (aspirin)
*streptomycin
sulfa drugs
*tobramycin
*vancomycin
*viomycin

Appendix VI

PARTS OF THE EARMOLD

DESCRIPTIONS

Tubing Types:

Canal—Canal portion only.

Canal-Lock—Canal with one half of concha rim.

Half-Shell—Same as Shell but with bowl extending only half way to helix.

High Frequency—One that allows the maximum volume of air between the receiver nub, or tubing connection, and the tympanic membrane.

Non-Occluding—One that leaves the ear canal open to the outside air. Often called an "open mold."

Shell—Consists of canal and a thin shell covering bowl of ear. May be with or without helix.

Skeleton—Consists of canal, complete concha rim and bridge. May be without helix.

¾ Skeleton—Same as the Skeleton but with the central portion of the concha rim removed.

Semi-Skeleton—Consists of canal, bridge, and helix. No concha rim.

Direct Coupled Type:

Receiver—Full solid mold with metal snap ring or other attachment to hold a receiver directly onto the earmold.

All-In-The-Ear—Designed to hold an all-in-the-ear instrument in the ear.

PARTS OF THE EARMOLD:

Anti-Helix—That part of the earmold that extends into the anti-helix of the ear.

Bowl—That part of a Shell mold covering the bowl of the ear.

Bridge—That part extending from the canal to the junction of the concha rim and the helix.

Canal—That part that goes into the ear canal.

Concha Rim—That part of the Skeleton mold that extends from the canal to the helix and fits into the concha of the ear.

Flare—A funnel-shaped enlargement of the sound bore at the end of the canal.

Heel—That part lying between the tragus and the anti-tragus.

Helix—That part extending into the helix of the ear.

Receiver Base—That part on which the base of the receiver rests.

Receiver Cavity—The sound chamber directly beneath the receiver nub.

Sound Bore—The hole extending through the canal to the tubing connection on the receiver nub.

Vent—Any hole giving free passage of air to the sound bore or to the ear canal.

Small Vent—One with a diameter of .040".

Medium Vent—One with a diameter of .082".

Large Vent—One with a diameter of .128".

Diagonal Vent—A vent that enters the sound bore below the tubing or receiver nub.

External Vent—An external groove or opening leading from the outside air to the ear canal.

Parallel Vent—A vent that does not enter the sound bore, but terminates at the end of the earmold canal.

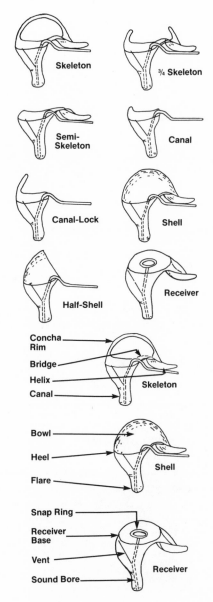

SYRINGE METHOD OF EARMOLD IMPRESSIONS

Courtesy of Robert Hocks, Hocks Laboratories and
National Association of Earmold Laboratories.

THE SYRINGE METHOD . . .
varies from the hand method in that you use the material in a softer state and that you use a syringe to inject the material rather than by hand. Place the liquid into the cup or bowl and add the powder. Spatulate until the liquid and powder have formed a soupy mix and then transfer immediately into the barrel of the syringe which can be done with a "stir pack" or spatulate. The ability to use the material while it is still extremely soft will partially help eliminate the problem of distorting a flexible ear. It should be pointed out that the softer material is obtained by mixing the material for less duration than in the hand method, not by using more liquid or less powder. NEVER CHANGE THE RECOMMENDED PRO-PORTIONS OF MATERIAL.

IMPRESSION . . .
should be allowed to remain in the ear for a minimum of 10 minutes.

TO REMOVE THE IMPRESSION . . .
grasp the bulk of the material with one hand, and with the other hand, begin to press or peel the edges of the ear back and away from the impression. Slowly begin to rotate the top of the impression forward towards the nose which will disengage the concha and helix area. This forward motion should also be accompanied with a outward motion away from the head. This removal should be slow so as to not stretch or tear the canal portion or form a vacuum. The cottom dam should come out attached to the end of the canal section. If the cotton dam should remain in the ear, proceed to remove it by using the thread attached to the cotton. Always use your otoscope for a final inspection of the ear before dismissing the client.

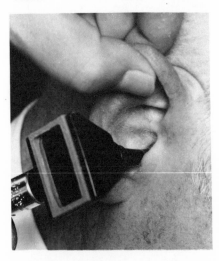

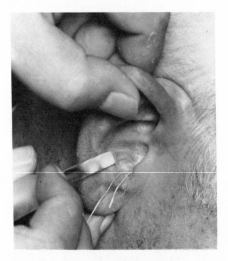

Step I
Make a thorough inspection of the ear with an otoscope.

Step II
A cotton block of correct size is an absolute necessity when using the syringe. Set the cotton block just past the second bend.

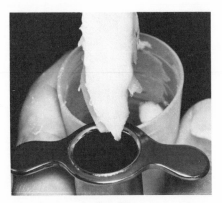

Step III

Thoroughly mix impression material and place in the barrel with the spatula while it is still "soupy". The quicker you can use the material, the better the impression.

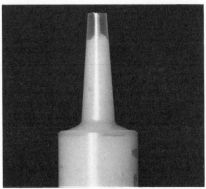

Step IV

Insert the plunger and force the material to within ¼" of the end of the nozzle to eliminate air pockets.

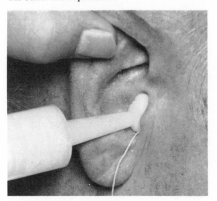

Step V

Place the tip of the nozzle ¼" into the canal entrance and force the material through the syringe into the canal.

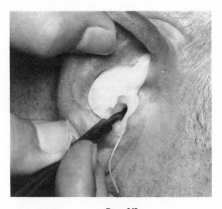

Step VI

After filling the canal and conch and helix, the little finger or "stir-pack" tool can be used to fully pack the canal if needed.

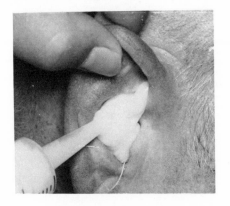

Step VII

"Shoot" the remaining material into the conch, helix and tragus area.

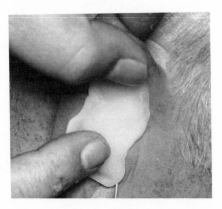

Step VIII

Lightly firm the material into the ear with the fingers to eliminate air pockets. Be careful not to distort the ear or the impression.

AMERICAN SPONDAIC AND PB WORD LISTS

Modern speech tests evolved largely from word lists developed during World War II for use in Army and Navy Aural Rehabilitation Centers. Auditory Test No. 9 was standardized for this purpose in the Psycho-Acoustic Laboratory (PAL) of Harvard University during 1943-1944. Report No. 2802 of the Office of Scientific Research and Development (OSRD) contained the results of this study.

J. P. Egan used that report as the basis for an article, "Articulation Testing Methods", which appeared in *Laryngoscope*, Vol. 58: 955-991, 1948. Included were two lists of 42 words each:

PAL SPONDEE LIST 1

1. airplane	15. doorstep	29. oatmeal
2. armchair	16. dovetail	30. outlaw
3. backbone	17. drawbridge	31. playground
4. bagpipe	18. earthquake	32. railroad
5. baseball	19. eggplant	33. shipwreck
6. birthday	20. eyebrow	34. shotgun
7. blackboard	21. firefly	35. sidewalk
8. bloodhound	22. hardware	36. stairway
9. bobwhite	23. headlight	37. sunset
10. bonbon	24. hedgehog	38. watchword
11. buckwheat	25. hothouse	39. whitewash
12. coughdrop	26. inkwell	40. wigwam
13. cowboy	27. mousetrap	41. wildcat
14. cupcake	28. northwest	42. woodwork

PAL SPONDEE LIST 2

1. although	15. hotdog	29. playmate
2. beehive	16. housework	30. scarecrow
3. blackout	17. iceberg	31. schoolboy
4. cargo	18. jackknife	32. soybean
5. cookbook	19. lifeboat	33. starlight
6. daybreak	20. midway	34. sundown
7. doormat	21. mishap	35. therefore
8. duckpond	22. mushroom	36. toothbrush
9. eardrum	23. nutmeg	37. vampire
10. farewell	24. outside	38. washboard
11. greyhound	25. padlock	39. whizzbang
12. footstool	26. pancake	40. woodchuck
13. grandson	27. pinball	41. workshop
14. horseshoe	28. platform	42. yardstick

At the Central Institute for the Deaf (CID) in St. Louis, MO, 36 of the more familiar words were selected from the 84 in the PAL lists and scrambled into six lists for Auditory Tests W-1 and W-2. These tests were developed under contracts with the Office of Naval Research and the Veterans Administration. Alphabetically, the words so selected were:

SPONDEES USED IN AUDITORY TESTS W-1 AND W-2

1. airplane	13. greyhound	25. padlock
2. armchair	14. hardware	26. pancake
3. baseball	15. headlight	27. playground
4. birthday	16. horseshoe	28. railroad
5. cowboy	17. hotdog	29. schoolboy
6. daybreak	18. hothouse	30. sidewalk
7. doormat	19. iceberg	31. stairway
8. drawbridge	20. inkwell	32. sunset
9. duckpond	21. mousetrap	33. toothbrush
10. eardrum	22. mushroom	34. whitewash
11. farewell	23. northwest	35. woodwork
12. grandson	24. oatmeal	36. workshop

Phonograph records containing the scrambled lists are available from Technisonic Studios, Inc., 1201 So. Brentwood Blvd., Richmond Heights, MO 63117. Auditory Test W-1 was recorded at a constant level of intensity with the carrier phrase at a 10 dB higher level than the words themselves. The intensity level of every three words in the recording of Auditory Test W-2 is reduced three dB from the preceding three words.

The W-1 lists A and B (with the exception of the word "airplane") are available on reel tape from the Los Angeles Foundation of Otology, 2130 W. Third St., Los Angeles, CA 90057. These tape recordings are commonly referred to as "LAFO speech test tapes."

Cassette tapes of the LAFO recordings are available from the Audiotone Division of Lear Siegler Industries, P.O. Box 2905, Phoenix, AZ 85062. One side has W-1 lists A and B. The other side has four selections from the W-22 PB word lists. The speaker on the LAFO tapes is Richard Hughes, PhD.

A cassette tape also available from Audiotone contains the multiple-choice sentence tests of discrimination developed by Kenneth W. Berger, PhD. The speaker on these tapes is James H. Delk.

Word lists for discrimination tests as well as threshold tests were also prepared by the Psycho-Acoustic Laboratory. These lists formed the basis for the Auditory Test W-2, also developed at the Central Institute for the Deaf under contracts with the Office of Naval Research and the Veterans Administration.

Four sets of 50 one-syllable familiar words were selected and arranged in such a manner that all the speech sounds of American English appear in about the same ratio as they would in ordinary conversation. These so-called "phonetically-balanced" word lists have been randomized and are those commonly used to determine speech discrimination scores (SDS) or the "PB-Max".

J. P. Egan, in his original work, presented 20 phonetically balanced lists, each containing 50 one-syllable words. These lists, however, have been largely supplanted by the CID lists.

The following are the words used at the Central Institute for the Deaf, St. Louis, MO for Auditory Test No. W-22:

PB LIST 1

1. ace	11. day	21. it	31. owl	41. toe
2. ache	12. deaf	22. jam	32. poor	42. true
3. an	13. earn (urn)	23. knees	33. ran	43. twins
4. as	14. east	24. law	34. see (sea)	44. yard
5. bathe	15. felt	25. low	35. she	45. up
6. bells	16. give	26. me	36. skin	46. us
7. carve	17. high	27. mew	37. stove	47. wet
8. chew	18. him	28. none (nun)	38. them	48. what
9. could	19. hunt	29. not (knot)	39. there (their)	49. wire
10. dad	20. isle (aisle)	30. or (oar)	40. thing	50. you (ewe)

PB LIST 2

1. ail (ale)	11. dumb	21. ill	31. off	41. that
2. air (heir)	12. ease	22. jaw	32. one (won)	42. then
3. and	13. eat	23. key	33. own	43. thin
4. bin (been)	14. else	24. knee	34. pew	44. too (two, to)
5. by (buy)	15. flat	25. live (verb)	35. rooms	45. tree
6. cap	16. gave	26. move	36. send	46. way (weigh)
7. cars	17. ham	27. new (knew)	37. show	47. well
8. chest	18. hit	28. now	38. smart	48. with
9. die (dye)	19. hurt	29. oak	39. star	49. yore (your)
10. does	20. ice	30. odd	40. tare (tear)	50. young

PB LIST 3

1. add (ad)	11. done (dun)	21. is	31. out	41. this
2. aim	12. dull	22. jar	32. owes	42. though
3. are	13. ears	23. king	33. pie	43. three
4. ate (eight)	14. end	24. knit	34. raw	44. tie
5. bill	15. farm	25. lie (lye)	35. say	45. use (yews)
6. book	16. glove	26. may	36. shove	46. we
7. camp	17. hand	27. nest	37. smooth	47. west
8. chair	18. have	28. no (know)	38. start	48. when
9. cute	19. he	29. oil	39. tan	49. wool
10. do	20. if	30. on	40. ten	50. year

PB LIST 4

1. aid	11. clothes	21. his	31. ought (aught)	41. through
2. all (awl)	12. cook	22. in (inn)	32. our	42. tin
3. am	13. darn	23. jump	33. pale (pail)	43. toy
4. arm	14. dolls	24. leave	34. save	44. where
5. art	15. dust	25. men	35. shoe	45. who
6. at	16. ear	26. my	36. so (sew)	46. why
7. bee (be)	17. eyes (ayes)	27. near	37. stiff	47. will
8. bread (bred)	18. few	28. net	38. tea (tee)	48. wood (would)
9. can	19. go	29. nuts	39. than	49. yes
10. chin	20. hang	30. of	40. they	50. yet

Phonograph and tape recordings of Auditory Test W-22 are available from the same sources as were noted above for Auditory Tests W-1 and W-2.

The PAL recordings available from the Technisonic Studios are voiced by Rush Hughes. Ira Hirsh is the speaker on the CID W-22 lists. Additional word tests will be found in the appendices to:

Hearing and Deafness, edited by Hallowell Davis and S. Richard Silverman (New York, Holt, Rinehart and Winston, 4th Ed.)

Audiology, Hayes A. Newby (New York, Appleton-Century-Crofts, 4th Ed.)

Appendix IX

SPEECH DISCRIMINATION TESTS

By presently accepted definition, all 50 words of a W-22 list must be voiced in order to get an accurate maximum speech discrimination score. Since this is often a tiring experience, a shorter monosyllabic, phonetically-balanced, word list to be used as a speech discrimination test was developed by Lawrence J. Deutsch, PhD, and Barbara Kruger, MA.

The abstract of the article, "The Clinical Use of 25 Word Auditory Discrimination Tests" for *The Journal of Auditory Research* reads as follows:

"A point biserial correlation technique was employed to systematically select 25 monosyllables which will approximate the whole list W-2 Score. Twenty-five word lists were derived from W-22 lists 1C and 2C using a clinical population (N = 75); the derived lists correlated .97 and .98 with the original lists. The whole and derived lists were then administered to a new clinical population (N = 34); main difference of less than one percent and correlation coefficients of .95 and .88 were found."

DERIVED LIST 1C-25

1. true	8. toe	15. us	22. none (nun)
2. give	9. felt	16. poor	23. stove
3. as	10. yard	17. ran	24. what
4. skin	11. could	18. carve	25. me
5. jam	12. twins	19. deaf	
6. east	13. earn	20. knees	
7. she	14. ace	21. you (ewe)	

DERIVED LIST 2C-25

1. smart	8. dumb	15. tree	22. else
2. off	9. flat	16. yore (your)	23. ease
3. does	10. star	17. by (buy)	24. gave
4. one (won)	11. well	18. rooms	25. show
5. move	12. send	19. own	
6. way (weigh)	13. die (dye)	20. cars	
7. oak	14. key	21. cap	

Appendix X

PBK WORD LISTS

To facilitate speech discrimination testing with young children, Harriet L. Haskins (formerly of Johns Hopkins Hospital) developed special word lists as part of her Master's thesis at Northwestern University. They are presented here through her cooperation.

The PBK Lists are a phonetically balanced test of speech discrimination for children, developed according to Egan's formula of phonetic composition and vocabulary items common to the International Kindergarten Union List and the Harvard PB-50 Test. They were studied for effectiveness in developing an articulation curve and were calibrated against the Harvard List 13 which has the best degree of phonic balance of that group. All lists were found to meet the requirements of an articulation curve.

For expediency in clinical use with young patients the following lists of 50 items have been divided according to phonetic balance formula and randomized into two equal lists of 25 words.

PBK List 1

1. please	26. smile
2. great	27. bath
3. sled	28. slip
4. pants	29. ride
5. rat	30. end
6. bad	31. pink
7. pinch	32. thank
8. such	33. take
9. bus	34. cart
10. need	35. scab
11. ways	36. lay
12. five	37. class
13. mouth	38. me
14. rag	39. dish
15. put	40. neck
16. fed	41. beef
17. fold	42. few
18. hunt	43. use
19. no	44. did
20. box	45. hit
21. are	46. pond
22. teach	47. hot
23. slice	48. own
24. is	49. bead
25. tree	50. shop

PBK List 2

1. this	26. toe
2. ma	27. south
3. pick	28. rest
4. glove	29. tongue
5. gun	30. best
6. forth	31. reach
7. trade	32. slide
8. each	33. food
9. ask	34. new
10. wake	35. ball
11. calf	36. three
12. rope	37. closed
13. night	38. kept
14. chew	39. off
15. guess	40. sick
16. wave	41. thread
17. cloud	42. day
18. good	43. feel
19. barn	44. wood
20. left	45. pig
21. shoe	46. crack
22. flag	47. dime
23. rode	48. wash
24. hook	49. and
25. front	50. look

PBK List 3

1. laugh	26. path
2. falls	27. feed
3. paste	28. next
4. plow	29. wreck
5. page	30. waste
6. weed	31. crab
7. gray	32. peg
8. park	33. freeze
9. wait	34. race
10. fat	35. bud
11. ax	36. darn
12. cage	37. fair
13. knife	38. sack
14. turn	39. got
15. grab	40. as
16. rose	41. grew
17. lip	42. knee
18. bee	43. fresh
19. bet	44. tray
20. his	45. cat
21. sing	46. on
22. all	47. camp
23. bless	48. find
24. suit	49. yes
25. splash	50. loud

PBK List 4

1. tire	26. most
2. seed	27. thick
3. purse	28. if
4. quick	29. them
5. room	30. sheep
6. bug	31. air
7. that	32. set
8. sell	33. dad
9. low	34. ship
10. rich	35. case
11. those	36. you
12. ache	37. may
13. black	38. choose
14. else	39. white
15. nest	40. frog
16. jay	41. bush
17. raw	42. clown
18. true	43. cab
19. had	44. hurt
20. cost	45. pass
21. vase	46. grade
22. press	47. blind
23. fit	48. drop
24. bounce	49. leave
25. wide	50. nuts

Appendix XI

SPANISH WORDS

A selection of Spanish monosyllabic and bisyllabic words, courtesy of Audiotone International, P.O. Box 6708, Metairie, LA 70009.

BISILABOS

1. carta	14. regla	27. tretas	40. cinco
2. huevo	15. rancho	28. luna	41. salsa
3. lado	16. galgo	29. sombra	42. costa
4. baile	17. granja	30. mano	43. doce
5. hambre	18. multa	31. frente	44. ostras
6. trampa	19. tanque	32. verdad	45. pasta
7. modo	20. finca	33. agua	46. culpa
8. burro	21. queso	34. veinte	47. rosca
9. guerra	22. hombro	35. boca	48. brusco
10. mesa	23. lengua	36. cestos	49. clima
11. caso	24. turno	37. pipas	50. joven
12. tema	25. sano	38. blusa	
13. bosque	26. broma	39. once	

MONOSILABOS

LISTA 1

1. den	26. lo
2. tras	27. ser
3. le	28. tan
4. ir	29. ve
5. un	30. das
6. nos	31. mis
7. soy	32. pan
8. ya	33. luz
9. vid	34. gris
10. voz	35. fin
11. dan	36. muy
12. tus	37. los
13. ver	38. des
14. se	39. flor
15. el	40. vas
16. san	41. del
17. ni	42. bar
18. don	43. te
19. la	44. con
20. res	45. es
21. paz	46. can
22. tres	47. di
23. por	48. sol
24. mal	49. mes
25. club	50. ton

LISTA 2

1. mil	26. dos
2. cruz	27. va
3. las	28. si
4. vez	29. les
5. da	30. gran
6. fe	31. ven
7. tu	32. tal
8. van	33. en
9. sin	34. pon
10. ron	35. mar
11. hay	36. ti
12. sur	37. me
13. pez	38. tos
14. gas	39. mas
15. no	40. sed
16. sus	41. col
17. yo	42. tren
18. flan	43. han
19. voy	44. su
20. dar	45. hoy
21. son	46. cal
22. vil	47. sud
23. par	48. rey
24. de	49. plan
25. sal	50. mi

Appendix XII

FRENCH WORDS

A selection of French words from the list used by audiologists at the Hotel-Dieu de Saint-Jerome of the Province of Quebec, Canada, and published with their permission.

AUDIOMETRIE VOCALE (ADULTES)

Liste de mots dissyllabiques

1. bouteille	13. chanteur	25. orange
2. serviette	14. servante	26. vaisselle
3. parole	15. fromage	27. farine
4. cousine	16. voiture	28. lavage
5. programme	17. journal	29. tambour
6. bataille	18. notaire	30. ceinture
7. village	19. valise	31. passable
8. dentelle	20. jalouse	32. chaloupe
9. sacoche	21. chasseur	33. rancune
10. cerise	22. chaussette	34. depart
11. fourchette	23. carotte	35. couloir
12. courir	24. docteur	36. horloge

Listes de mots PB (Adultes)

Liste A

1. bar	14. orgue	27. cogne	40. fourbe
2. gel	15. moule	28. prince	41. trouve
3. celle	16. joute	29. piece	42. cruche
4. creme	17. foungue	30. plus	43. bigle
5. guepe	18. fume	31. racle	44. style
6. cor	19. neige	32. phrase	45. crime
7. laide	20. chaude	33. quatre	46. brique
8. juche	21. cil	34. charme	47. trombe
9. pose	22. fiche	35. sable	48. grande
10. taupe	23. soeur	36. solde	49. voile
11. pour	24. rance	37. forte	50. ruine
12. coq	25. chatte	38. borne	
13. vole	26. mise	39. bourse	

Liste B

1. base	14. coute	27. poil	40. morte
2. chic	15. bouche	28. transe	41. sport
3. mince	16. douze	29. blonde	42. parle
4. range	17. toque	30. grippe	43. charge
5. veuf	18. loge	31. griffe	44. casque
6. bile	19. face	32. cirque	45. boucle
7. ligue	20. vague	33. givre	46. lettre
8. chose	21. gare	34. prune	47. clair
9. dome	22. meche	35. brute	48. plaire
10. sauf	23. cerf	36. couple	49. niece
11. ruche	24. herbe	37. course	50. rogne
12. mule	25. homme	38. snob	
13. doute	26. fuite	39. flore	

Liste de mots dissyllabiques (Enfants)

1. camion	13. soulier	25. citron
2. chapeau	14. raisin	26. fourneau
3. bateau	15. poulet	27. radis
4. toupie	16. agent	28. auto
5. bouchon	17. croissant	29. cochon
6. oiseau	18. manteau	30. tricot
7. fourmi	19. jambon	31. bouton
8. savon	20. lunettes	32. jardin
9. ciseau	21. bobine	33. crayon
10. marin	22. passoire	34. pliant
11. ballon	23. torchon	35. buffet
12. maison	24. tapis	36. couteau

Listes de mots PB (Enfants)

1. balle	14. broc	27. glace	40. soeur
2. bras	15. fleur	28. vase	41. yeux
3. noix	16. bleu	29. poire	42. peigne
4. pomme	17. sel	30. col	43. canne
5. seau	18. clef	31. faux	44. rape
6. feuille	19. nappe	32. meuble	45. poele
7. feu	20. bas	33. deux	46. coq
8. pelle	21. pois	34. fraise	47. dos
9. lait	22. botte	35. arbre	48. oeuf
10. bague	23. eau	36. tasse	49. queue
11. mat	24. beurre	37. boite	50. verre
12. doigt	25. noeud	38. bol	
13. brosse	26. chaise	39. pot	

Appendix XIII

GERMAN WORDS

A selection of German words, which appeared in an article by David F. Barr, PhD, "Speech Audiometry Materials," *Audecibel*, Summer 1969, pp. 115-117. Published with the permission of the author.

German spondee word list

Sonntag	Einfall	Ausgang	Stadtrat
Fernglas	Treibholz	Denkbar	Ruckblick
Rotkraut	Beispiel	Unfall	Landwirt
Vorhang	Ordnung	Bahnhof	Antwort
Fussball	Weinacht	Zeitung	Rundfunk

German PB word list

Mensch	Zug	manch	strich
Frau	Chor	Haus	trotz
Geld	von	nur	Zorn
Tisch	noch	kann	trost
mit	darf	Schuld	Weh
vier	Bett	Fest	gern
rot	Stamm	trub	bald
Saal	aus	fort	Sinn
Ruf	Blatt	Gast	Herz
rund	Bein	kaum	wohl
Larm	Platz	wohl	kund
frei	Seit	tief	Angst
Bahn	Wut		

Appendix XIV

PORTUGUESE WORDS

A selection of Portuguese monosyllabic words, courtesy of Prof. Pedro Luiz Mangabeira Albernaz, Av. Brig. Faria Lima, 830-3 andar-Conj. 31-01.452-Sao Paulo, Brazil.

MONOSSÍLABOS

Lista 1	Lista 2	Lista 3	Lista 4
1. til	1. chá	1. dor	1. jaz
2. jaz	2. dor	2. boi	2. cão
3. ról	3. meu	3. til	3. cal
4. pus	4. tom	4. fól	4. boi
5. faz	5. zum	5. gim	5. nu
6. gim	6. mel	6. cal	6. faz
7. rir	7. til	7. nhá	7. gim
8. boi	8. gim	8. chá	8. pus
9. vai	9. dil	9. tom	9. seis
10. mel	10. nu	10. sul	10. nhá
11. nu	11. pus	11. tem	11. meu
12. lhe	12. nhá	12. pus	12. tem
13. cal	13. sul	13. nu	13. zum
14. meu	14. jaz	14. cão	14. til
15. tem	15. ról	15. vai	15. lhe
16. dil	16. tem	16. mel	16. sul
17. dor	17. faz	17. rir	17. chá
18. chá	18. lhe	18. jaz	18. ról
19. zum	19. boi	19. zum	19. mel
20. nhá	20. cal	20. meu	20. dor
21. cão	21. rir	21. lhe	21. vai
22. tom	22. cão	22. ler	22. dil
23. seis	23. ler	23. faz	23. tom
24. ler	24. vai	24. seis	24. rir
25. sul	25. seis	25. dil	25. ler

Appendix XV

ARABIC AND HEBREW WORDS

Fig. 1 PHONETICALLY BALANCED WORD LISTS IN ARABIC AND HEBREW

Arabic	Hebrew	
1. בנת (ילדה)	מס	דבש
2. נום (חצי)	צחוק	צל
3. אח (ידיד)	דוד	סל
4. ראח (הלך)	עד	חוף
5. סבוע (סבוע)	איש	כס
6. יום (יום)	ג'א	סוג
7. עיד (חג)	יש	גן
8. שו (מה)	כר	גוש
9. כיף (איך)	דב	גר
10. צ'ורה (תמונה)	אם	כיס
11. בית (בית)	רק	זבוב
12. מו (יש)	גיר	יום
13. סף (כהה)	לול	תום
14. ג'מב (על יד)	גן	גז
15. מליח (טוב)	פין	דלי
16. כתאב (ספר)	סוס	עב
17. חוז (פח)	דן	סם
18. לוח (לוח)	בת	כרוך
19. ארד (רצפה)	כבר	כת
20. כאן (היח)	גבול	אך
	כלום	הן
	סהם	רוק
	סתיו	כלי
	דת	פרי
	גז	פתיל

Appendix XVI

GLOSSARY OF COMPUTER TERMINOLOGY

adder. an electronic circuit that provides a sum and carry when adding two numbers.

address. a pattern of characters that identifies a unique memory location.

algorithm. term used to specify the procedures by which a given result is obtained.

alphanumeric. a generic term for alphabet letters, numerical digits, and special characters that are machine-processable.

ALU. arithmetic and logic unit. A subsystem that can perform arithmetic and logical operations on data sent to it.

analog. analog circuitry; the term "linear" circuitry is also used. Circuitry that varies the intensity of the electricity continuously over a specific range. Analog computers are used in industry to measure or monitor fluid pressures, etc., as opposed to digital computers used for manipulating digitized information. In data communications using telephone lines, digital information is converted to analog to be carried on the telephone lines.

application program. a program designed to satisfy a user's requirements.

ASCII. pronounced "as key," an acronym for American Standard Code for Information Interchange. An eight-level code (seven bits plus parity bit).

assembler. a computer program that creates a machine language program from a user's symbolic language program.

asynchronous transmission. a transmission of data method by which each character is synchronized by a start and stop character. This method is a relatively slow procedure.

backup. software, hardware, or data retained in reserve in case one or more parts of a system fail or become lost.

base address. a beginning address from which a final address is derived by adding a relative (to zero) address.

BASIC (Beginners All-purpose Symbolic Instruction Code). a high-level language developed for ease of use. Easy to learn, BASIC has become a standard for mini-computers.

baud. a unit of signaling speed. Speed as expressed in bauds is equal to the number of bits passed per second.

bit. the smallest unit of information in a binary system of notation. A bit is either zero or one.

branch. a "go to" or branch instruction directs execution of an instruction other than the next sequential instruction.

buffer. a memory device or procedure used as intermediate storage to compensate for the differences in speeds between devices. Normally the input is much faster than the output. The input is called in to fill the buffer only when the data have been expended from the buffer to the slower output.

bug. an error in a program. It can be either incorrect coding or incorrect logic flow. To debug is to find and correct the bug.

bus. connectors that are parallel between components allowing faster data transfer than serial connectors.

byte. a group of bits acted upon by the computer as the smallest unit, usually eight bits. Larger computer systems use 16 or 32 bit bytes.

COBOL (Common Business Oriented Language). a higher level language for business applications using everyday English-like phrases. Requires more memory than BASIC.

CPU (Central Processor Unit). a section within the computer system containing the arithmetic unit, main storage (memory), and special registers. It performs and controls instruction processing and arithmetic functions.

CPS (characters per second). a measure of speed for input and output devices of a computer. The term is used to specify the handling speed of the device.

CRT (cathode ray tube). used to display images like a television. The CRT is used in conjunction with a keyboard to form a terminal device for the computer.

default. a condition which will exist from start-up or power-on unless specifically altered; i.e., a computer will assume that a printer is not attached at start-up. The computer must be told when the printer is available; therefore, the default for the printer is no (or off).

disk or **disc.** a magnetic plate-like medium used for storing information. The plate rotates much like a phonograph record but faster. Read/write heads can be positioned to transfer data in the form of magnetized bits. Many different types and sizes are available, with capacities in the millions of bytes.

digital. information in quantized or discrete form, not continuous or linear as in analog.

floppy disk. a flexible disk, 5″ or 8″ in diameter, in a heavy paper envelope. Slots allow reading and writing while the disk spins within the cushioned envelope. For-

---

Jack M. Delk, Director of Data Processing, Warren County, New York

merly known as a diskette. Normally used as a storage medium for minicomputers and as an input medium for larger computers. Storage capacity can be up to 1.2 million characters depending on type, and costs as little as $3.00.

full duplex. a device capable of transmitting and receiving at the same time. Usually requires four wires, two for transmission and two to receive.

gigo. short for "garbage in, garbage out," meaning that if you feed the computer misinformation, you'll get misinformation in return.

half duplex. a device capable of transmitting and receiving, but not at the same time. Two wires can be used instead of four.

handshaking. an exchange of predetermined signals used for establishing control between a computer and another device such as a terminal.

hard copy. machine-printed document or report.

hardware. the physical electronic and mechanical system including the computer, printer, disk drives, etc.

hexidecimal. a computer numbering system which is base 16, as opposed to base 10 for decimal:

8 4 2 1		value of bits	
		hexi-	
		decimal	decimal
0 0 0 0	=	0	0
0 0 0 1	=	1	1
0 0 1 0	=	2	2
0 0 1 1	=	3	3
0 1 0 0	=	4	4
0 1 0 1	=	5	5
0 1 1 0	=	6	6
0 1 1 1	=	7	7
1 0 0 0	=	8	8
1 0 0 1	=	9	9
1 0 1 0	=	A	10
1 0 1 1	=	B	11
1 1 0 0	=	C	12
1 1 0 1	=	D	13
1 1 1 0	=	E	14
1 1 1 1	=	F	15

Maximum value of four bits is F_{16} or 15_{10}. Maximum value of an eight-bit byte is FF_{16} or 255_{10}, or 256 separate numbers, letters, and special characters can be placed in an eight-bit byte.

host. a computer used as the main source of computation or data for satellite devices drawing upon it.

indexing. a method of indirectly addressing data. In an indexed table of data, the index pointers are relative to the first position of the table. In an indexed disk storage file, the index is a separate item containing a key of a wanted record and its address location on the disk.

integrated circuit. IC. a small component with electrical terminals containing a chip of silicon. The silicon surface is processed to form up to thousands of transistors, capacitors, resistors, and diodes connected to form an electronic circuit. The IC can be preprogrammed to be a microprocessor.

interface. v. to connect devices. n. a device used to allow unlike devices to communicate with each other.

job turn-around time. the time required to process a job from initial submission to final output.

kilobyte. usually expressed as "K" to denote memory capacity, and "KB" to denote capacity of a storage medium or its speed. One kilobyte is equivalent to 1024 bytes. The smallest of the microcomputers usually has a 4K memory—4096 bytes.

memory. the portion in the central processor unit where data and instructions can be stored and retrieved.

microcomputer. a small computer that uses a microprocessor for its CPU (central processor unit).

microprocessor. one or more ICs that can be programmed with stored instructions. The ICs contain at least a controller, some registers, and ALU being the basic components of a CPU.

minicomputer. a small computer system most often used for a specific application.

MODEM. a contraction of MOdulator/ DEModulator. A device that allows data to be transmitted and received using telephone lines. A MODEM is placed between a computer and the telephone lines at one end. At the other end is another MODEM, then another computer, terminal, or other device.

on-line system. a computer system that allows its input to be directly entered from a terminal device. Sometimes considered interactive conversation between a computer and a terminal.

operating system. a set of programs that monitors and controls user programs. Also known as a supervisor.

parity check. a system that tests to ensure that the number of ones or zeros in an array of binary digits is consistently odd or even.

program. a set of computer instructions put together to satisfy an end result.

RAM. random access memory—where data or instructions may be written to or read from.

register. circuitry within the CPU used for accumulation of digits or address modification.

response time. the time a computer takes to react to a specific act; e.g., how long it takes to answer a question.

ROM read only memory—contains data or instructions that are permanently stored and cannot be written over. Generally the information is placed in ROM at the time of manufacture. Some of the instructions are executed when the computer is powered up to orient itself and its environment.

software. programs used to direct the computer in its execution.

supervisor. an operating system that monitors and controls user programs.

synchronous transmission. a transmission method in which the synchronizing of characters is controlled by timing signals generated at the transmitting and receiving devices. Both devices are frequency aligned. This is much faster than asynchronous transmission. Synchronous is also called bi-sync or binary synchronous.

terminal. any device capable of sending or receiving data. Normally a CRT (TV-type screen) is used for display and a typewriter-type keyboard is attached.

update. to modify a program or data file with new information.

video monitor. a CRT device used by an operating system to display the status of the computer and the jobs being processed.

word. a group of bits as a unit that can be stored at a certain memory address.

word processing. a computer system that allows letter composition and text editing. The information can be updated at any time and printed at the user's discretion.

Appendix XVII

GLOSSARY OF TELECOMMUNICATIONS TERMS

acoustic coupler. the interface device between a teletypewriter and telephone which converts the teletypewriter signals into tones compatible with the voice band of the telephone lines, and vice versa at the receiving end. Also called modem (for modulator-demodulator); terminal unit, TU cradle—the part of the acoustic coupler in which the telephone handset rests.

ACU. automatic control unit. A device tied into the acoustic coupler that, after from 2 to 12 rings, automatically turns on the acoustic coupler and TTY so that messages may be left on machines when the recipient is not at home.

ASR. automatic send and receive. The type of TTY in which a message may be prepunched on tape for later sending through the transmitter of the machine.

contacts. a series of metal strips which are operated by the keyboard to give appropriate signals over the telephone line. It has been said that 90% of poor reception by the receiving machines is due to dirty or improperly adjusted contacts in the transmitting machine.

CRT. cathode ray tube. Readout is on a TC screen.

CUL. see you later.

DDD. direct distance dialing. A system that permits people to make long distance telephone calls without operator assistance.

88. love and kisses.

GA. go ahead. The typists signal that the person typing has finished what they were saying and for the party on the other end of the line to begin typing.

HD. hold; to put a conversation on hold.

keyboard. that part of the TTY which the sender operates to transmit messages.

KSR. keyboard send and receive. The type of TTY which operates by keying only.

LED. light emitting diode. Readout is on single unit characters that move across a screen as typing proceeds.

MCU. message control unit. A device operating in conjunction with an ACU, which causes the TTY to type out an identification message. Can only be used with ASR machines.

monitor lamp. the lamp on the terminal unit that indicates where the unit is receiving a ringing telephone, a busy signal, or other electrical impulse from the telephone line.

OIC. oh, I see.

page printer. the type of TTY in which a sheet of paper containing the message feeds out of the top of the machine.

platen. the roller over which the paper passes on a page printer.

power lamp. the lamp which indicates that the acoustic coupler is tuned and ready for use.

range finder. a lever operating over a scale which is adjusted to get the best reception of messages. If in good adjustment, it will be set in the middle of a range of 75-80 units on the scale.

RO. receive only. The type of TTY that has no keyboard and can receive messages but not send them.

SK. send-kill. A "sign off" message indicating that the person typing has finished their call and is ready to hang up. This should be acknowledged by the other party also typing. SK is an indication that they agree with the termination of the call. This term comes from usage by railroad telegraphers.

strip printer. the type of TTY in which the message is on a narrow strip of paper feeding out of the left side of the machine.

TDD. telecommunications device for the deaf. An all-inclusive term embracing all types of compatible devices by which deaf people communicate over the telephone networks, such as TTYs, CRTs, LEDs. (Credit for this term goes to Betty Broeker of Philadelphia Community College).

TDI. Telecommunications for the Deaf, Inc.

telephone ring relay. the device that actuates a light when the telephone rings, alerting the deaf recipient of a telephone call. Also called Signaller.

teletypewriter. the basic name of the device sending printed messages over wires from one station to another to another. Also called teleprinter. Teletype is the trade-marked product of the Teletype Corporation, and is always written with a capital T.

typing unit. that part of the TTY by which the message is printed on paper.

TTY. generally used abbreviation for teletypewriter.

INTERNATIONAL STANDARD MANUAL ALPHABET

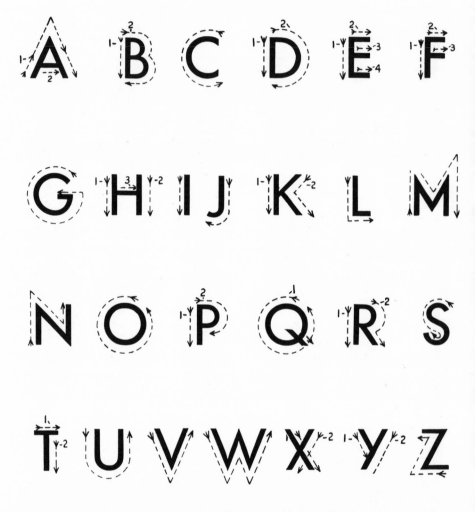

Anyone who can print simple block letters can make immediate use of the alphabet shown above in communicating with most deaf-blind persons. Dotted lines, arrows, and numbers indicate proper direction, sequence, and number of strokes. Print only in the palm area. Do not try to connect letters. Complete one, pause, then complete the next on the same palm area. Pause longer at the end of a word. Faster communication is often possible with the One Hand Manual Alphabet, but it must be memorized and practiced often.

Appendix XIX

ONE HAND MANUAL ALPHABET

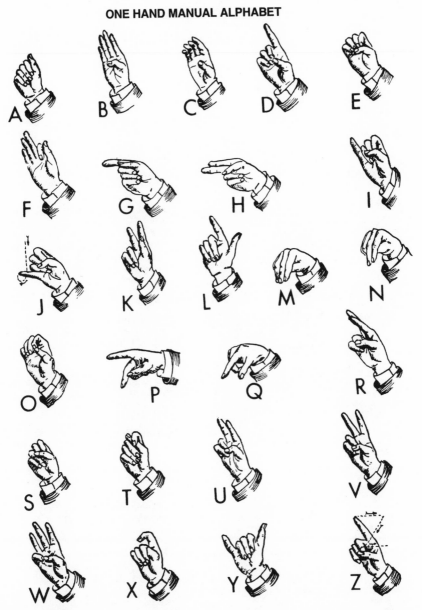

International Standard Manual Alphabet—courtesy of The Industrial Home for the Blind, 57 Willoughby Street, Brooklyn, New York 11201.

Communication with a deaf-blind person who knows the above alphabet can be quite rapid. The finger positions are formed within his cupped hand. Certain letter formations are closely related, and it often speeds memorizing if they are learned in the following groups and in the order given: (A C E O S T) (D G H I J L X Z) (K P) (M N Q) (B F R U V W Y)

Appendix XX

BIBLIOGRAPHY

The following are some periodicals of interest to members of the hearing healthcare profession.

AMERICAN ANNALS OF THE DEAF
Outreach Services Pre-college Program,
publisher
800 Florida Avenue, NE
Washington, DC 20002
Feb., Jun., Aug., Oct., Dec.

AMERICAN JOURNAL OF AUDIOLOGY
A journal of clinical practice
American Speech-Language-Hearing Association,
publisher
10801 Rockville Pike
Rockville, MD 20852
Quarterly

AMERICAN JOURNAL OF OTOLARYNGOLOGY,
HEAD AND NECK MEDICINE AND
SURGERY
W.B. Saunders Co., publisher
The Curtis Center
Independence Square West
Philadelphia, PA 19106-3399
Bimonthly

AMERICAN JOURNAL OF OTOLOGY, THE
Decker Periodicals, Inc., publisher
One James Street South
P.O. Box 620, LCD1
Hamilton, Ontario
Canada L8N 3K7
Bimonthly

ANNALS OF OTOLOGY, RHINOLOGY, AND
LARYNGOLOGY
Annals Publishing Co., publisher
4507 Lacleed Avenue
St. Louis, MO 63108
Monthly

ARCHIVES OF OTOLARYNGOLOGY
American Medical Association, publisher
515 North State Street
Chicago, IL 60610
Monthly

ASHA
American Speech-Language-Hearing Association,
publisher
10801 Rockville Pike
Rockville, MD 20852
Monthly

AUDECIBEL
National Hearing Aid Society, publisher
20361 Middlebelt
Livonia, MI 20852
Quarterly

AUDIOLOGISCHE AKUSTIK-AUDIOLOGICAL
ACOUSTICS
Hans-Jurgen von Killisch-Horn, publisher
Hauptstrasse 64
Postfach 103964
6900 Heidelberg 1, Germany

AUDIOLOGY - JOURNAL OF AUDITORY
COMMUNICATION
S. Karger AG, publisher
P.O. Box 4009
Basel, Switzerland
Bimonthly

AUDIOLOGY TODAY, Bulletin of the American
Academy of Audiology
University of Texas Medical School, publisher
6431 Fannin
Houston, TX 77225
Bimonthly

AURICLE, THE
Auditory-Verbal International, Inc., publisher
505 Cattell Street
Easton, PA 18042
Quarterly

AUSTRALIAN JOURNAL OF AUDIOLOGY
National Acoustic Laboratories, publisher
5 Hickson Road
Sydney, Australia

BRITISH JOURNAL OF AUDIOLOGY
Published for the British Society of Audiology by
Academic Press
24-28 Oval Road
London NW1 7DX, United Kingdom
Quarterly

BROADCASTER, THE
The National Association of the Deaf, publisher
814 Thayer Avenue
Silver Spring, MD 20910
Monthly

BULLETIN OF THE AMERICAN ACADEMY OF
OTOLARYNGOLOGY-HEAD AND
NECK SURGERY
American Academy of Otolaryngology-Head and
Neck Surgery, Inc., publisher
One Prince Street
Alexandria, VA 22314
Monthly

CAHIERS DE L'AUDITION
F. Fontanez, publisher
5, rue du Mal-Joffre
06400 Cannes, France

EAR AND HEARING
Official journal of the American Auditory Society
Williams & Wilkins, publisher
428 E. Preston Street
Baltimore, MD 21202
Bimonthly

EAR, NOSE AND THROAT JOURNAL
International Publishing Group, publisher
4959 Commerce Parkway
Cleveland, OH 44128
Monthly

HEARING CONSERVATION NEWS
National Hearing Conservation Association,
publisher
900 Des Moines Street, Suite 200
Des Moines, IA 50309
Quarterly

HEARING INSTRUMENTS
Edgell Communications, Inc., publisher
P.O. Box 6019
Duluth, MN 55806
Monthly

HEARING JOURNAL, THE
The Laux Company, Inc. publisher
63 Great Road
Maynard, MA 01754
Monthly

HEARING RESEARCH
Elsevier Science Publisher B.V., publisher
P.O. Box 211, 1000 AE
Amsterdam, The Netherlands
Monthly

JOURNAL OF THE ACOUSTICAL SOCIETY OF
AMERICA
Acoustical Society of America, publisher
500 Sunnyside Boulevard
Woodbury, NY 11797
Monthly

JOURNAL OF THE AMERICAN ACADEMY OF
AUDIOLOGY, THE
Decker Periodicals Publishing, Inc., publisher
320 Walnut Street, Suite 400
Philadelphia, PA 19106
Quarterly

JOURNAL OF REHABILITATION OF THE DEAF
American Deafness and Rehabilitation Association,
publisher
P.O. Box 251554
Little Rock, AR 72225

JOURNAL OF SPEECH AND HEARING
RESEARCH
American Speech-Language-Hearing Association,
publisher
10801 Rockville Pike
Rockville, MD 20852
Bimonthly

LANGUAGE, SPEECH, AND HEARING
SERVICES IN THE SCHOOLS
American Speech-Language-Hearing Association,
publisher
10801 Rockville Pike
Rockville, MD 20852
Quarterly

LARYNGOSCOPE
The Laryngoscope Co., publisher
9216 Clayton Road, Suite 18
St. Louis, MO 63124

NEWSOUNDS
Alexander Graham Bell Association for the Deaf,
Inc., publisher
3417 Volta Place NW
Washington, DC 20007-2778
Published 10 times a year

OTOLARYNGOLOGIC CLINICS OF
NORTH AMERICA
W. B. Saunders Co., publisher
The Curtis Center
Independence Square West
Philadelphia, PA 19106-3399
Bimonthly

OTOLARYNGOLOGY–HEAD AND NECK
SURGERY
Mosby Yearbook, publisher
11830 Westline Industrial Drive
St. Louis, MO 63146
Monthly

SEMINARS IN HEARING
Thieme Medical Publishers, Inc., publisher
381 Park Avenue South
New York, NY 10016

SHHH JOURNAL
Self Help for Hard of Hearing People, Inc., publisher
7800 Wisconsin Avenue
Bethesda, MD 20814
Bimonthly

SOUND & VIBRATION
Acoustical Publications, Inc., publisher
P.O. Box 40416
Bay Village, OH 44140

VOICE, THE
Voice International Publications, Inc., publisher
723 Upper N. Broadway #522,
Corpus Christi, TX 78403-2663
Bimonthly

VOLTA REVIEW, THE
Alexander Graham Bell Association for the Deaf,
Inc., publisher
3417 Volta Place NW
Washington, DC 20007
Published 7 times a year